HEALTH
and Health Care Delivery in Canada

ELSEVIER evolve

YOU'VE JUST PURCHASED
MORE THAN A TEXTBOOK!

Evolve Student Resources for *Health and Health Care Delivery in Canada*, Second Edition, include the following:

- Glossary
- Review Questions
- Suggested Readings
- Web Resources

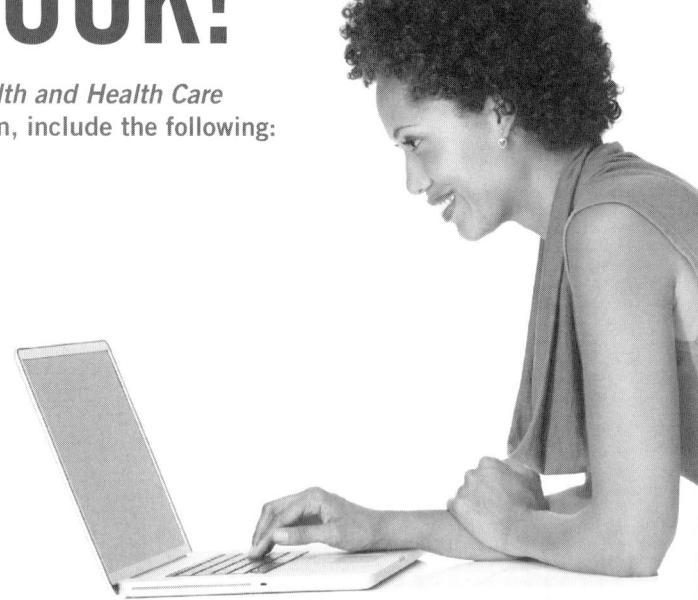

Activate the complete learning experience that comes with each textbook purchase by registering at

http://evolve.elsevier.com/Canada/Thompson/Health/

REGISTER TODAY!

HEALTH
and Health Care Delivery in Canada

Second Edition

Valerie D. Thompson, RN, PHC, NP
Former Professor, School of Health & Life Sciences
and Community Services
Conestoga Institute of Technology and Advanced Learning

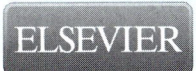

ELSEVIER

Copyright © 2016 Elsevier Canada, a division of Reed Elsevier Canada, Ltd.

All rights reserved. No part of this publication may be reproduced or transmitted in any form or by any means, electronic or mechanical, including photocopy, recording, or any information storage and retrieval system, without permission in writing from the publisher. Reproducing passages from this book without such written permission is an infringement of copyright law.

Requests for permission to make copies of any part of the work should be mailed to College Licensing Officer, access ©, 1 Yonge Street, Suite 1900, Toronto, ON M5E 1E5. Fax: (416) 868-1621. All other inquiries should be directed to the publisher.

Every reasonable effort has been made to acquire permission for copyrighted material used in this text and to acknowledge all such indebtedness accurately. Any errors and omissions called to the publisher's attention will be corrected in future printings.

Notices

Knowledge and best practice in this field are constantly changing. As new research and experience broaden our understanding, changes in research methods, professional practices, or medical treatment may become necessary.

Practitioners and researchers must always rely on their own experience and knowledge in evaluating and using any information, methods, compounds, or experiments described herein. In using such information or methods they should be mindful of their own safety and the safety of others, including parties for whom they have a professional responsibility.

With respect to any drug or pharmaceutical products identified, readers are advised to check the most current information provided (i) on procedures featured or (ii) by the manufacturer of each product to be administered, to verify the recommended dose or formula, the method and duration of administration, and contraindications. It is the responsibility of practitioners, relying on their own experience and knowledge of their patients, to make diagnoses, to determine dosages and the best treatment for each individual patient, and to take all appropriate safety precautions.

To the fullest extent of the law, neither the Publisher nor the authors, contributors, or editors assume any liability for any injury and/or damage to persons or property as a matter of products liability, negligence or otherwise, or from any use or operation of any methods, products, instructions, or ideas contained in the material herein.

The Publisher

Library and Archives Canada Cataloguing in Publication

Thompson, Valerie D., 1948-, author
    Health and health care delivery in Canada / Valerie D. Thompson,
RN, PHC, NP, Conestoga Institute of Technology and Advanced Learning.
—Second edition.

Includes bibliographical references and index.
ISBN 978-1-927406-31-1 (pbk.)

    1. Medical care—Canada. 2. Public health—Canada. 3. Medicine,
Preventive—Canada. I. Title.

RA449.T46 2015   362.10971   C2015-901272-4

Vice President, Publishing: Ann Millar
Managing Editor: Roberta A. Spinosa-Millman
Developmental Editor: Joanne Sutherland
Publishing Services Manager: Deborah L. Vogel/Patricia Tannian
Project Manager: Pat Costigan/Sharon Corell
Copy Editor: Cathy Witlox
Cover Design: George Kirkpatrick
Interior Design: Brett J. Miller, BJM Graphic Design & Communications
Book Designer: Ashley Miner
Cover Image: Don Farrall/Digital Vision/Getty Images
Typesetting and Assembly: Toppan Best-set Premedia Limited
Printing and Binding: Edwards Brothers Malloy

Elsevier Canada
420 Main Street East, Suite 636,
Milton, ON Canada L9T 5G3
416-644-7053

3 4 5   19 18 17

E-book ISBN: 978-1-927406-65-6

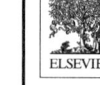

Working together to grow libraries in developing countries

www.elsevier.com • www.bookaid.org

To the little ones in my life—Gregory, Severin, Russell, Colton, Penelope, Lillian, and Bridgit—in the hopes that our health care system will remain sustainable and effective for their lifetimes.

To all the students entering the health care field, as well as existing health care professionals, who work tirelessly, adapt to continuous change, improvise, and overcome obstacles to ensure that health care in Canada is the best it can be.

Preface

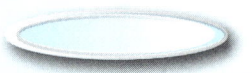

Individuals working in any facet of health care must understand the components of health and wellness and how health care is delivered in Canada. This unique text will provide a valuable overview of and foundation for understanding these important and challenging concepts.

While by no means exhaustive, *Health and Health Care Delivery in Canada*, Second Edition, discusses many components of health and health care delivery. After introducing the concepts of health and illness, the book builds on population health principles in order to methodically examine the cost, structure, and function of the Canadian health care system at the federal, provincial, and municipal levels. The text also looks at human health resources, legal and ethical aspects of health care, and the future of health care in Canada.

The book's content has been carefully selected in order to highlight essential material. Each chapter relates to and expands on ideas in the previous chapter so that common threads are carried throughout the book and material flows in an orderly and understandable manner.

By the end of this book, students will be able to say, "I understand health care issues in Canada and how different levels of government operate in terms of health care delivery. I understand how our health care system is funded and the future issues facing health and health care in Canada," and, most important, "I understand the system that I am choosing to work in." Intended to accompany postsecondary introductory courses in Canadian health care delivery, this book offers students a foundation with which they can easily move forward to other, more specifically focused courses.

CONTENT

Chapter 1 (The History of Health Care in Canada) provides the reader with a summary of the highlights in the history of our health care system. These include the events leading up to the implementation of the *Canada Health Act*, which is the foundation of the health care system in Canada. Students are encouraged to examine the principles of this Act in terms of their relevance in the twenty-first century. Chapter 2 (Health and the Individual) sets the stage for the rest of the book by providing the student with an understanding of the key concepts of health, wellness, illness, disease, and disability. Among other things, students are encouraged to examine their own health beliefs and health behaviours and to consider how these contribute to maintaining health. Chapter 3 (Population Health: Introduction and Principles) explains how the government and other health care stakeholders evaluate the health of Canadians, identify risk factors, implement strategies to deal with current health problems, and predict problems that are likely to arise in the future.

Chapter 4 (The Law and Health Care) analyzes legal issues, clarifying provincial, territorial, and federal boundaries in terms of legislation and the law. Considerable discussion is devoted to current laws regarding confidentiality and consent to treatment. Chapter 5 (Ethics and Health Care) highlights ethical principles and points out that health care professionals are held to a higher level of ethical accountability than are those in many other professions. This chapter also discusses the fine line that sometimes divides ethics and health-related legal issues. The student will learn why this boundary is so fragile and how to practise in a moral and ethical manner.

Chapter 6 (The Role of Health Canada and Other Federal and International Health Agencies) and Chapter 7 (The Role of Provincial and Territorial Governments in Health Care) focus on the division of powers and the implementation of health care from federal and provincial or territorial levels. Chapter 7 follows two families who have recently immigrated to Canada, highlighting some variations in the provincial and territorial health care plans and how these differences affect the families. Instructors are encouraged to expand on health care delivery in their own jurisdictions while comparing it with those of other jurisdictions. Chapter 8 (The Dollars and "Sense" of Health Care Funding) looks critically at where the money for health care comes from and where it goes, and also examines what "strings" the federal government attaches to its funding for the provinces and territories. The chapter focuses on the cost of health care in general, as well as on the cost of specific procedures. It examines the sobering fact that real-life health care decisions are made based on who qualifies for treatment under a provincial or territorial plan and who does not—and who will opt to pay for services out-of-pocket.

Chapter 9 (Practitioners and Practice Settings) provides the student with a clear picture of our human health resources—who delivers the care, in what setting, and under what circumstances. It examines how primary health care reform is changing the way in which health care is delivered across Canada.

Chapter 10 (Current Issues and Future Trends in Health Care in Canada) discusses important challenges currently facing Canada's health care system, such as the state of mental health services, managing care for Canada's aging population, the shortage of human health resources, and the increasing need for home care services. This chapter also contains an expanded discussion on the health of Aboriginal Canadians, disparities that affect their health and well-being, the challenges they face, and health care services available for this unique segment of the Canadian population.

Additionally, this chapter explores other issues that will impact the future of health care in Canada. How can Canada maintain adequate health care services in the face of complex medical problems, increasingly expensive drugs, advancing and costly technology, and less funding? Will electronic medical records and electronic health records be implemented at a national level, and how and when will this implementation take place? Although no concrete answers exist, the student will be prepared to look ahead, aware of the significant obstacles that we as a nation must overcome if we are indeed to salvage publicly funded health care for all.

Learning Features

Each chapter contains several unique features meant to stimulate student interest. Learning outcomes outline the objectives for the chapter. Key terms define challenging concepts. Chapter summaries and review questions underscore key elements.

Additional features include general interest, "Thinking It Through," "In the News," and "Case Example" boxes. These features encourage the student to think through facts, points of interest, and actual situations and to answer questions that promote exploration of personal views, general discussion, and, in some cases, further investigation. Additional Evolve® online resources to accompany the text can be found at http://evolve.elsevier.com/Canada/Thompson/health.

Acknowledgements

Writing a book of this nature cannot possibly occur in isolation. I owe a great deal to so many people, from those working with the Canadian Institute for Health Information—particularly Jennie Hoekstra, Barbara Loh, Angela Allain-Levasseur, and Angela Baker—and provincial and territorial governments to colleagues representing individual professions. Those listed below have contributed essential information to this book and confirmed that information in their area of expertise is both correct and relevant:

Dr. Don Nixdorf
Executive Director
British Columbia Chiropractic Association

Dr. S. Brooke Milne
Department of Archeology
University of Manitoba

Richard Baker
Founder
Timely Medical Services

Dr. Richard Wedge
Director of Medical Programs
Prince Edward Island Department of Health

Nadeem Esmail
Director, Health System Performance Studies
Fraser Institute

Keith Walls
Manager, Population Health Fund Section
Public Health Agency of Canada

I would like also to acknowledge and thank Elsevier's reviewers, who provided helpful comments, constructive criticism, and suggestions for improvements during various stages of the manuscript. I am grateful for the advice and recommendations provided to me, much of which was used to prepare this second edition.

Dianne Brown, RN, BScN, MN
Educator and Instructional Designer
Red River College

Michael W. K. Chan, MBA, BSc OT
Dip. Hospital Departmental Management
Professor, Faculty of Health Sciences
Mohawk College

Stephanie Clack, CHIM
Instructor, School of Health and Public Safety
SAIT Polytechnic: Southern Alberta Institute of Technology

Sandra Cotton, BA, CHIM
Health Information Management Program Coordinator
Centre for Distance Education

Shalene Creighton, MRT(R)
Instructor, Medical Radiologic Technology
Northern Alberta Institute of Technology

Dianna Fong Lee, MA, OT(C)
Program Coordinator and Professor, Occupational Therapist Assistant
and Physiotherapist Assistant Program, School of Health Sciences
Conestoga College Institute of Technology and Advanced Learning

Laurie Kenward, BHRS, CHIM
Coordinator, HIM Program
Douglas College

Keltie MacDonald, RN, HBA, BEd, MSc
Professor, Pre-Health Science Program
Confederation College

Alisha Renshaw
Physiotherapist/Occupational Therapist Assistant, Fitness & Health Promotion
MOAWC Instructor, Medical Office Administrator/Ward Clerk (MOAWC)
Willis College

Wade Sharpe, BSc, MRT(N), MEd
Professor, Medical Radiation Sciences
(Nuclear Medicine)
Michener Institute of Applied Health Sciences

Kathy F. Spurr, BSc, RRT, MHI, FCSRT
Assistant Professor, School of Health Sciences
Dalhousie University

Melissa Wiman, BSc, MSc, PhD
Adjunct Professor, School of Human Kinetics
Laurentian University

I also owe a debt of gratitude to clear language consultant Susan Milne for her ongoing assistance in keeping me organized and in ensuring that the language of each chapter was clear and concise prior to the publisher's edit. Also thanks to Lynda Cranston and Jennifer McIntyre for their guidance on content organization. I'd also like to acknowledge Carla Shapiro for her legal review of Chapter 4. As well, I cannot thank the editors from Elsevier—Ann Millar, Joanne Sutherland, Roberta A. Spinosa-Millman, and Cathy Witlox—enough for their expert advice, endless reviews, and constructive suggestions. Elsevier is an outstanding company to work with, and the result of its attention to detail is well evident in this publication.

Valerie D. Thompson
February 2015

Contents

Preface	vi
Special Features	xviii

Chapter 1

The History of Health Care in Canada — 1

Learning Outcomes — 1
Key Terms — 2

Evolution of Health Care: An Overview — 3
  Division of Responsibilities for Health — 3
  The Origins of Medical Care in Canada — 4
  Aboriginal Medicine and the Shaman — 4
  The Concept of Public Health Is Introduced — 5
  The Role of Volunteer Organizations in Early Health Care — 6
  The Role of Nursing in Early Health Care — 9
  The Development of Hospitals in Canada — 9

The Introduction of Health Insurance — 11
  First Attempts to Introduce National Health Insurance — 11
  Post–World War II: The Political Landscape — 12
  Progress Toward Prepaid Hospital Care — 12
  Progress Toward Prepaid Medical Care — 13

Significant Events Leading Up to the *Canada Health Act* — 15
  Events Following the Introduction of the *EPF Act* — 17

The *Canada Health Act* (1984) — 18
  Criteria and Conditions of the *Canada Health Act* — 19
  Interpreting the *Canada Health Act* — 24
  Additional Components of the Act — 25

After the *Canada Health Act*: Commissioned Reports and Accords — 26
  Social Union — 28
  Commissioned Reports — 29
  Accords — 33

Summary — 36
Review Questions — 37
References — 38

Chapter 2

Health and the Individual — 39

Learning Outcomes — 39
Key Terms — 40

Health, Wellness, and Illness: Key Concepts — 41
  Health — 41
  Wellness — 41
  Illness — 46
  Disease — 46
  Disability — 47

Health Models — 48
  Medical Model — 49
  Holistic Model — 49

Wellness Model ... 49
International Classification of Functioning Disability and Health ... 50

Changing Perceptions of Health ... 50

The Psychology of Health Behaviour ... 52
Transtheoretical Model ... 52
Social–Ecological Model ... 53
Protection Motivation Theory ... 53
Health Belief Model ... 53

The Health–Illness Continuum ... 55
Sick Role Behaviour ... 57
Stages of Illness: Influence on Patient Behaviour ... 60
Self-Imposed Risk Behaviours ... 61

The Health of Canadians Today ... 62
Leading Causes of Death in Canada ... 63

Summary ... 66

Review Questions ... 67

References ... 68

Chapter 3

Population Health: Introduction and Principles ... 69

Learning Outcomes ... 69

Key Terms ... 70

Population Health Approach ... 70

Key Determinants of Health ... 71
1. Income and Social Status ... 72
2. Social Support Networks ... 74
3. Education and Literacy ... 75
4. Employment and Working Conditions ... 75
5. Social Environment ... 76
6. Physical Environment ... 77
7. Personal Health Practices and Coping Skills ... 77
8. Healthy Child Development ... 78
9. Biology and Genetic Endowment ... 78
10. Health Services ... 79
11. Gender ... 79
12. Culture ... 80

Introduction of Population Health to Canada ... 80
The Lalonde Report, 1974 ... 81
Alma-Ata Conference, 1978 ... 81
Ottawa Charter for Health Promotion, 1986 ... 83
The Epp Report, 1986 ... 83
The Public Health Program Initiative ... 83
Toward a Healthy Future: The First *Report on the Health of Canadians,* 1996 ... 84
National Forum on Health, 1994–1997 ... 85

Partners in Population Health Action ... 86
Health Canada ... 87
Public Health Agency of Canada ... 87
The Canadian Institutes of Health Research ... 87
Canadian Institute for Advanced Research ... 88
Canadian Policy Research Networks ... 89
Statistics Canada ... 89
The Canadian Institute for Health Information ... 89

The Public Health Agency of Canada Template ... 90
Measure the Population Health Status ... 90
Analyze the Determinants of Health ... 93

Use Evidence-Informed Decision Making	93
Employ Upstream Investments	94
Use Multiple Strategies	94
Engage the Public	95
Think Intersectoral Collaboration	95
Demonstrate Accountability for Health Outcomes	96

Population Health Promotion Model 96

Population Health in Canada and Abroad 97

Summary 98

Review Questions 99

References 99

Chapter 4

The Law and Health Care 101

Learning Outcomes 101

Key Terms 102

Laws Used in Health Care Legislation 103

Constitutional Law	103
Statutory Law	104
Regulatory Law	104
Common (Case) Law and Civil Law in Canada	105
Classifications of Law: Public and Private Law	105

Federal and Provincial Jurisdictional Framework 111

Workplace Safety	111
Drugs and the Law	112
Health Canada's Emergency Powers	118

Health Care as a Right 120

Medically Necessary: What Does It Mean?	120
The Canadian Charter of Rights and Freedoms	121
The Law, the Constitution, and End-of-Life Issues	123

The Legality of Private Services in Canada 124

Physicians' Opting Out of the Public Plan	125
Independent Health Care Facilities	125

Informed Consent to Treatment 127

Types of Consent	129
Who Can Give Consent	131

The Health Record 132

The Importance of Accurate Recording	133
Ownership of Health Information	133
Storage and Disposal of Health Information	134
Federal Legislation and Privacy Laws	135
Confidentiality	136
Security	138
Electronic Health Information Requirements	138

Health Care Professions and the Law 140

Regulated Health Care Providers	140
Nonregulated Health Care Providers	142

Other Legal Issues in Health Care 142

The Use of Restraints	142
Patient Self-Discharge From a Hospital	143
Good Samaritan Laws	143
Whistleblowing	144

Summary 145

Review Questions 146

References 146

Chapter 5

Ethics and Health Care 149

Learning Outcomes 149

Key Terms 150

What Is Ethics? 151
Morality and Morals 151
Values 153
Sense of Duty 155

Ethical Theories: The Basics 155
Teleological Theory 156
Deontological Theory 156
Virtue Ethics 156
Divine Command 157

Ethical Principles and the Health Care Profession 158
Beneficence and Nonmaleficence 158
Respect 158
Autonomy 159
Truthfulness 159
Fidelity 160
Justice 160

Patients' Rights in Health Care 161
Duties and Rights 164
Autonomy and the Patient 165
Truthfulness 166
Parental Rights, Ethics, and the Law 167
Rights and Mental Competence 169

Ethics at Work 169
The Code of Ethics 170

End-of-Life Issues 174
Euthanasia 174
The Right to Die 176
Palliative Care 178

Allocation of Resources 179
Organ Transplantation 179
Finances and Resources 180
Northern Access to Health Care 182

Other Ethical Issues in Health Care 182
Abortion 182
Genetic Testing 184
Patenting Genes 185

Summary 187

Review Questions 188

References 188

Chapter 6

The Role of Health Canada and Other Federal and International Health Agencies 191

Learning Outcomes 191

Key Terms 192

Health Canada: Objectives and Responsibilities 193

Health Canada Organization: Ministry Level 195

Branches of Health Canada 197
Internal Services 197
External Services 199

Agencies of Health Canada 208
Canadian Institutes of Health Research 208
Hazardous Materials Information Review Commission 209
Patented Medicine Prices Review Board 209
Public Health Agency of Canada 210
Assisted Human Reproduction Canada 211

International Health Agencies Working With Health Canada 211
World Health Organization 211
Pan-American Health Organization 218

    Organisation for Economic
      Co-operation and Development 218

Summary   218

Review Questions   220

References   220

Chapter 7

The Role of Provincial and Territorial Governments in Health Care   221

Learning Outcomes   221

Key Terms   222

Provincial and Territorial Health Care Plans   223
    Division of Powers   223
    Structure of the Health Plans:
      An Overview   224

Regionalization Initiatives Across Canada   226
    British Columbia   227
    Alberta   227
    Saskatchewan   228
    Manitoba   228
    Ontario   228
    Quebec   229
    New Brunswick   229
    Nova Scotia   230
    Prince Edward Island   230
    Newfoundland and Labrador   231
    Northern Regions   231

Health Care: Who Pays for It?   234
    Health Care Premiums   234
    Payroll Tax   235
    Other Sources of Funds   236
    Distribution of Funds   236

Health Insurance   237
    Provincial Insurance Plans   237
    Insured and Uninsured Services   241

Drug Plans   249

Summary   251

Review Questions   252

References   252

Chapter 8

The Dollars and "Sense" of Health Care Funding   255

Learning Outcomes   255

Key Terms   256

Funding Versus the Delivery of Health Care   257

Levels of Health Care Funding   257
    Federal Health Transfer Payments   258
    Negotiating Funds: Health Accords   260
    Federal Government Costs for
      Direct Health Care   260
    Provincial and Territorial Costs
      for Direct Health Care   261
    Indirect Costs of Poor Health   262

Expenditures for Hospitals   263
    Hospital Funding Mechanisms   264
    Cost-Reduction Strategies   269

Long-Term Care Accommodation   274

The Rising Cost of Drugs   277
    Major Cost Drivers for Drug
      Expenditures   277
    Drug Insurance   277
    Brand-Name and Generic Drugs   278
    Controlling the Cost of Patented
      Drugs   279

Human Health Resources   279
    How Physicians Are Paid: Billing
      Options   280

Other Health Care Cost Drivers   283
    Technology   283
    Outsourcing   284
    Electronic Health Records   284

Conclusion   285

Summary	286
Review Questions	287
References	287

Chapter 9

Practitioners and Practice Settings — 289

Learning Outcomes	289
Key Terms	290
Categories of Health Care Providers	**291**
Conventional Medicine	293
Complementary and Alternative Medicine (CAM)	293
Regulation of Health Care Professions	**296**
Title Protection	300
Controlled Acts	301
Delegated Acts	302
Complaint Process	304
Educational Standards	304
Licence to Practise	304
Nonregulated Professions and Occupations	304
Conventional Health Care Providers	**306**
Physicians	306
Nurses	310
Physician Assistants	312
Pharmacists	313
Midwives	313
Optometrists and Opticians	314
Osteopathic Physicians	314
Podiatrists (Chiropodists)	315
Personal Support Workers	315
Psychologists	316
Speech-Language Pathologists and Audiologists	316
Respiratory Therapists	317
Physiotherapists	318
Occupational Therapists	318
Administrative Roles	319
Laboratory and Diagnostic Services	321
Volunteer Caregivers	321
Practice Settings	**321**
Clinics	322
Primary Health Care Reform	**324**
Primary Health Care Groups	325
Telephone Helplines	327
Community Health Centres	329
Health Service Organizations	329
Summary	330
Review Questions	331
References	331

Chapter 10

Current Issues and Future Trends in Health Care in Canada — 333

Learning Outcomes	333
Key Terms	334
Mental Health	**335**
Structure and Implementation of Services	335
The Stigma of Mental Illness	336
Common Mental Health Disorders	337
Challenges	338
The Future of Mental Health Care	340
Health Care Costs and an Aging Population	**341**
Associated Concerns	341
Predictions for the Future	343
Human Health Resources	**344**
Availability of Regulated Nurses	344
Strategies to Attract and Retain Nurses	345
Shortage of Doctors	346

Home and Continuing Care — 348
- The Problem — 348
- Recipients of Home Care — 349
- Accessing Home Care Services — 349
- The Impact of Home Care — 349
- Funding — 349
- The Future — 350

Drug Coverage — 351
- Funding — 351
- The Future — 351

Wait Times and Access to Medical Care — 352
- Improving Wait Times — 352
- Improving Emergency Department Wait Times — 354

Aboriginal Health Care — 355
- Status Versus Non-Status Indians — 356
- The Challenges — 357
- Systems of Health Care Delivery for Aboriginals — 363
- Strategies for Improvement — 366

Information Technology and Electronic Health Records — 367
- Security and EHRs — 370
- Advantages of Electronic Charts — 370
- Challenges for EHR Sustainability — 371

The Future of Primary Health Care — 372
- The Financial Sustainability of Health Care in Canada — 373

Summary — 374

Review Questions — 375

References — 375

Glossary — 379

Appendix: *Declaration of Alma-Ata* — 397

Index — 401

Special Features

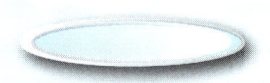

Chapter 1

Box 1.1 Innovation in Newfoundland: The Cottage Hospital System (p. 10)
Box 1.2 Legislation Leading Up to the *Canada Health Act* (p. 15)
Box 1.3 Tax Points Explained (p. 16)
Box 1.4 Eligibility for Health Care Under the *Canada Health Act* (p. 18)
Box 1.5 The Primary Objective of Canadian Health Care Policy (p. 18)
Box 1.6 The *Canada Health Act*: Criteria and Conditions (p. 19)
Box 1.7 New Brunswick Leads the Way in Community Care (p. 27)
Box 1.8 Three Major Reports on the Status of Health Care in Canada (p. 29)
In the News Selling Plasma for a Profit (p. 7)
In the News Doctors Striking for Autonomy (p. 26)
In the News Not Criminally Responsible? (p. 35)

Chapter 2

Box 2.1 Health: An Evolving Definition (p. 42)
Box 2.2 People With Disabilities: Rights Are Formally Recognized (p. 48)
Box 2.3 Stages of Illness (p. 60)
In the News Do You Know Who Terry Fox Is? (p. 43)
In the News Landmark Ruling on Physician-Assisted Suicide (p. 56)

Chapter 3

Box 3.1 Population Health Versus Public Health (p. 71)
Box 3.2 The SES Gradient (p. 73)
Box 3.3 Landmark Studies Support the Link Between Employment and Health Status (p. 75)
Box 3.4 Alma-Ata Definition of *Primary Health Care* (p. 81)
Box 3.5 Strategies for Improving the Health of Canadians (p. 85)
Box 3.6 Epidemiology Explained (p. 92)
Box 3.7 An Aging Population: An Example of Population-Based Surveillance (p. 93)
In the News Angelina Jolie's Medical Choice (p. 79)
In the News The World Health Organization: In Support of Primary Health Care (p. 82)
In the News Health Research Model (p. 88)

Chapter 4

Box 4.1 Equality of Care for Hearing Impaired People (p. 106)
Box 4.2 Strategies for Avoiding Legal Problems (p. 109)
Box 4.3 Supervised Use of Controlled Drugs (p. 117)
Box 4.4 Landmark Court Challenge: *Chaoulli v. Quebec* (p. 121)
Box 4.5 Confidentiality: An Age-Old Concept (p. 137)
In the News Nondisclosure: A Criminal Offence? (p. 109)
In the News A Significant Drug Problem: Who Should Assume Responsibility? (p. 114)

Chapter 5

Box 5.1 A Modern Version of the Hippocratic Oath (p. 165)

In the News Watered-Down Chemotherapy Drugs (p. 154)
In the News Should Age Be a Factor? (p. 162)
In the News Wait Lists: Do They Work? (p. 164)
In the News Rights of the Individual Versus Medical Advice (p. 168)
In the News When Does a Child Have a Right to Autonomy? (p. 170)
In the News The Latimer Tragedy (p. 175)
In the News Patents on "Products of Nature" Invalid (p. 186)

Chapter 6

Box 6.1 The First Ever Food Guide for First Nations, Inuit, and Métis (p. 202)
Box 6.2 CIHR Institutes Across Canada (p. 208)
Box 6.3 The World Health Organization: The Six-Point Agenda (p. 212)
Box 6.4 WHO 2013 Four-Phase Alert System (p. 214)
In the News Failed Refugee Applicants and the Provision of Health Care (p. 195)
In the News Revolutionary Eyewear Gives Visually Impaired People a New "Look" at Life (p. 203)
In the News Agreement Reduces the Cost of Generic Drugs (p. 210)

Chapter 7

Box 7.1 The *Constitution Act*: A Clarification (p. 223)
Box 7.2 Regional Health Authorities: A Definition (p. 226)
Box 7.3 Reciprocal Agreement (p. 240)
Box 7.4 Private Clinics: Concerns (p. 243)
Box 7.5 Uninsured (Chargeable) Versus Insured Physician Services (p. 245)
In the News Funding to Improve Care to Remote First Nations Communities (p. 232)

Chapter 8

Box 8.1 Equalization Payments Embedded in the Canadian Constitution (p. 259)

Chapter 9

Box 9.1 Regulated Professions: Common Elements (p. 300)
In the News Treatment Versus Risk: What Are the Facts? (p. 295)
In the News Yukon Finally Licenses Nurse Practitioners (p. 311)

Chapter 10

Box 10.1 The Sioux Lookout Meno Ya Win Health Centre (p. 365)
In the News Clara's Big Ride (p. 337)
In the News Inadequate Mental Health Care in Prisons: The Consequences (p. 339)
In the News Métis and Non-Status Indians Seek Recognition as Status Indians (p. 357)

CHAPTER ONE

The History of Health Care in Canada

Learning Outcomes

1.1 Summarize the early evolution of health care in Canada.
1.2 Discuss the introduction of health insurance.
1.3 Describe significant events and legislation shaping health care from 1960 until the introduction of the *Canada Health Act* (CHA).
1.4 Describe the criteria and conditions of the *Canada Health Act*.
1.5 Explain the events that have occurred since the implementation of the *Canada Health Act*, including commissioned reports and accords.

KEY TERMS

Aseptic technique, p. 10
Block transfer, p. 16
Canada Health Act, p. 18
Catastrophic drug costs, p. 31
Delisted, p. 17
Eligible, p. 18
Extra billing, p. 17
First ministers, p. 28
Health accord, p. 32
Medically necessary, p. 24
Medicare, p. 13
Palliative care, p. 31
Prepaid health care, p. 13
Primary health care reform, p. 27
Quarantine, p. 3
Refugee claimants, p. 4
Royal assent, p. 18
Social movements, p. 12
User charges, p. 25

"It isn't so much that this country needs a good and caring health care system; our health care system needs a good and caring country" (Wynne-Jones, 2002). What does this quote mean to you? Do you agree with it? Keep these words in mind as you read this chapter and as you answer the questions that appear at the end of it.

This chapter will teach about the evolution of our health care system since before Confederation and about the struggles of the Canadians who built the system into what it is today. Affected by social, economic, and technological growth, health care in Canada has transformed dramatically over the past 200 years. Every decade has brought changes to where and how people live, their views of and responses to illness, and the kind of treatment they expect. The level and quality of health care have, for the most part, adjusted accordingly, but change has not come easily.

As you read this chapter, note continuing parallels between the needs of the population and the adaptation and growth of health care services. When you reach the end, think about the criteria and conditions of the *Canada Health Act* in particular, and ask yourself if the Act still meets the needs of Canadians. Is health care universal? Is health care accessible to all? Is it provided to all Canadians on uniform terms? Is it delivered in a timely fashion to all? Continued debate about the quality and availability of our health care has generated repeated demands for system improvements and for increases in dedicated funds. Does the *Canada Health Act* need to be changed, or do the expectations and attitudes of Canadians need adjustment, as the opening quote suggests? Jot down your thoughts about these questions before you continue reading, and then compare your thoughts with those shared in this chapter.

EVOLUTION OF HEALTH CARE: AN OVERVIEW

With the passage of the *British North America Act* in 1867 (renamed the *Constitution Act* in 1982), Confederation became a reality. The Dominion of Canada consisted of Ontario and Quebec (formerly Upper and Lower Canada, respectively), New Brunswick, and Nova Scotia, and Sir John A. Macdonald was the Dominion's prime minister. Each province had its own representation in government, its own law-making body (which evolved into a provincial government), and its own Lieutenant Governor to represent the Crown. The *British North America Act* also established a federal government comprising the House of Commons and the Senate—the same structure in place today. The first census for the new Dominion, in 1871, showed a population of 3,689,257—a large enough number to warrant closer attention to people's health care needs. Legislation regarding responsibilities for health care was vague at best, but, even at this early stage, responsibilities were divided between the federal and provincial governments.

DIVISION OF RESPONSIBILITIES FOR HEALTH

Health matters received little attention in the *British North America Act*. The federal government was charged with responsibilities for the establishment and maintenance of marine hospitals, the care of Aboriginal populations, and the management of **quarantine**. Relatively common, quarantines were imposed to prevent outbreaks of such diseases as cholera, diphtheria, typhoid fever, tuberculosis (TB), and influenza (Health Canada, 2006).

Provinces were responsible for establishing and managing hospitals, asylums, charities, and charitable institutions. Many of the provinces' responsibilities regarding health care—including social welfare, which, broadly speaking, encompassed health and public health matters—were assumed by default since they were not clearly outlined in the Act as federal responsibilities. Today, the federal government retains responsibility for health care for Aboriginal communities, some members of the RCMP and the armed forces, people detained by Correctional Services, and veterans. As well, under the Interim Federal Health Program (IFHP), the federal government pays for temporary health insurance for selected **refugee claimants**, discussed in more detail in Chapter 7.

Quarantine
The enforced isolation of people having or suspected of having a contagious disease.

Refugee claimants
People who, feeling unsafe in their home country, seek protection in another country.

In 1919, the federal government created the Department of Health, largely to assume its health-care-related responsibilities, which included working collaboratively with the provinces and territories in health care matters and promoting new health care initiatives. (From 1867 to 1919, federal health concerns were managed by the Department of Agriculture.) Early projects undertaken by this new department reflected the issues faced by Canadians at that time—specifically, the increase in sexually transmitted infections (STIs) and the recognition of the importance of keeping children healthy and safe. In response, venereal disease clinics were established across the country, and campaigns promoting child welfare were launched.

In 1928, the Department of Health became known as the Department of Pensions and National Health. The name changed again in 1944 to the Department of National Health and Welfare, and federal responsibilities expanded to include food and drug control, the development of public health programs, health care for members of the civil service, and the operation of the Laboratory of Hygiene (a precursor to Canada's current Laboratory Centre for Disease Control). In 1993, the department was renamed Health Canada. The federal government also retains responsibility for health coverage for certain population groups (discussed in Chapter 6).

THE ORIGINS OF MEDICAL CARE IN CANADA

With the European settlers (primarily from England and France) came the first doctors in Canada, a combination of civilian and military physicians. These doctors cared for the sick at home and then in hospitals once they were built. In the eighteenth century and early nineteenth century, only the wealthier settlers were able to afford medical attention from a doctor and to seek care in a hospital when required. The less fortunate received care through religious and other charitable organizations or from family and friends, who provided in-home care using botanical remedies and other natural medicines shared with them by the Aboriginals.

Canada's first medical school was established in Montreal in 1825. By the time of Confederation, the country had a steadily increasing number of doctors, hospitals, and medical schools, resulting in medical and hospital care that was more accessible to all sectors of the population.

ABORIGINAL MEDICINE AND THE SHAMAN

The medicine practised by Aboriginal peoples in North America (i.e., First Nations, Métis, Inuit) has a long and rich history. Sometimes referred to as shamans or medicine men (note, however, the role of healer was not exclusive to men; in many Aboriginal cultures, women have long been recognized as equally powerful healers), traditional Aboriginal practitioners were believed to have a strong connection to the spirit world and to Mother Earth. Many of the shaman's teachings and remedies attempted to maintain balance and harmony among spiritual and natural elements and the human populations that depended on these elements for survival. Current issues and trends related to Aboriginal health are discussed in Chapter 10.

Like many traditions, an understanding of healing and the use of herbal medicines was passed down through generations via oral teachings and observances. While attributing some ailments to the presence of evil spirits, traditional healers nevertheless knew how to use local plants, herbs, roots, and fungi to remedy common sicknesses that are still prevalent today. For example, Aboriginal healers used willow bark (which contains salicylic acid, one of the base elements in Aspirin) to treat headaches, blood-wort with rosebuds to treat sore throats, and dandelion to treat skin irritation and rashes. Today, many traditional medicines have been incorporated into contemporary Western medicinal practices.

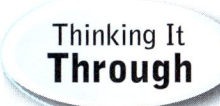

Traditions still play a significant role in Aboriginal health care and will affect how an individual responds to a diagnosis as well as to a treatment plan. Research some of the significant traditions of an Aboriginal population in your geographic area. Bearing these traditions in mind, how could you enhance the delivery of culturally sensitive health care?

THE CONCEPT OF PUBLIC HEALTH IS INTRODUCED

At the beginning of the nineteenth century, the prevalence of infectious diseases peaked. In 1834, William Kelly, a British Royal Navy physician, suspected a relationship between sanitation and disease and deduced that water was possibly a major contaminant. Although how disease spread was not clearly understood, many recognized the effectiveness of quarantine practices in limiting the spread.

Upper and Lower Canada each established a board of health, in 1832 and 1833, respectively. These boards of health enforced quarantine and sanitation laws, imposed restrictions on immigration (to prevent the spread of disease), and stopped the sale of spoiled food. Some health care measures met tremendous public opposition. For example, in the mid-1800s, a doctor in Nova Scotia attempted to introduce a smallpox vaccine, which had been discovered and proven successful in England around the turn of the century. Public resistance was strong despite proof that the vaccine protected individuals from the disease. Consequently, the value of smallpox vaccinations was not fully appreciated until the 1900s.

In the early 1900s, the provinces began establishing formal organizations to manage public health matters. A bureau of public health was established in Saskatchewan in 1909 and became a government department in 1923. The provinces of Alberta, Manitoba, and Nova Scotia likewise established departments of health in 1918, 1928, and 1931, respectively. These public health units assumed responsibility for public health matters, including activities such as pasteurizing milk, testing cows for tuberculosis, managing TB sanatoriums, and controlling the spread of STIs. Maternal and child health care became a focus of public health initiatives at the beginning of the twentieth century. Both doctors and nurses actively promoted such things as immunization clinics and parenting education.

The Role of Volunteer Organizations in Early Health Care

In the eighteenth and early nineteenth centuries, Canadians' health care needs were attended to largely by volunteer organizations, which were also relied upon heavily for raising funds for health care. Some of these groups are discussed below. Many will be familiar because they still function today.

The Order of St. John

The Order of St. John (later known as St. John Ambulance) was introduced to Canada in 1883 by individuals from England with knowledge of first aid, disaster relief, and home nursing. The organization and its volunteer responsibilities expanded over the years, providing invaluable assistance and health care to Canadians. Today, members provide health care services at public events and participate in community health initiatives across Canada (St. John Ambulance, 1995).

The Canadian Red Cross Society

The Canadian Red Cross Society was founded in 1896. In the early 1900s, the Red Cross established a form of home care designed to keep families together during times of illness. The Red Cross gradually became involved in other public health initiatives, establishing outpost hospitals, nursing stations, nutrition services, and university courses in public health nursing (Canadian Red Cross, 2008).

For over 40 years, the Canadian Red Cross Society also supervised the collection of blood from volunteer donors across Canada. However, the society was stripped of this responsibility in the late 1990s, following the contaminated blood crisis: from 1980 to 1985, at least 2000 people who had received blood and blood products contracted HIV; another 30,000 people were infected with hepatitis C between 1980 and 1990.

After the 1997 report prepared by Mr. Justice Krever, *Final Report: Commission of Inquiry on the Blood System in Canada*, a new national blood authority, Canadian Blood Services, was created. On September 26, 1998, Canadian Blood Services assumed full responsibility for the Canadian blood system outside of Quebec (in Quebec, Héma-Québec), and it continues in that role today (Canadian Blood Services, n.d.; Krever Commission, 2004; Krever Inquiry, n.d.).

Traditionally, giving blood has been voluntary, with no cost to those receiving transfusions of blood or blood products. More recently, the sale of some blood products has been sanctioned by Health Canada, but not without controversy from both an ethical and safety perspective (In the News: Selling Plasma for a Profit).

Today the Canadian Red Cross is part of a worldwide humanitarian network providing emergency aid and disaster relief at home and abroad. The organization also offers educational courses including those in cardiopulmonary resuscitation (CPR), first aid, and water safety and provides Canadians with a variety of community support services.

In the News — Selling Plasma for a Profit

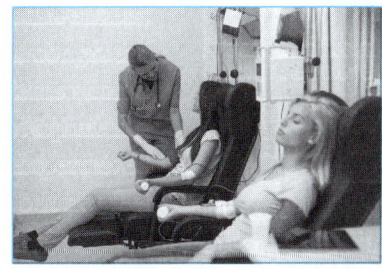

Plasma is used to make pharmaceutical products such as albumin (for burn and trauma patients), clotting factors (for those who have hemophilia), and immune globulin (for those with immune disorders and some infections). Canadian Blood Services collects plasma from volunteers, but not nearly enough to meet Canadian demands. Therefore, Canada imports many of these products, mostly from the United States and obtained from paid donors.

A private company (Canadian Plasma Resources) has opened a clinic in Toronto and plans to open more across Canada to collect blood plasma—and to pay the donors. In March 2014, Ontario introduced legislation to prevent the Toronto company from collecting plasma from paid donors. So the company instead offers donors $25 in the form of a donation to a charity or a nontransferable visa voucher as compensation for their time. Health Canada has the authority to grant licences to approved clinics, but each province and territory has the right to allow or disallow the practice of paying donors for blood and blood products. The practice is allowed in Manitoba, for example, but not in Quebec.

Continued on next page

Concerns include that, with the offer of paying people for blood or plasma, the number of volunteer donors will diminish and contaminated products may enter the blood supply. Canadian Blood Services and the Canadian Hemophilia Society, however, both support the initiative and believe it is safe.

Sources: Health Canada. (2013). *Backgrounder paper: Plasma donations in Canada.* Retrieved from http://www.hc-sc.gc.ca/dhp-mps/consultation/biolog/plasma-consult-disc-eng.php; Canada Plasma Resources. (n.d.) *About us.* Retrieved from http://www.giveplasma.ca/about-us; Frketich, J. (2014, March 21). Ontario moves to halt pay-for-plasma clinics. *Hamilton Spectator.* Retrieved from http://www.thespec.com/news-story/4424277-province-moves-to-halt-pay-for-plasma-clinics/; CBC News. (2013, February 24). Payment for blood donors comes to Canada. *CBC.* Retrieved from http://www.cbc.ca/news/health/payment-for-blood-donors-comes-to-canada-1.1312896; Ferguson, R. (2014, March 18). Plasma clinic plans to open in Toronto in defiance of promised Ontario ban. *Toronto Star.* Retrieved from http://www.thestar.com/news/queenspark/2014/03/18/plasma_clinic_plans_to_open_in_toronto_in_defiance_of_promised_ontario_ban.html; Grant, K. (2014, March 14). Ontario tries to ban blood-buying before clinics open. *The Globe and Mail.* Retrieved from http://www.theglobeandmail.com/life/health-and-fitness/health/ontario-tries-to-ban-blood-buying-before-clinics-open/article17506642/.
Photo credit: © Can Stock Photo Inc. / 4774344sean.

Victorian Order of Nurses

The Victorian Order of Nurses (VON) was founded in 1897 and was one of the first groups to identify the health care needs of the population, particularly of women and children, in remote areas of the country and to provide services to these groups. Today, the VON is the largest national provider of home care services. Its other services include health promotion and educational services (e.g., prenatal education), well-baby clinics, school health services, palliative care services, and continuing care programs in First Nations communities.

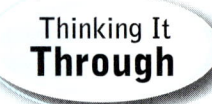

Volunteers have played a major role in the development of health care in Canada over the years. Today, in the face of widespread shortages in health care services, both in hospitals and in the community, the health care system increasingly depends on volunteers.

1. What roles do volunteers continue to play in health care? Identify four areas that would benefit from the contributions of volunteers.

2. How do you think social and demographic trends will affect the roles of volunteers and volunteer organizations?

Children's Aid Society

The Children's Aid Society of Toronto, created in 1891, was the first of many such volunteer organizations to be established across Canada over the next ten years (Ontario Association of Children's Aid Societies, 2008). Originally, Children's Aid Society volunteers acted as board members and assumed duties that paid professionals perform today. The Children's Aid Society initially focused on providing food and shelter to disadvantaged children, with little thought given to maintaining the family unit. Children at risk for harm or abuse and needing protection were removed from the family environment and placed in foster homes or orphanages. Today, the provision of a secure and caring environment for the child is still paramount, but keeping families together is also a priority.

THE ROLE OF NURSING IN EARLY HEALTH CARE

Nursing care has been an essential element of the Canadian health care system since the 1600s, when the Hôtel-Dieu Hospital in Quebec launched the first structured training for North American nurses in the form of a nursing apprenticeship (Canadian Museum of Civilization, 2004).

In 1873, the first school of nursing was established at Mack's General and Marine Hospital in St. Catharines, Ontario (Mount Saint Vincent University, 2005). Another nursing school opened at Toronto General Hospital in 1881. Over the next 50 years, many hospital-based schools of nursing were established, and, in 1919, the University of British Columbia offered the first university degree program for nurses.

The Canadian National Association of Trained Nurses (CNATN) became Canada's first formal nursing organization in 1908, with a mandate to provide support for nurses graduating from formal programs. In the early 1970s, in most jurisdictions, education for nurses was moved from hospitals to colleges and universities.

THE DEVELOPMENT OF HOSPITALS IN CANADA

An order of Augustinian nuns from France who worked as "nursing sisters" established Canada's first hospital, the Hôtel-Dieu de Quebec, which opened in Quebec City in 1639. The nuns set up several other hospitals in the days before Confederation. In fact, with government funding often limited and unreliable, all of Canada's early hospitals were charitable institutions that relied on financial support from wealthy people and well-established organizations. It was not until the already-established Toronto General Hospital closed from 1867 to 1870 due to lack of funds that the Ontario government passed an act providing yearly grants to hospitals and other charitable institutions, laying the groundwork for the present-day provincial government funding of hospitals.

Aseptic technique
A procedure performed under sterile conditions to reduce the risk of infection.

Hospitals of the early 1800s were crowded places focused on treating infectious diseases primarily among people of the poorer classes, who could not afford private care. By contrast, the wealthier segment of the population avoided hospitals, instead hiring doctors, who would visit patients' homes to provide treatment. With the introduction of anaesthesia, the **aseptic technique**, and improved surgical procedures in the 1880s, however, hospitals were finally regarded as places to go to get well, and the use of hospital facilities increased.

In the early 1900s, tuberculosis sanitariums were developed to isolate and care for tuberculosis patients. The disease was difficult to treat, with surgical removal of diseased organs often the only viable cure, and many tuberculosis patients died in hospital. Special institutions to care for mentally ill people were also established. Because of the shame associated with mental illness at the time, those who suffered from it were often forcibly admitted to these institutions by family members. Most patients never emerged.

With grants from federal and provincial governments and advances in medical care, the number of hospitals increased over the next several decades. Physician and hospital services remained out-of-pocket expenses for patients, although some had insurance protection through their employers. Charitable and religious organizations continued to assist those who could not afford care.

During this time, governments made some efforts to improve access to medical care and to provide an affordable fee structure for it (Box 1.1).

Box 1.1   Innovation in Newfoundland: The Cottage Hospital System

In the 1930s, approximately 1500 communities in Newfoundland were scattered across 7000 miles of coastline. To service these communities, in 1934, the provincial government developed the Cottage Hospital and Medical Care Plan, which funded the building of a network of small hospitals and paid doctors and nurses to travel to port communities along the extensive coastline. One hospital was even built on a boat.

Intended primarily to provide outpatient care, these small hospitals were equipped with minimal inpatient facilities (20 to 30 beds), an operating room, diagnostic facilities, and a well-equipped emergency department. Outpatient services offered included immunizations, prenatal and infant care, and patient follow-up at home. The hospitals were staffed mostly by physicians and nurses with surgical and emergency care experience, and an annual fee of $10 provided a family with health care and use of the cottage hospitals, including transfer to the nearest base hospital when necessary.

Not only was Newfoundland's cottage hospital system innovative and progressive for its time; to this day, provincial and territorial systems draw on some of its key elements, such as small clinics for rural communities.

Source: Connor, J. H. T. (2007). Twillingate: Socialized medicine, rural doctors and the CIA. *Newfoundland Quarterly, 100*(424). Retrieved from http://www.newfoundlandquarterly.ca/issue424/twillingate.php.

THE INTRODUCTION OF HEALTH INSURANCE

Concerned about the continued shortage of physicians within their community, in 1914, without government approval, the residents of the small municipality of Sarnia, Saskatchewan, devised a plan to offer a local doctor $1500 (from municipal tax dollars) as an incentive to practise medicine in the community rather than join the army. The scheme proved successful and, over the next several years, attracted a number of doctors to the area. In 1916, the provincial government passed the *Rural Municipality Act*, formally allowing municipalities to collect taxes to raise funds for retaining physicians and administering and maintaining hospitals. By 1931, 52 municipalities in Saskatchewan had enacted similar plans. Not long afterward, the provinces of Manitoba and Alberta followed suit.

In 1919, the first federal attempt to introduce a publicly funded health care system formed part of a Liberal election campaign. However, once in power, the Liberals were unsuccessful in their negotiations for joint funding with the provinces and territories, so the plan was not carried out.

In the aftermath of the Depression in the 1930s, public pressure for a national health program mounted. Canadians had realized that a more secure, affordable, and accessible health care system was necessary.

First Attempts to Introduce National Health Insurance

In 1935, the Conservative government of R. B. Bennett pledged to address social issues such as minimum wage, unemployment, and public health insurance. Bennett's government proposed the *Employment and Social Insurance Act* on the advice of the Royal Commission on Industrial Relations. Under the Act, the federal government would gain the right to collect taxes to provide social benefits. The Act, however, was declared unconstitutional by the Supreme Court of Canada and the Privy Council of Great Britain on the grounds that it violated provincial and territorial authority.

Although employment and social insurance were deemed the responsibility of provincial and territorial governments in 1937, the federal government began shortly thereafter to secure some gains in overseeing social programs. In 1940, under Prime Minister Mackenzie King, the provincial and federal governments agreed to amend the *British North America Act* to allow the introduction of a national unemployment insurance program. By 1942, this program was fully operational. Two years later, in 1944, the federal government passed another piece of legislation introducing family allowances for each child aged 16 and under (often referred to as "the baby bonus"), paving the way for more social programs, the modification of existing ones, and formalized health insurance.

Post–World War II: The Political Landscape

Major changes in Canada's political landscape followed World War II. Provinces and territories began to exercise more authority over the social and economic lives of their populations. A shift in thinking, largely due to the devastating effects of the Depression, resulted in the idea that governments were responsible for providing citizens with a reasonable standard of living and acceptable access to basic services, such as health care. Canadians wanted the security and equity that a publicly funded health care system would bring.

Canadians, particularly the middle class, had felt the impact of not having access to appropriate health care. The rich could afford proper care; the poor could turn to charities. The expanding middle class was caught in between.

At the same time, medical discoveries were advancing treatment, care, and diagnostic capabilities. A shift from home- to hospital-based care, particularly when complex medical procedures were involved, created a perceived need for a more organized approach to health care. Various **social movements** advanced this agenda because people believed the involvement of the federal government would result in more stable and equitable funding, which would, in turn, support and promote medical discoveries and treatment options.

> **Social movements**
> Advancements by a collective of people to promote a common interest by acting together to influence public policy.

In 1948, the federal government set up a number of grants to fund the development of health care services in partnership with the provinces. In 1952, these grants were supplemented by a national old-age security program for individuals 70 years of age or older. That same year, the provinces and territories introduced financial aid for people between the ages of 60 and 69, provided on a cost-sharing basis with the federal government. In 1954, legislation permitted the federal government to finance allowances for adults who were disabled and unable to work. All of these measures contributed to Canadians' health and well-being.

Yet, despite increasing public requests for a nationally funded health care system, the provinces, the territories, and the federal government continued to struggle over how the system would be implemented. Who would be in charge of what, and how much power would the federal government hold over matters under provincial and territorial control?

Looking for a workable solution, the federal government ultimately decided to offer funds to the provinces and territories to help pay for health care costs; however, it also set restrictions on how the funds could be spent.

Progress Toward Prepaid Hospital Care

The National Health Grants Program of 1948 marked the first step the federal government took into the provincial and territorial jurisdictions of health care.

Through this program, the federal government offered the provinces and territories a total of $30 million to improve and modernize hospitals, to provide training for health care providers, and to fund research in the fields of public health, tuberculosis, and cancer treatments. Welcomed in all jurisdictions, these grants resulted in a hospital building boom that lasted nearly 30 years.

The next decade saw little progress in the introduction of comprehensive insurance plans in the provinces and territories. Then, in 1957, the federal government under John Diefenbaker introduced the *Hospital Insurance and Diagnostic Services Act*. The Act proposed that any province or territory willing to implement a comprehensive hospital insurance plan would receive federal assistance in the form of 50 cents on every dollar spent on the plan, literally cutting in half the province's or territory's expenses for insured services—an appealing offer indeed! Five provinces, along with the Northwest Territories and Yukon, bought into the plan immediately. All remaining jurisdictions were on board by 1961.

Even with the financial aid of the federal government, some provinces and territories were not able to implement comprehensive services, primarily because of population distribution. To rectify this problem, the federal government introduced an equalization payment system through which richer provinces would share revenue with poorer provinces to ensure all could offer equal services.

The *Hospital Insurance and Diagnostic Services Act* stated that all residents of a province or territory were entitled to receive insured health care services upon uniform terms and conditions. The Act provided residents with full care in an acute care hospital for as long as the physician felt necessary. It also included care provided in outpatient clinics, but not in tuberculosis sanitariums, mental institutions, or homes for the aged.

Services for some allied health workers (e.g., physiotherapists) and other non-medical professionals, as well as diagnostic procedures, were covered by provincial and territorial health insurance plans only if the care was provided in a hospital setting and under the direction of a physician. This coverage paved the way for a huge increase in hospital admissions, some more necessary than others. If **prepaid health care** was available with no out-of-pocket fee in the hospital, why would a patient go elsewhere, where he or she would have to pay? As a result, spending for hospital services increased dramatically.

Progress Toward Prepaid Medical Care

Tommy Douglas, known as the father of **medicare** (although this remains controversial—Justice Emmett Hall is also sometimes referred to as Canada's father of medicare), was the premier of Saskatchewan from 1944 to 1961 (Tommy Douglas Research Institute, n.d.). Douglas long campaigned for a combined comprehensive

Prepaid health care
Access to "medically necessary hospital and physician services on a prepaid basis, and on uniform terms and conditions" (Health Canada, 2005).

Medicare
The informal name for Canada's national health insurance plan. Note that the term's use in Canada differs from that in the United States, where *Medicare* refers to a federally sponsored program for individuals over the age of 65 (Health Canada, 2004).

hospital and medical insurance plan that everyone could afford. He firmly believed that the implementation of a social health insurance plan was a government responsibility and that private insurance plans, while useful, discriminated against those with lower incomes, disabilities, and serious health issues.

In 1939, the Saskatchewan government enacted the *Municipal and Medical Hospital Services Act*, permitting municipalities to charge either a land tax or a personal tax to finance hospital and medical services—a precursor to comprehensive hospital insurance in the province. Eight years later, in 1947, Tommy Douglas's government passed the *Hospital Insurance Act*, guaranteeing Saskatchewan residents hospital care in exchange for a modest insurance premium payment.

Then, in 1960, Douglas was ready to take the next step of providing Saskatchewan citizens with comprehensive, publicly funded medical care in addition to hospital insurance. His initial attempts to introduce medical care insurance inspired fierce opposition from Saskatchewan doctors, who worried they would be controlled by the province. Douglas fought an election campaign with a platform promising to introduce the health insurance program and was re-elected in 1960. The following year, Douglas left Saskatchewan to lead the New Democratic Party in Ottawa. Under his successor, Premier Woodrow Lloyd, the *Saskatchewan Medical Care Insurance Act* was passed in 1961 and took effect in July 1962.

On the day the medicare law came into effect, the doctors in Saskatchewan launched a province-wide doctors' strike. The provincial government recruited doctors from Great Britain and the United States to cope with the emergency. Fortunately, the strike was short-lived, lasting only 23 days, but it left bitterness and discontent in its wake.

In early August of 1962, the Saskatchewan government revised the *Medical Care Insurance Act* in an attempt to repair the relationship with the province's doctors. One amendment allowed doctors the option of practising outside the medical plan. By 1965, however, most doctors were working within the plan, finding it the easier route to follow. (Billing patients separately and collecting money owed proved expensive and time-consuming and resulted in only a marginal difference in remuneration.) Most other provinces and territories adopted similar plans over the next few years.

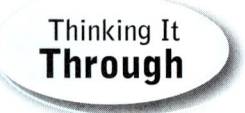

The *Saskatchewan Medical Care Act*, which enforced socialized medicine and imposed fee schedules, prompted outrage and strike action among Saskatchewan's doctors. Even today, with changes in fee structures and fee-for-service remuneration, some physicians feel a threat to their independence.

Continued on next page

Assume that you were a physician in Saskatchewan in 1962, self-employed in a sector that was considered free enterprise. Feeling that your independence as a health care provider was threatened, what would you do in response to the medicare proposals? Would you go on strike? How else might you respond?

SIGNIFICANT EVENTS LEADING UP TO THE *CANADA HEALTH ACT*

The federal government remained committed to a comprehensive health insurance program. Box 1.2 summarizes the Hall Report, the *Medical Care Act*, and the *Established Programs and Financing (EPF) Act*, all of which played a significant role leading up the *Canada Health Act*.

Box 1.2 **Legislation Leading Up to the *Canada Health Act***

The Hall Report (1960)—*Royal Commission on Health Services*

- Investigated the state of health care in Canada and was instrumental in passing the *Medical Care Act* of 1966
- Supported the introduction of a national medicare
- Suggested the construction of new medical schools and hospitals
- Recommended that the number of physicians in Canada be doubled by 1990
- Recommended that private health insurance companies in the country be replaced by ten provincial public health insurance plans
- Recommended the federal government retain strong control over health care financing but allow provinces and territories some authority over the implementation of their health care services

The *Medical Care Act* (1966)

- Implemented on July 1, 1968, and accepted by all provinces and territories by 1972
- Allowed all jurisdictions to administer the plan as they saw fit as long as they adhered to the criteria of universality, portability, comprehensive coverage, and public administration (mirroring the *Canada Health Act*)
- Covered only in-hospital care and physicians' services
- Caused the federal government, provinces, and territories to recognize the need for community-based care and restructuring of the funding formula because of soaring costs of physician and hospital care

Continued on next page

The *Established Programs Financing Act* (1977)

- Introduced a new funding formula to allocate money to health care and to postsecondary education
- Replaced the previous 50/50 cost-sharing formula with a **block transfer** of both cash and tax points (Box 1.3)
- Reduced restrictions on how jurisdictions could spend money, allowing them to fund community-based services
- Provided more transfer money for an extended health care services program, which covered intermediate care in nursing homes, ambulatory health care, residential care, and some components of home care

Block transfer
One payment from the federal to the provincial and territorial governments to cover all services.

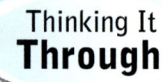

Thinking It Through

With the implementation of the *Medical Care Act*, health care costs rose dramatically, fuelling the claim that health care in Canada is consumer-generated—meaning that because health care is perceived as being free, many have sought care indiscriminately, going to the doctor for almost any complaint.

1. Do you think consumers should bear more responsibility for system costs by being more discriminating about when and why they access health care?

2. Do you think Canadians as a whole regard health care as "free," without recognizing they are paying for it (indirectly or otherwise)?

Box 1.3 Tax Points Explained

Provinces and territories get tax points with the federal government, calculated as a percentage of selected taxes collected in a jurisdiction. These points reduce the amount the federal government taxes the province or territory and, in turn, allow the province or territory to increase its taxes by the amount of its tax points and then use the money earned to pay for health care services. The result is that individuals pay the same amount in taxes but the tax money is distributed differently. For example, if the federal government taxes a province's population $200,000 less, that province can tax its residents an additional $200,000 (in place of what the residents would have had to pay the federal government) and use that money for health care services.

Sources: Government of Canada. (2002). *The transfer of tax points to provinces under the Canada health and social transfer.* Retrieved from http://dsp-psd.tpsgc.gc.ca/Collection-R/LoPBdP/BP/bp450-e.htm; Department of Finance Canada. (2008). *Tax points transfer.* Retrieved from http://www.fin.gc.ca/transfers/taxpoint/taxpoint-eng.asp.

Events Following the Introduction of the *EPF Act*

In the few years following the introduction of the *EPF Act*, health care spending continued to increase dramatically, resulting in provincial and territorial overspending and necessitating cuts to health care. Hospitals had to make cuts—some staff were let go, some medical services were either **delisted** or cut altogether, and doctors' fees were capped. In response, in 1978, outraged doctors began billing patients over and above what the provincial or territorial plan paid (in accordance with the negotiated fee schedule). For example, if the public insurance plan paid $25 for a doctor's visit, the doctor added an extra amount—say $10—and asked the patient to pay out-of-pocket for that service. This practice was called **extra billing** and contravened the principles of the *Medical Care Act*.

Opposition to extra billing was swift, with the public claiming that the fees unfairly limited access to health care. Tensions rose between physicians and the public sector. Once again, Justice Emmett Hall was asked to lead a health care services review, with the assistance of Dr. Alice Girard from Quebec. The mandate was to scrutinize issues that had risen since the previous Hall Report, including the legality of extra billing.

Hall's conclusions were released in 1980 in a report called *Canada's National–Provincial Health Program for the 1980s*. The report stated that extra billing violated the principles of the *Medical Care Act* and created a barrier for those who could not afford to pay. Hall recommended an end to extra billing and suggested that, instead, doctors be allowed to operate entirely outside of the *Medical Care Act*. That way, patients had the choice of avoiding a doctor who was not working within the boundaries of the provincial or territorial insurance plan.

Physicians opting out of the public insurance plan would bill patients directly for their services; patients would then have to collect money from their provincial or territorial insurance plan. Alternatively, the doctor could bill the plan for services, the plan would pay the patient, and the patient would pay the doctor with the money received, plus any amount the doctor charged above the plan's allowances. It was a lengthy and cumbersome process.

Hall also advised that national standards be created to uphold the principles and conditions of the *Medical Care Act*, that the criterion of accessibility be added to the Act, and that an independent National Health Council be established to assess health care in Canada and to suggest policy and legislative changes when needed.

The recommendations from the second Hall Report were taken seriously but put on hold until the Parliamentary Task Force on Federal–Provincial Arrangements completed its review the following year. This task force was to review the funding arrangements under the *EPF Act* and the other subsidies the federal

---

Delisted

The removal of an item from a list or a registry. In Canada, the term is frequently used when a medical service is no longer considered medically necessary and is removed from the government's list of insured services (CBC News, 2009; Sibbald, 2002).

Extra billing

An additional fee, considered a contravention of the *Canada Health Act*, charged to the user by a health care provider for a service covered under the terms of a provincial or territorial health insurance plan.

government provided to the provinces and territories. The task force's recommendations included adjusting equalization payments, introducing federal responsibility for income distribution, and separating health care funding from higher education funding.

Together, the Hall Report and the report of the Parliamentary Task Force on Federal–Provincial Arrangements prompted the *Canada Health Act*, new and comprehensive legislation that replaced both the *Hospital Insurance and Diagnostic Services Act* and the *Medical Care Act*.

THE *CANADA HEALTH ACT* (1984)

The ***Canada Health Act*** became law in 1984 under Prime Minister Pierre Trudeau's Liberal government. It received **royal assent** in June 1985 and is still in place today, governing and guiding—and perhaps limiting—our health care delivery system. The Act's primary goal is to provide equal, prepaid, and accessible health care to **eligible** Canadians (Box 1.4) and thereby meet the objectives of Canadian health care policy (Box 1.5).

> **Canada Health Act**
> Legislation passed in 1984 that governs and guides the delivery of equal, prepaid, and accessible health care to Canadians.
>
> **Royal assent**
> The final stage a bill passes through before becoming law. Largely symbolic in nature, this approval is given by the Governor General as a representative of the Crown.
>
> **Eligible**
> Qualified for inclusion because of meeting certain criteria or requirements.

Box 1.4   Eligibility for Health Care under the *Canada Health Act*

To be eligible for health care in Canada, a person must be a lawful resident of a province or territory. The *Canada Health Act* defines a resident as "a person lawfully entitled to be or to remain in Canada who makes his home and is ordinarily present in the province, but does not include a tourist, a transient or a visitor to the province" (*Canada Health Act*, 1985, s. 2). Each province or territory determines its own minimum residence requirements.

Source: *Canada Health Act*, R.S.C., c. C-6 (1985).

Box 1.5   The Primary Objective of Canadian Health Care Policy

"To protect, promote and restore the physical and mental well-being of residents of Canada and to facilitate reasonable access to health services without financial or other barriers."

Source: Health Canada. (2004). *What is the* Canada Health Act*?* Retrieved from http://www.hc-sc.gc.ca/hcs-sss/medi-assur/cha-lcs/overview-apercu-eng.php.

CRITERIA AND CONDITIONS OF THE CANADA HEALTH ACT

The *Canada Health Act* established criteria and conditions for the delivery of health care. To qualify for federal payments, the provinces and territories must adhere to the five criteria discussed below, as well as to two additional conditions (Box 1.6).

Box 1.6 — **The *Canada Health Act*: Criteria and Conditions**

Criteria
1. Public administration
2. Comprehensive coverage
3. Universality
4. Portability
5. Accessibility

Conditions
1. Information
2. Recognition

Source: Library of Parliament. (2005). *The* Canada Health Act: *Overview and options.* Retrieved from http://www.parl.gc.ca/information/library/PRBpubs/944-e.pdf.

Public Administration

The *Canada Health Act* stipulates that each provincial and territorial health insurance plan be managed by a public authority on a nonprofit basis. That is, the health insurance plan must not be governed by a private enterprise and must not be in the business of making a profit. The public authority answers to the provincial or territorial government regarding its decisions about benefit levels and services and must have all records and accounts publicly audited.

To meet the criteria of the Act, health plans must be overseen by the Ministry of Health, the Department of Health, or the equivalent provincial or territorial government department. Services provided under the umbrella of the relevant department are distributed via different vehicles, primarily via regional health authorities or the equivalent.

Comprehensive Coverage

Provincial and territorial health insurance plans allow eligible persons with a medical need to access prepaid, medically necessary services provided by physicians and hospitals. Select services offered by dental surgeons, when delivered in the hospital setting, are also covered. Services included under the provincial or territorial plan must be equally available to all insured residents of the province or territory; there must be no barriers to access (Case Example 1.1).

Case Example 1.1

Alois goes to his doctor to have a wart on his hand removed. The procedure may or may not be covered, depending on what province Alois lives in. For example, it is covered in Newfoundland and Labrador, so, as a resident of that province, Alois would have the procedure covered. In Ontario, though, wart removal on the hand is not a prepaid service, so if Alois lived there, he would have to pay for the procedure himself (or through supplementary insurance).

Each province or territory has the latitude to select which services will be covered under its specific plan. Coverage may include components of home care or nursing home care, chiropractic care, eye care under specific conditions, and pharmacare for designated population groups. Comprehensive coverage of these provincially or territorially tailored services must be offered to every eligible resident in the jurisdiction.

Universality

All eligible residents of a province or territory are entitled, on uniform terms and conditions, to *all* of the insured health services that are provided under the provincial or territorial health insurance plan.

The federal government allowed the provinces and territories to decide whether they would charge their residents insurance premiums. Where premiums were charged, however, a citizen's inability to pay could not prevent his or her access to appropriate medical care. The province or territory, then, would be able to subsidize premiums for those with low incomes but could not discriminate on any basis—for example, on the individual's previous health record, current health status, race, or age. *Universality* means that no matter how young or old or rich or poor a person is or what his or her health condition is, that person is eligible for the same insured health services as anyone else (Case Example 1.2).

Case Example 1.2

Juan requires surgery. He lives in British Columbia, a province that charges health care premiums. However, Juan cannot afford to pay the premiums. Universality requires that the province subsidize his premium payments so that Juan can have his surgery and any other health care he needs. Premiums aside, even if Juan were very rich and required surgery for which there was a long wait list, he would not be able to buy his way to the top of the list.

Portability

Canadians moving from one province or territory to another are covered for insured health services by their province of origin during any waiting period in the province or territory to which they have moved. Most jurisdictions enforce a three-month wait before public health insurance becomes active. Under the Act, the waiting period cannot exceed three months. Individuals moving to Canada may also have to endure a waiting period of up to three months and are, therefore, encouraged to have private insurance in place in the interim.

Canadians who leave the country will continue to be insured for health services for a prescribed period of time. Every province or territory sets its own time frame (usually six months less a day, or 183 days). Ontario states that a person may be out of the country for a maximum of 212 days in any given year, while Alberta, British Columbia, Manitoba, and New Brunswick state that a person must remain in the province for at least six months to retain coverage. In Nova Scotia, with permission and under certain conditions, a temporary absence of up to one year is allowed. Newfoundland and Labrador offers out-of-province coverage for individuals who remain in the province for only four months of the calendar year—the lowest residency requirement of all jurisdictions, in part, due to the number of migrant workers in the province. As well, every jurisdiction offers coverage for special situations, such as absences for educational or work purposes. Although Canadian residents are covered for necessary care (i.e., urgent or emergency care) while absent from their home province (e.g., for business or a vacation), they are not permitted to seek elective surgeries or other planned care in another province or territory. In some cases, prior approval for coverage may be granted for elective nonemergency surgery (Case Example 1.3).

Case Example 1.3

At 69 years old, Nancy is booked for elective hip replacement surgery in six months in her home province of Nova Scotia. However, she decides to visit her sister in British Columbia and have her hip replaced there because surgical wait times are shorter. To ensure that the Nova Scotia government will cover the cost of Nancy's surgery in British Columbia, she has to contact the Nova Scotia Department of Health for prior approval. If Nancy has the surgery without requesting approval from the Nova Scotia Department of Health, or if she is denied approval, she will have to pay for the surgery out-of-pocket.

However, if Nancy falls down the stairs and breaks her hip while she is visiting her sister, the surgery would be done in British Columbia, and the total cost would be covered by her province of origin without question.

The Web sites of the provincial and territorial ministries of health offer information about the particulars of each jurisdiction's health care coverage.

Insured services received outside the person's province of origin will be paid at the host province's rate, except by Quebec (Case Example 1.4).

Case Example 1.4

Jeremy, a 20-year-old resident of Ontario, is visiting friends in Saskatchewan. While there, he develops a severe and persistent sore throat and pays a visit to a local doctor. Even if the cost of a visit to the family doctor is $20 in Saskatchewan but is only $15 in his home province of Ontario, the Ontario health plan will pay the full $20 required by the doctor in Saskatchewan.

Now, consider the situation if Jeremy is from Quebec. If the fee for the same doctor's visit is $15 in Quebec, the Quebec health plan will pay only $15 to the doctor in Saskatchewan, and Jeremy will have to pay $5. Quebec does not honour the host province's or territory's fee schedule if it is higher than its own.

Accessibility

The criterion of accessibility was added to the *Canada Health Act* in an attempt to ensure that eligible individuals in a province or territory have reasonable access to all insured health services on uniform terms and conditions. *Reasonable access* means access to services when and where they are available, as they are available. A service may not be available to a person because of where he or she lives—for example, in a more remote community (Case Example 1.5). Or a service may be unavailable because of a shortage of beds or lack of health care providers to supply the service (Case Example 1.6). Individuals needing a service that is not available must be granted access to that service in the closest location it is offered—whether in another town or city, in another province, or in the United States.

Accessibility applies to wait times as well. Some jurisdictions have established maximum wait times for certain procedures. If a person has to wait for a procedure (e.g., a hip replacement) beyond that set time limit, the province or territory will send the person somewhere else for the procedure (Case Example 1.3). Note, however, that a province or territory would pay for a patient to receive an available service only at the closest alternative location, not a location farther afield or one that the patient prefers.

The interpretation of *reasonable access* is controversial. A person living in Churchill, Manitoba, will not have the same access to health care as a person living in Halifax, Toronto, or Vancouver. Today, service availability even varies between rural and urban settings. For the purposes of the *Canada Health Act*, accessibility has been interpreted as access to services where and when available. It does not, in the true sense of the word, guarantee "equality" of services across Canada.

Case Example 1.5

Monique is a 40-year-old woman living in Sioux Lookout, Ontario. She has just been diagnosed with breast cancer. Her community does not have access to radiation therapy, but this therapy is available in Thunder Bay, Ontario. In accordance with the accessibility criterion, Monique would be sent to Thunder Bay for her treatments. If radiation therapy was not available in Thunder Bay—or if the wait time was excessive—Monique would be sent to Winnipeg, Manitoba.

Case Example 1.6

Pang went into labour at 28 weeks gestation. Delivery was imminent, and it was concluded that no facilities in her home province of British Columbia or close by could provide the highly specialized care required for the premature baby (reasons for such service unavailability could include no bed being available or a shortage of nursing staff). Pang was transferred by air ambulance to a hospital in Washington. The baby stayed in hospital for three weeks until he was stable enough to be sent back to British Columbia. The B.C. Medical Care Plan covered all medical expenses.

The following two conditions were imposed upon provinces in the *Canada Health Act*:

- *Information.* Each province or territory must provide the federal government with information about the insured health care services and extended health care services for the purposes identified in the *Canada Health Act.*
- *Recognition.* The provincial and territorial governments must publicly recognize the federal financial contributions to both insured and extended health care services.

Interpreting the Canada Health Act

Medically necessary is a subjective term that has been hotly debated within the context of the *Canada Health Act* (also see Chapter 8). Typically, a physician or other health care provider eligible to bill the provincial or territorial plan makes a clinical judgement to provide the patient with specific "medically necessary" services, which usually include assessment, diagnostic tests, and treatment. Note, however, that some jurisdictions may not cover all diagnostic tests and treatments. Since the *Canada Health Act* does not detail which services should be insured, the range of insured services varies among provinces and territories.

Medical services (e.g., Caesarean section) must not be provided simply for the convenience of the patient or physician. And when more than one treatment is available, a physician must consider cost effectiveness. For example, when faced with two treatment options that have similar outcomes, a physician must recommend the less expensive option.

What one doctor considers medically necessary another doctor may not. Consider breast reduction: a surgeon in Manitoba might determine that this surgery is medically necessary for a particular patient with large breasts because of the backaches and muscle strains she suffers. Another surgeon may not think breast reduction is medically necessary for this patient, meaning that the patient would have to pay for the surgery since it would then be considered a cosmetic procedure.

> **Medically necessary**
> A clinical judgement made by a physician regarding the necessity of a service provided under a provincial or territorial health plan to maintain, restore, or palliate (i.e., ease symptoms, such as pain, without curing the underlying disease).

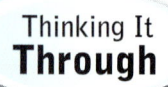

The term *medically necessary* appears in the *Canada Health Act* to identify procedures and services that are covered by provincial and territorial insurance.

1. Do you think that the term is too subjective?

2. Are there health services in your province or territory that you feel should be covered but are not?

Physicians, through their governing body, and government officials—usually from the Ministry or Department of Health—select which services are medically necessary and are, therefore, insured. At designated intervals, the provinces and territories review their lists of insured services, sometimes adding services, sometimes removing them.

A few years ago, for example, many jurisdictions removed elective newborn circumcision from the list of insured services because evidence showed no medical reason for this procedure and found other reasons (e.g., a belief that a circumcised penis is cleaner or that the baby should resemble his father) to be invalid. However, circumcision is still insured when a valid medical reason exists for doing it.

Also addressed in the *Canada Health Act* are extra billing and **user charges**. Under the Act, extra billing and user charges are not allowed because they create a barrier to seeking medical care. If a province or territory nevertheless permits extra billing or user charges, the federal government will total the amount of money the province or territory has collected and will deduct that amount from the next transfer of funds. Proponents of user charges believe they play a useful role in today's health care climate: for example, charging people who use the emergency department for nonurgent complaints (Case Example 1.7) may ultimately improve emergency department wait times.

> **User charges**
> A fee imposed for an insured health service that the provincial or territorial health care insurance plan does not cover.

Case Example 1.7

Miao, who lives in Alberta, went to the emergency department because she had a bad cold. The provincial plan would cover the cost of the visit, but the hospital charged Miao an additional $30 because she came to Emergency instead of going to her doctor. The $30 is a user charge.

ADDITIONAL COMPONENTS OF THE ACT

The *Canada Health Act* specifically outlines extended health care services that are considered medically necessary and are thus insured. Extended health care services insured under the Act include intermediate care in nursing homes, adult residential care services, home care services, and the services provided in ambulatory care centres.

A number of services, such as certain components of home care, however, are not covered under the Act and are subject to each province's or territory's health insurance plan. Some jurisdictions, for example, will provide a certain number of home care hours per week. Once the limit is reached, the patient must pay a home care agency for additional care. The legislation prohibiting user charges and extra billing, therefore, does not apply to extended health care services.

Each province and territory chooses which optional services (i.e., services that are not medically necessary) will be covered under its health plan. Optional services may include chiropody (i.e., foot care), massage therapy, physiotherapy, dental care, drug plans, and assistive devices coverage. (Note: Services supplied within a hospital or other insured facility are usually covered.)

The amount of coverage for optional services will vary. For example, a province's plan may cover up to $200 per month in physiotherapy services. Services in excess of this amount are subject to user charges and extra billing, which, as mentioned, are permitted for services deemed not medically necessary under the Act.

AFTER THE *CANADA HEALTH ACT*: COMMISSIONED REPORTS AND ACCORDS

Most of the resistance to the Act came from physicians and those affected directly by the restrictions set out in the Act. In 1986, Ontario physicians participated in a 25-day strike in opposition to the Act, arguing that the key issue was not money but professional freedom, a claim not well received by the public (In the News: Doctors Striking for Autonomy). That same year, the Canadian Medical Association opposed the implementation of the *Canada Health Act* on the grounds that it violated the *Constitution Act* of 1982. The case went to the Supreme Court of Canada but did not proceed.

In the News — Doctors Striking for Autonomy

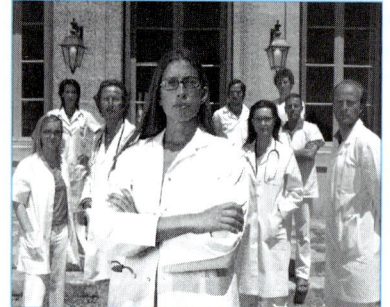

On June 12, 1986, Ontario doctors took strike action on the grounds that banning extra billing violated their right to contract directly with patients and undermined the quality of care. Doctors saw this ban as an end to their independence, a means of essentially turning them into civil servants. For the first time, Ontarians turned on the news to see militant doctors marching with picket signs in hand.

While the strike was supported by nearly all regions and specialties, a majority of doctors did not participate. Furthermore, public opinion remained firmly opposed to the doctors' arguments. In fact, the strike was widely viewed as a public relations disaster. The Ontario Medical Association later admitted that, to a large degree, hostile public opinion prompted the end of the strike.

Ultimately, the strike failed to stop the ban on extra billing. The true outcome? Bitter feelings that persist even today.

Sources: Kravitz, R. L., Shapiro, M. F., Linn, L. S., et al. (1989). Risk factors associated with participation in the Ontario Canada doctor's strike. *American Journal of Public Health, 79*, 1233–1277; Brennan, R. (1986, December 27). Doctor's strike memories linger. *The Windsor Star*, p. A3.
Photo credit: Ghislain & Marie David de Lossy/GetStock.

Just prior to the introduction of the Act, most of the provinces and territories had established some form of extra billing, user charges, or both as a result of events leading up to the implementation of the *Canada Health Act*. These extra fees could not be removed overnight. Over the next two years, the federal government imposed monetary penalties to noncompliant jurisdictions, again fuelling resentment and opposition. The federal government decided, however, to reimburse provinces that took corrective action against extra billing and user charges within three years. Most jurisdictions complied, but these practices were not entirely eliminated. Even today, some provinces and territories defy this part of the Act, resulting, each year, in withheld funding primarily related to user charges at private clinics deemed by the federal government to be operating outside of the law.

In the decade following the implementation of the *Canada Health Act*, the health care system in Canada experienced increasing difficulties that persist today. At first, hospitals had trouble functioning within their allotted budgets. Provinces and territories pushed for more money to sustain reasonable levels of care, yet federal funding continued to dwindle. In the early 1990s, hospitals restructured, downsized, redistributed beds, laid off staff, cut services, and closed. Doctors and nurses left the country, and fewer graduates pursued careers in these roles, leading to widespread staffing shortages.

Some provinces and territories responded proactively by establishing innovative and alternative health care strategies (Box 1.7). Home care became a priority across Canada; the concept of "health care teams" (i.e., the physician working with other health care providers to deliver more comprehensive, patient-oriented care) was introduced; access to primary care services (e.g., through after-hours clinics, telephone helplines, and extended office hours) was improved; and **primary health care reform** began to take place (Table 1.1).

Primary health care reform
Changes to the delivery of primary health care with the goal of providing all Canadians access to an appropriate health care provider 24 hours a day, 7 days a week, no matter where they live.

Box 1.7 New Brunswick Leads the Way in Community Care

New Brunswick was one of the first jurisdictions to predict the problems related to funding shortfalls, cutbacks, population changes, and an increased need for hospital beds. The province led the move toward community-based care, called "hospital without walls," and established the Extra-Mural Program, which focused on shortening hospital stays and providing the appropriate care and support to meet health care needs in home and community settings. This concept was actually introduced in 1979, five years before the *Canada Health Act* was passed.

Throughout the 1980s and 1990s, various provinces and territories completed investigations into the state of health care—the Royal Commission on Health Care

Continued on next page

in Nova Scotia (1989), Advisory Committee on the Utilization of Medical Services in Alberta (1989), Premier's Commission on Future Health Care in Alberta (1989), New Brunswick Commission on Selected Health Care Programs (1989), Commission on Directions in Health Care in Saskatchewan (1990), Premier's Council on Health Strategy in Ontario (1991), Royal Commission on Healthcare and Costs in British Columbia (1991), and the Health Services Review in British Columbia (1999).

National reports were also commissioned—for example, the first and second reports on the health of Canadians, released in 1996 and 1999, respectively, examined and summarized the health status of Canadians.

By 2002, public confidence in health care was at an all-time low, with health care topping the list of Canadians' concerns. Only recently have Canadians become more concerned about the environment than health care. Ironically, environmental concerns (e.g., pollution, contaminated drinking water, poor air quality) squarely interact with health care concerns.

Source: South East Regional Health Authority. (n.d.). *Extra-Mural Program.* Retrieved from http://www.serha.ca/extra_mural/htm/english/about_us.htm.

Table 1.1 The Goals of Primary Health Care Reform

Medical Model of Health Care	Primary Health Care Reform Goals
Physician-based care	Team-oriented care
Illness-focused	Emphasis on health
Hospital-based care	Community-based care
Curative (in relation to disease)	Focus on health promotion and disease prevention
Problems are isolated	Care is comprehensive and integrated (i.e., holistic)
Health care provider–dominated	Collaborative care involving patient, family, and loved ones

SOCIAL UNION

First ministers
The premiers of the provinces and territories.

In 1997, the provincial and territorial **first ministers** met with their federal counterparts to form a social renewal program that would bind all governments to a commitment to move forward collaboratively on what the first ministers called a social union (Social Union, 1999). First ministers from all jurisdictions, except Newfoundland and Quebec, gathered to press Ottawa for a funding increase. Over the next several months, negotiations became increasingly confrontational, with the federal government wanting a voice in how money would be spent and on what services (e.g., cancer treatments, improvements to emergency departments, long-term care). However, in 1999, Prime Minister Jean Chrétien put forth a plan that offered the provinces and territories more spending flexibility. On January 22, 1999, all of the provinces (including Quebec) and territories agreed to commit to the prime minister's proposals. Quebec, however, did not sign the final agreement on February 4, 1999 (Government of Canada, 1999). The province opposed any arrangements that implied the federal government would have any authority over provincial social policy. As well, Quebec was unwilling to sign any agreement that did not clearly support the province's right to unconditionally opt out of programs supported by or initiated by the federal government, which the social union did not provide for.

The social union was a significant move forward in harmonizing federal–provincial and federal–territorial relationships. The union's goal was to clarify the role of the federal government with respect to funding and commitment and to work collaboratively to improve health care and social programs for Canadians.

The union agreed to maintain the five criteria of the *Canada Health Act* and to work continuously to improve health care by sharing information and innovations. The ministers also pledged to report ongoing government activities to keep Canadians informed about their health status and public programs. The union was committed to working collaboratively with Aboriginal people, their governments, and their organizations to improve health care and social programs for Aboriginals. The federal government promised to boost health care spending by $11.5 billion over the next five years, starting in the 1999–2000 fiscal year.

Commissioned Reports

By the end of 2002, three major reports on the status of health care in Canada had been commissioned and released: the Mazankowski Report, the Kirby Report, and the Romanow Report. See Box 1.8 for the key points of each report.

Box 1.8 **Three Major Reports on the Status of Health Care in Canada**

The Mazankowski Report: *A Framework for Reform* (2001)

Commissioned by former Alberta premier Ralph Klein in August 2000 and chaired by Donald Mazankowski, former Cabinet member in the Mulroney government

Purpose: to provide strategic advice to the premier on the preservation and future enhancement of quality health services for Albertans

Continued on next page

Key Points:

- Supported private health care in that it recommended doctors be allowed to work in private health care venues after devoting a specific amount of time to the public sector
- Recommended, after review, delisting selected services currently covered under the provincial plan
- Recommended the implementation of province-wide electronic health records and electronic health cards
- Suggested that taxes be used as a source of increased revenue and that Albertans pay higher health premiums (not well received)

Significant Outcomes: By 2003, Alberta had implemented a province-wide electronic health record initiative, becoming the first Canadian province to do so.

The Kirby Report: *The Health of Canadians—The Federal Role* (2002)

Led by Senator Michael J. Kirby

Purpose: to examine the state of the Canadian health care system and the role of the federal government in it

Key Points:

- Bore important similarities to the Mazankowski Report
- Felt the health care system was unsustainable with existing levels of funding
- Recommended the implementation of new taxes or insurance premiums that were geared to income
- Recommended setting limits to wait times; once the limit was reached, stated the government should pay for the patient to receive treatment elsewhere, even in the United States if necessary
- Recommended a government-funded assistance plan for medications under certain circumstances related to the cost of medications proportionate to a person's (or a family's) income
- Recommended an immediate outlay of $2 billion for information technology, including the development of a national system for electronic health records, and another $2.5 billion over five years for advanced medical equipment
- Suggested government incentives encouraging health care providers to return to Canada and outlay of funds to recruit and train doctors and nurses

Significant Outcomes: This report was not as widely accepted as the Romanow Report. However, Ontario did adopt payment premiums for health care.

The Romanow Report: *Building on Values: The Future of Health Care in Canada* (2002)

Led by Roy Romanow, former premier of Saskatchewan and chair of the Commission on the Future of Health Care in Canada

Purpose: to present recommendations to ensure the survival of Canada's health care system and to consider health promotion and disease prevention initiatives

Key Points:

- Bore important similarities to the Mazankowski Report
- Gathered information and advice from Canadians through public forums and meetings held across the country
- Believed that health care was sustainable but that immediate action was necessary by all levels of government (funding and revision)
- Opposed privatization of health care, stating that any new plans creating private health care initiatives should be discouraged
- Recommended the creation of the Health Council of Canada to oversee improvements to health care, to conduct regular reviews of the health care system (e.g., home- and community-based care, primary care reform initiatives, human health resources, implementation of drug plans, wait times), and to report findings to the public
- Recommended that reform initiatives be paid for by the federal government's surplus or by raising taxes (e.g., the federal government could establish a dedicated cash-only Canada Health Transfer)
- Recommended adding the criterion of accountability to the *Canada Health Act*
- Recommended extending coverage for home care, diagnostic testing, **palliative care**, and mental health care
- Suggested that Employment Insurance benefits and job security be extended to family members and friends who choose to care for sick or dying loved ones at home
- Recommended that **catastrophic drug costs**, subject to certain terms and conditions (e.g., ability to pay), be covered
- Recommended that a national body control the price of drugs, provide a centralized list of drugs covered by public health plans, monitor the safety and cost of new drugs seeking federal approval for use, and review the efficacy and outcomes of drugs in use
- Recommended the establishment of another independent agency to review and approve prescription drugs and to ensure that Canadians have clear and concise information about the drugs they are taking
- Advocated the organization of a central body to monitor and streamline wait lists, but did not recommend a limit on wait times

Significant Outcomes: See Impact of the Romanow Report, below.

Sources: Mazankowski, D. (2001). *A framework for reform: Report of the Premier's Advisory Council on Health*. Retrieved from http://www.health.alberta.ca/resources/publications/PACH_report_final.pdf; Kirby, M. J. L. (2002). *The health of Canadians—The federal role. Final report*. Retrieved from http://www.parl.gc.ca/37/2/parlbus/commbus/senate/Com-e/soci-e/rep-e/repoct02vol6-e.htm; Romanow, R. (2002). *Building on values: The future of health care in Canada*. Retrieved from http://www.cbc.ca/healthcare/final_report.pdf.

Palliative care
Care for the dying. Palliative care services, offered in the home or another facility (e.g., palliative care unit in a hospital or a hospice), may include nursing care, counselling, and pain management and may involve those close to the patient.

Catastrophic drug costs
Prescription drug costs that cause undue burden on individuals with serious health conditions or illnesses.

Impact of the Romanow Report

Following the release of the Romanow Report, the federal government under Prime Minister Jean Chrétien stated that the report would provide the foundation for the direction of health care over the next several years. In 2004, the federal government earmarked $10 billion for health care to be distributed over a 10-year time frame to address the problems identified in the report.

Several of Romanow's recommendations have been implemented. On April 1, 2004, the Canada Health Transfer (CHT) and the Canada Social Transfer (CST) replaced the Canada Health and Social Transfer (CHST), a set amount of money (a block transfer payment) from the federal government to the provinces intended to pay for health care, postsecondary education, and welfare. See also Chapter 8.

Health promotion campaigns have been maintained and further promoted by all levels of government. Limits on wait times were implemented across the country, and current wait times were required to be posted on the Internet. The Health Council of Canada was created as a result of the 2003 First Ministers' Accord but was subsequently disbanded by the federal government in 2014. At the 2004 first ministers' meeting, Canada's first ministers agreed on more funding and initiatives for health care renewal, including funding for family members to remain at home to care for ill relatives. Primary health care reform initiatives have been tested, implemented, and revised across Canada. Funds have been made available for information technology and electronic health records in all jurisdictions. A national catastrophic drug plan (see Chapter 8) has not been implemented, although most jurisdictions now have one of their own.

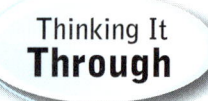
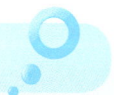

Introducing a national drug plan and increased coverage for home care, two of the recommendations made in the Romanow Report, would cost billions of dollars. To date, neither has been implemented.

1. Do you think that health care as we know it is sustainable?

2. Are Canadians expecting too much, or do Canadians need to change their expectations?

3. Do you think a national paid-for drug plan and increased coverage for home care would be cost effective?

Accords

The following summaries of first ministers' meetings highlight the most recent **health accords** between the federal government and the provincial and territorial governments.

First Ministers' Meeting, 2000

In September 2000, the first ministers met and agreed to work together to identify the significant issues facing health care in each province and territory, to prioritize these concerns, and to pledge to work collaboratively to address these concerns on both a provincial or territorial and national level.

The major issues identified at this meeting included the following (First Ministers, 2000):

- Timely access to health care
- Health promotion and disease prevention
- The structure and function of primary care services (access and wait times)
- The shortage of health care providers across Canada
- The cost and availability of home and community health care services
- The cost and management of medications, health information, and electronic health records
- The inadequacy of diagnostic equipment
- The lack of accountability to Canadians regarding the implementation and function of health care services

A number of meetings followed. Agreements were achieved, commitments were made, and funding was pledged to address concerns. The renewed commitment at each subsequent meeting built on the promises made at the September 2000 first ministers' gathering. Each meeting addressed the same general concerns but extracted more specific promises regarding various health care services and federal funding.

First Ministers' Accord on Health Care Renewal, 2003

In February 2003, the prime minister and the premiers of seven provinces met in Ottawa to outline the immediate direction for health care in Canada. The overriding commitment made was to preserve universal health care under the current *Canada Health Act* (First Ministers, 2003).

A key component of this accord was the outlining of standards of care for Canadians, including access to health care providers 24 hours a day, 7 days a week; prompt access to diagnostic services and treatments; the implementation

> **Health accord**
> A legal agreement between the federal and provincial and territorial governments on health care funding.

of a nationwide electronic health record system; and financial assistance for those who needed medications but could not afford them.

Created at this meeting, the Health Reform Fund, over a five-year time frame, would channel money into primary care, a catastrophic drug plan, and home care services. The federal government would transfer money to the provinces and territories so that they could address the specific needs of their residents.

The ministers also addressed the unique needs of Aboriginal people. The federal government pledged to work more closely with provincial and territorial governments and Aboriginal leaders to bring health care services for Aboriginal people on par with those provided to other Canadians.

The equalization payment program was re-examined to ensure that all provinces had adequate funding to provide comparable health care services to their citizens. As previously mentioned, it was through this accord that the Canada Health Transfer was created, separating the funding formula that had combined federal funding for both health care and postsecondary education.

In this accord, the federal government also pledged to introduce a compassionate care benefit package through the Employment Insurance program, along with job protection through the Canada Labour Code (as recommended in the Romanow Report), to provide financial security and job protection for individuals who temporarily leave their place of employment to care for a seriously ill or dying parent, spouse, or child. This recommendation was implemented in 2012.

First Ministers' Meeting on the Future of Health Care, 2004

The First Ministers' Meeting on the Future of Health Care was convened to follow up on agreements made in 2003, discuss progress, and move forward with other proposals (First Ministers, 2004). At this meeting, the prime minister and premiers signed a second agreement, with the federal government pledging $41 billion for health care services over a 10-year time frame. Once again, the first ministers renewed their commitment to building on the criteria of the current *Canada Health Act* and to working together in a constructive and open manner. They promised to share information and to be more accountable to the public about progress being made. The Health Council of Canada was given increased responsibilities to report to Canadians on health outcomes.

The prime minister, first ministers, and Aboriginal leaders established the Aboriginal Health Transition Fund, which provided $200 million for improving Aboriginal health care services to meet the needs of Aboriginal people across Canada.

Annual Conference of Ministers of Health, 2005

At the Annual Conference of Ministers of Health in 2005, particular consideration was given to the catastrophic drug coverage mentioned at previous meetings. The ministers of health discussed measures to move forward with previous recommendations to standardize the price of drugs across Canada and pledged to have better control over the pharmaceutical industry's relationship with provincial and territorial health insurance plans (First Ministers, 2005).

The Kelowna Accord, 2006

The first ministers met again in Kelowna, British Columbia, where the federal government promised to spend $5 billion over five years to improve health, housing, and education for Aboriginal people (Kelowna Accord, 2006). The ministers also established the *Blueprint on Aboriginal Health*, a plan aimed to bring the health outcomes of Aboriginal people in line with those of the general Canadian population—although provinces and territories have yet to commit to the plan.

A few days later, the Paul Martin minority Liberal government fell, and the promises outlined in the Kelowna Accord were never met.

The Mental Health Commission of Canada (MHCC), 2007

The Standing Senate Committee (the Kirby Report) recommended the creation of a mental health commission to focus attention on mental health in Canada. The MHCC identifies problems related to mental health and makes recommendations for improvement. Such problems include inmates with mental health issues, housing, health care, and supporting individuals with mental illness as well as their families (In the News: Not Criminally Responsible?).

In the News — Not Criminally Responsible?

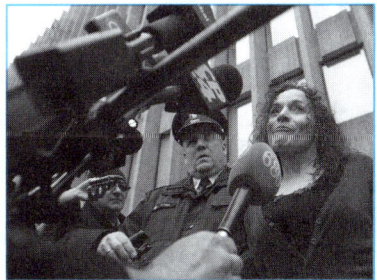

Richard Kachkar, 64, killed Toronto police officer Sgt. Ryan Russell, running him over with a snowplow in 2011. He was charged with murder in the first degree. The defence claimed that Mr. Kachkar was mentally ill at the time of the incident, thus not responsible for his actions. His behaviour before and leading up to the incident was erratic. Three psychiatrists testified that they believed Mr. Kachkar to be psychotic at the time. In April 2013, the jury found Mr. Kachkar to be not criminally responsible for his actions.

In early 2014, the Ontario Review Board granted Mr. Kachkar escorted passes into the community despite a doctor's claim that his condition was not well understood and the fact that he had not begun treatment. If, during periodic reviews, he is deemed no longer a danger to the public, Kachkar could be released. Opposition to the decision to allow him escorted passes was fierce. Christine Russell, the victim's wife, has pledged to appear at each review and to fight to

Continued on next page

keep Mr. Kachkar from being released. Had Mr. Kachkar been found responsible for his actions, despite his mental illness, he would have been sent to a penitentiary, possibly without any treatment. What good would that have done?

Sources: Small, P. (2013, March 27). Richard Kachkar found not criminally responsible in Sgt. Ryan Russell's snowplow death. *Toronto Star*. Retrieved from http://www.thestar.com/news/crime/2013/03/27/richard_kachkar_found_not_criminally_responsible_in_police_officers_snowplow_death.html; Mandel, M. (2014, January 11). Bid to stop freedom for Sgt. Ryan Russell's killer. *Toronto Sun*. Retrieved from http://www.torontosun.com/2014/01/11/bid-to-stop-cop-killers-freedom.
Photo credit: The Canadian Press/Nathan Denette.

The 2014 Health Accord

The 2004 Health Accord expired in 2014. In 2012, Prime Minister Stephen Harper announced his plan for the 2014 Health Accord. Provisions for financing under this accord are effective until 2024. Under the plan, federal transfers will increase by 6% until 2017 and be tied to the gross domestic product (GDP) after that.

SUMMARY

1.1 Health care in Canada evolved from European settlers' bringing doctors and nurses (many of them with the military) to the country in the 1500s and 1600s and integrating many of their practices with those of the Aboriginal peoples. In the 1700s and early 1800s, volunteer organizations played a key role in the delivery of health care. The concept of public health emerged in the early 1800s, and, with the passage of the *British North America Act* in 1867, federal and provincial governments shared responsibilities for health care, which, over time, became more structured and formalized. As a result, some government funding of hospitals began around this time, and the first school of nursing was established in 1873 in St. Catharines, Ontario.

1.2 The road toward health insurance began with the first federal attempt to introduce a publicly funded health care system in 1919. Following World War II, governments began thinking that they had an obligation to provide Canadians with a better standard of living, including access to quality health care. Prepaid hospital care was introduced in 1948 and was well received by all jurisdictions. Shortly afterward, Saskatchewan spearheaded an organized push to integrate both medical and hospital care into the public health care system.

1.3 With the federal government committed to a comprehensive national health care system, a number of reports and pieces of legislation followed. The Hall Report, the *Medical Care Act*, and the *Established Programs and Financing Act* all played significant roles leading up to the *Canada Health Act*. In 1957, the federal government introduced the *Hospital Insurance and Diagnostic Services Act*, which was the precursor to prepaid health care for all Canadians. Prepaid health care as we know it today came into effect in 1984 with the passage of the *Canada Health Act*.

1.4 The five criteria established by the *Canada Health Act* of 1984 for the delivery of health care are public administration, comprehensive coverage, universality, portability, and accessibility. The two conditions included in the Act are information and recognition. The *Canada Health Act* specifically outlines extended health care services that are considered medically necessary and are thus insured. *Medically necessary* is a subjective term that has been debated within the context of the *Canada Health Act*; *extra billing* and *user charges* are permitted only for services deemed not medically necessary under the Act.

1.5 There was some opposition to the *Canada Health Act* by physicians and the Canadian Medical Association on the grounds that it restricted extra billing and user charges and violated professional freedom. In the decade that followed the implementation of the Act, increasing difficulties in the health care system led some provinces and territories to establish innovative health care strategies, and primary health care reform began to take place. In 1997, the first ministers met with the federal government to work toward a social union and clarify the role of the federal government with respect to funding. By the end of 2002, three major reports on the status of health care in Canada had been commissioned and released: the Mazankowski Report, the Kirby Report, and the Romanow Report. Several first ministers' meetings over the past 15 years have resulted in the creation of new health accords.

REVIEW QUESTIONS

1. What were the health care responsibilities of the federal and provincial governments outlined in the *British North America Act*?
2. What organizations attended to the health care needs of Canadians in the eighteenth and nineteenth centuries?
3. How and when was health insurance first introduced in Canada?
4. How and when was the concept of prepaid hospital care introduced in Canada?
5. List and describe three pieces of legislation that played significant roles leading up to the creation of the *Canada Health Act*.
6. List and describe the criteria and conditions of the *Canada Health Act*.
7. What is meant by the terms *medically necessary*, *extra billing*, and *user charges*, and how do they relate to each other in the context of the *Canada Health Act*?
8. What are the goals of primary health care reform?
9. List and describe three major reports on the status of health care in Canada.

References

Canada Health Act. (1985). RSC, c. C-6.

Canadian Blood Services. (n.d.). *Media questions & answers*. Retrieved from http://www.blood.ca/Web/bloodcatest.nsf/page/Questions+and+Answers?OpenDocument.

Canadian Museum of Civilization. (2004). *A brief history of nursing in Canada from the establishment of New France to the present*. Retrieved from http://www.civilization.ca/cmc/exhibitions/tresors/nursing/nchis01e.shtml.

Canadian Red Cross. (2008). *Historical timeline 1900–1950*. Retrieved from http://www.redcross.ca/article.asp?id=7834&tid=019.

CBC News. (2009). No delisting of health services for now: Alberta health minister. *CBC*. Retrieved from http://www.cbc.ca/news/canada/edmonton/no-delisting-of-health-services-for-now-alberta-health-minister-1.803655.

First Ministers. (2000). *Details of the first ministers' conference, Ottawa*. Retrieved from http://www.scics.gc.ca/cinfo00/800038004_e.html.

First Ministers. (2003). *First ministers' accord on health care renewal, Ottawa*. Retrieved from http://www.hc-sc.gc.ca/hcs-sss/delivery-prestation/fptcollab/2003accord/nr-cp_e.html.

First Ministers. (2004). *First minister's meeting on the future of health care 2004: A 10-year plan to strengthen health care*. Retrieved from http://www.hc-sc.gc.ca/hcs-sss/delivery-prestation/fptcollab/2004-fmm-rpm/index-eng.php.

First Ministers. (2005). *Annual conference of federal-provincial-territorial ministers of Health, Toronto, Ontario*. Canadian Intergovernmental Conference Secretariat [News release]. Retrieved from http://www.scics.gc.ca/cinfo05/830866004_e.html.

Government of Canada. (1999). *Intergovernmental relations—social union issues*. Prepared by Jack Stilborn, Political and Social Affairs Division. Retrieved from http://dsp-psd.pwgsc.gc.ca/Collection-R/LoPBdP/BP/prb9937-e.htm.

Health Canada. (2004). *Canada's health care system (medicare)*. Retrieved from http://www.hc-sc.gc.ca/hcs-sss/medi-assur/index-eng.php.

Health Canada. (2005). Canada Health Act. *Frequently asked questions*. Retrieved from http://www.hc-sc.gc.ca/hcs-sss/medi-assur/res/faq-eng.php.

Health Canada. (2006). *Health care system: Background*. Retrieved from http://www.hc-sc.gc.ca/hcs-sss/pubs/system-regime/2005-hcs-sss/back-context-eng.php.

Kelowna Accord. (2006). *Aboriginal roundtable to Kelowna Accord: Aboriginal policy negotiations, 2004–2005*. Retrieved from http://parl.gc.ca/information/library/PRB-pubs/prb0604-e.htm.

Krever Commission. (2004). *Final report: Commission of inquiry on the blood system in Canada*. Retrieved from http://www.hc-sc.gc.ca/ahc-asc/activit/com/krever-eng.php.

Krever Inquiry. (n.d.). In *The Canadian Encyclopedia*. Retrieved from http://www.thecanadianencyclopedia.com/index.cfm?PgNm=TCE&Params=A1ARTA0009152.

Mount Saint Vincent University. (2005). *Formal training for nurses, the beginning*. Retrieved from http://www.msvu.ca/library/archives/nhdp/history.htm.

Ontario Association of Children's Aid Societies. (2008). *History of child welfare*. Retrieved from http://www.oacas.org/childwelfare/history.htm.

Sibbald, B. (2002). BC takes ax to budget of a health system "in danger." *Canadian Medical Association Journal*, *166*(4). Retrieved from http://www.cmaj.ca/cgi/content/full/166/4/492.

Social Union. (1999). *A framework to improve the social union for Canadians: An agreement between the Government of Canada and the governments of the provinces and territories*. Retrieved from http://socialunion.gc.ca/news/020499_e.html.

St. John Ambulance. (1995). *Our history*. Retrieved from http://www.kwsja.com/history.html.

Tommy Douglas Research Institute. (n.d.). *Achievements*. Retrieved from http://www.tommydouglas.ca/tommy/achievements/.

Wynne-Jones, T. (2002). Whose health: Who cares? [Editorial]. *Canadian Medical Association Journal*, *167*(2). Retrieved from http://www.cmaj.ca/cgi/content/full/167/2/156.

Chapter Two

Health and the Individual

Learning Outcomes

2.1 Describe the key concepts of health, wellness, illness, disease, and disability.

2.2 Explain the main models of health.

2.3 Understand changing perceptions of health.

2.4 Examine the psychology of health behaviour.

2.5 Describe the health–illness continuum and the impact of self-imposed risk behaviours.

2.6 Identify the leading causes of morbidity and mortality in Canada.

Key Terms

Aboriginal Canadians, p. 63
Cardiovascular disease, p. 65
Cerebrovascular disease, p. 66
Compensation, p. 55
Culture, p. 54
Disability, p. 47
Disease, p. 46
Etiology, p. 45
Exacerbation, p. 47
Health behaviour, p. 52
Health beliefs, p. 53
Health–illness continuum, p. 55
Health model, p. 48
Holistic, p. 49
Infant mortality, p. 63
Life expectancy, p. 62
Morbidity, p. 41
Mortality, p. 41
Remission, p. 47
Self-imposed risk behaviours, p. 49
Sick role behaviour, p. 57
Signs, p. 60
Symptoms, p. 60
Wellness, p. 41

Anyone entering a health care profession, either as a hands-on health care provider or as a contributor of administrative or technical expertise, will find it helpful to understand the concepts of health and wellness. It is also important to know what makes Canadians ill. Many of the medical conditions most health care workers encounter in their career are, to a large extent, preventable. Why, then, do people engage in risky behaviours—those that cause disease and illness or lead to disability? For one thing, many people take good health for granted until they are faced with illness or another incapacitating event.

Understanding patients' health beliefs and health behaviours, as well as their corresponding response to treatment, enables health care providers to maximize patients' health outcomes. Some patients will consider themselves well despite the presence of health problems. Others readily succumb to even minor alterations in their health state and require more intervention, understanding, and support.

Definitions of *health, wellness, illness, disease,* and *disability* evolve constantly, along with social consciousness, the delivery of health care, the affordability of health care services, and medical science. This chapter will explore these issues, provide information on the leading causes of **morbidity** and **mortality** in Canada, and discuss the impact of self-imposed risk behaviours on the individual and on the health care system in terms of disease and cost. It will also explain that the health care provider's goal, as part of the health care team, is to help his or her patients maintain their existing health, assist them in coping with illness, and support them on the road to recovery. Understanding health belief models, the psychology of health behaviour, and the ways individuals respond to illness will assist those pursuing careers in health care in supporting their patients.

HEALTH, WELLNESS, AND ILLNESS: KEY CONCEPTS

For a long time, *healthy* meant "not sick," and *sick* meant "not well." Today, the key concepts of health, wellness, and illness are defined in less black-and-white, either–or terms. Health care providers should understand the evolution of these definitions—how they have changed to become more multifaceted and inclusive over time.

HEALTH

The word *health* developed from the Old English word *hælth*, which meant a state of being sound and generally suggested a soundness or wholeness of the body. Initially, one was considered to be in good health if the body was in good functioning order. Over time, the meaning expanded to include a good or healthy state of mind. Thus, an individual must have both a healthy state of mind and physical well-being to be considered in good health.

In 1948, the World Health Organization (WHO) took the important step of acknowledging that health is multidimensional, and not merely the presence or absence of disease. While a vast improvement over previous definitions, WHO's definition (Box 2.1) has not formally changed since 1948.

WELLNESS

Although *wellness* and *health* are often used interchangeably, the two words are not synonymous; however, they share similar concepts. **Wellness** goes beyond having good physical and mental health. It considers how a person feels about his or her health and quality of life. For example, people may judge themselves to be well despite the presence of disease, sickness, sensory impairment, or physical disability (In the News: Do You Know Who Terry Fox Is?). This personal perception reflects how individuals adapt to, cope with, and accept their state of health and, in turn, defines their view of wellness.

Morbidity
The occurrence of disease or impairment resulting from accidents or environmental causes—for example, the number of people injured in a multiple-vehicle accident or the number of people who have a particular disease, such as cancer (but who have not died).

Mortality
The occurrence of deaths resulting from disease, accidents, or environmental causes—for example, the number of people killed in a multiple-vehicle accident or the number of people who died from a particular disease, such as cancer.

Wellness
Good health and a sense of well-being on many levels (i.e., emotional as well as physical) as described or experienced by an individual.

> **Box 2.1** **Health: An Evolving Definition**
>
> In 1948, the World Health Organization originally defined *health* as "a state of complete physical, mental, and social well-being and not merely the absence of disease or infirmity."
>
> As perceptions of health evolved, this definition came into question. For instance, some suggested that the word *complete* is unrealistic: How many people can claim to be completely healthy—and what does *completely healthy* mean? The ambiguity of this term is particularly evident today, with individuals living much longer, sometimes with serious ailments, such as heart disease or respiratory disease, or with physical limitations. Many health care providers struggled with this definition because it fails to include holistic concepts, such as spiritual wellness. Nurses, for example, must be aware of and respect the spiritual needs of their patients (e.g., by ensuring patients have access to a religious leader) when establishing a nursing diagnosis and implementing nursing interventions. As a result, WHO revised its concept of health to recognize the strong link between individuals and their environment, stating that it encompasses "the ability to identify and to realize aspirations, to satisfy needs, and to change or cope with environment. Health is therefore a resource for everyday life, not the objective of living. Health is a positive concept emphasizing social and personal resources, as well as physical capabilities" (World Health Organization, 1986).
>
> Sources: World Health Organization. (1948). *Preamble to the constitution of the World Health Organization as adopted by the International Health Conference.* New York; World Health Organization. (1986). *Health promotion: Concepts and principles in action—A policy framework.* Copenhagen: WHO Regional Office for Europe.

From a holistic perspective, to achieve wellness, a person must take responsibility for his or her own health by leading a balanced lifestyle and avoiding self-imposed risk behaviours. The path toward wellness is not static; it is continuous and must be a lifelong pursuit. Wellness develops from the decisions people make about how to live their lives with quality, good health (remember, good health is relative), and meaning. It is important to note that whether called the dimensions of health or the dimensions of wellness, each model may include dimensions that other models do not.

Dimensions of Wellness

The concept of wellness embraces several holistic elements, including, but not necessarily limited to, physical, emotional, intellectual, spiritual, and social health. Some models have more recently added environmental and occupational wellness.

In the News: Do You Know Who Terry Fox Is?

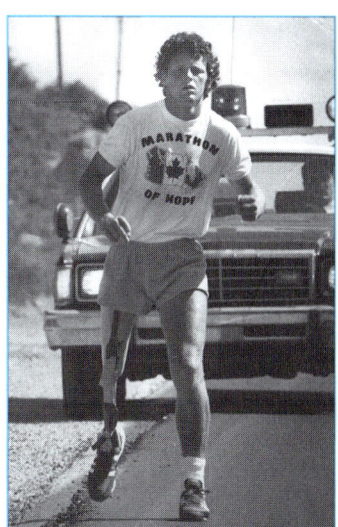

Terry Fox was born in Winnipeg, Manitoba, in 1958 and later moved to Port Coquitlam, British Columbia. A recognized athlete in high school, at 18 years old, Terry was diagnosed with bone cancer, which eventually resulted in the need for amputation of his right leg just above the knee.

Despite Terry's physical disability, he made the astonishing decision to run across Canada to raise money for cancer research. He began his run—his "Marathon of Hope"—on April 12, 1980, in St. John's, Newfoundland. As it continued, it attracted more and more media attention and support from the public. After 143 days and 5373 km, Terry ended his run near Thunder Bay, Ontario, when shortness of breath, fatigue, and chest pains forced him to seek medical attention. Doctors discovered that the cancer had spread to his lungs, and Terry died on June 28, 1981, one month short of his twenty-third birthday.

Before he died, Terry received the Order of Canada. He is considered by many to be Canada's greatest hero. The Terry Fox Run continues annually in Canada and in more than 60 countries around the world, raising millions of dollars every year. By May 2012, $650 million had been raised for cancer research in Terry's name.

Terry was a remarkable person who accepted his disability and did not allow it to dictate what he could or could not do. Although his physical health was threatened by cancer, he still felt well enough to put aside his personal pain in an effort to help others suffering with the disease. Terry's outlook stressed the wellness model of health.

Sources: Terry Fox Foundation. (n.d.). *Terry Fox*. Retrieved from http://www.terryfox.org/TerryFox/T_Fox.html; Terry Fox Foundation. (n.d.). *Facts*. Retrieved from http://www.terryfox.org/TerryFox/Facts.html.
Photo credit: Boris Spremo/GetStock.com.

A fine line exists between some of these holistic categories, so various wellness models may group or label them differently. As well, some literature refers to the "dimensions of health" rather than the "dimensions of wellness" but are similar in that they consider more than physical and mental health (Figure 2.1).

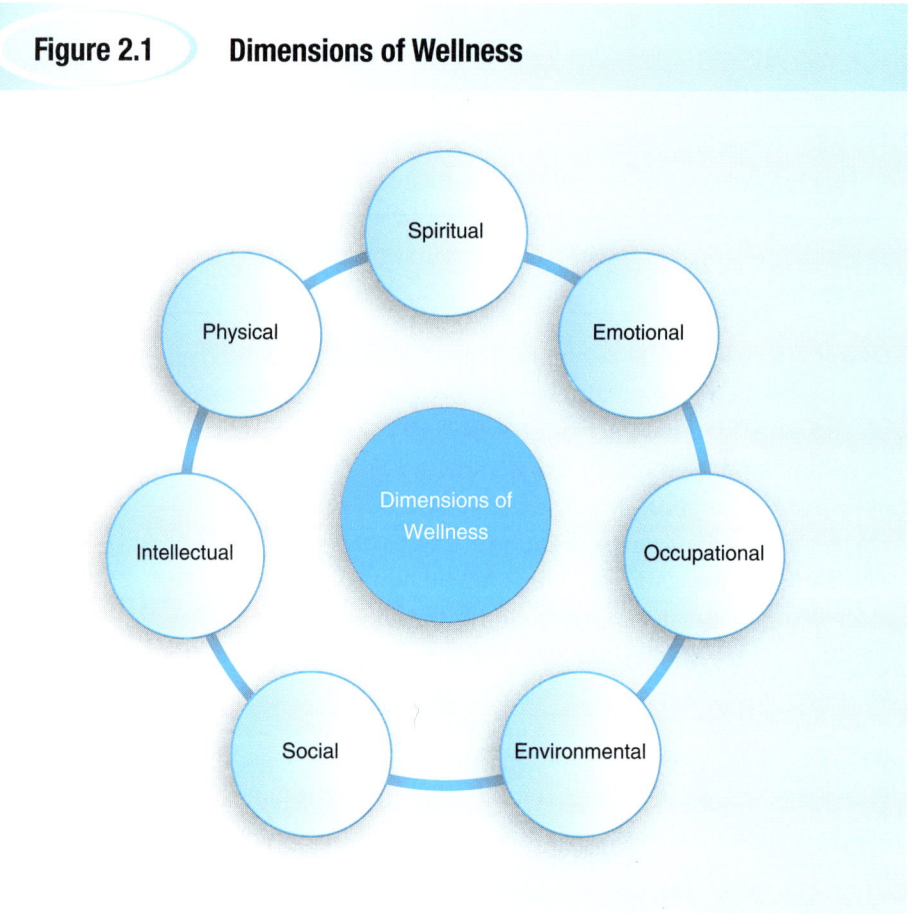

Figure 2.1 Dimensions of Wellness

Physical Wellness

The dimension of physical wellness entails maintaining a healthy body by eating a nutritious, balanced diet; exercising regularly; making intelligent, informed decisions about one's health; and seeking medical care when necessary. To do this, people must understand how lifestyle choices affect physical health.

Emotional Wellness

Emotional wellness and mental health are often but not necessarily interdependent entities. Emotional wellness includes people's ability to understand themselves, to recognize their strengths and limitations, and to accept who they are. The emotionally adapted person effectively handles and controls his or her emotions, communicates well, and seeks support when needed.

Good mental health allows a person to react proactively when things go wrong—to view adversity as an opportunity to learn and grow. Emotional health very much contributes to this ability. Mental illnesses, such as schizophrenia, bipolar disease, and depression, can affect a person's capacity to deal with situations effectively, especially when a situation poses challenges or problems. Mental illnesses usually have a physiological **etiology** and require treatment by a health care provider.

Etiology
The study of causes. In medicine, *etiology* refers to the origin or cause of a disease.

Intellectual Wellness

Intellectual wellness reflects people's ability to make informed decisions that are appropriate for and beneficial to themselves. From their experiences and learnings, intellectually well people are able to gather information throughout their lifespan and to use that information to make the best of situations. Moreover, these people apply critical thinking skills, prioritize data, and keep informed on current health research, treatments, and health-related issues.

Intellectual wellness may also include occupational health—personal satisfaction from one's career and the ability to balance career with other activities like family and leisure time.

Spiritual Wellness

Spiritual wellness may include a commitment to a religion or some higher power that evokes a sense of belonging to something greater than self. The spiritually well person seeks to contribute to society, plays an active role within the community, and displays gratitude and generosity. Spirituality may also involve solitude and reflection—focusing inward and reflecting upon feelings, actions, experiences, and ideas.

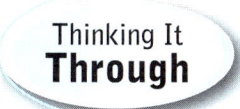

Spirituality has been linked to good health and general wellness, from fewer illnesses to faster recovery from illness and an enhanced ability to deal with stress.

1. What does *spirituality* mean to you?

2. Why do you think spirituality may contribute to better health?

Social Wellness

Social wellness is about relating effectively to others, including being able to form close, loving relationships, to laugh, to communicate effectively and empathically, to be a good listener, and to respond appropriately. Socially well individuals work agreeably in groups and within the community, are tolerant and accepting of others, and can form friendships and supportive networks. Confident and flexible, socially well people contribute to the welfare of others.

Environmental Wellness

Newer models of wellness take into account one's relationship with the environment (environmental wellness). An environmentally well person is one who engages in a lifestyle that is friendly to the environment. Friendliness to the environment entails consciousness about preserving the external world—walking or biking (instead of driving), recycling, choosing products that are less harmful to the environment (e.g., less packaging), and so on. It may also include creating a safe internal environment—for example, by protecting one's eyesight (e.g., using good lighting when reading or working) or limiting loud noises (e.g., controlling music volume).

Occupational Wellness

Occupational wellness occurs when a person feels secure, confident, and valued in his or her workplace setting. Occupationally well people manage work-related stress effectively, grow professionally, and balance the demands of their job with their personal lives. Whether people enjoy their job or hate it affects most aspects of their lives—and those of the people around them.

Illness

The term *illness*, often used to denote the presence of disease, can also refer to how a person feels about his or her health, whether or not a disease is present. Despite the absence of pathology or disease, a person may feel ill as a result of tiredness, stress, or both. Although this state differs from feeling healthy and energetic, by definition, it is not a disease.

Disease

> **Disease**
> A disorder or medical condition affecting a system or organ. The condition can be mental, physical, or genetic in origin. *Disease* also refers to a deviation from how the body normally functions.

Disease typically refers to a condition in which a person's bodily or mental functions are different from normal. Usually biological in nature, disease may affect various organs of the body and have symptoms that are either observable or difficult to detect. Causes of diseases include the presence of organisms such as bacteria, a virus, or a fungus. An example of a disease in which mental functions are affected is schizophrenia, which results in behavioural or psychological alterations and has a biological or biochemical explanation.

The term *disease* may be used, too, to describe a group of symptoms (more accurately called a *syndrome*) that are not related to a clear-cut disease process.

Disease is often used interchangeably with the vague words *ailment*, *disorder*, *condition*, or *dysfunction*. *Disease* is also sometimes used incorrectly to refer to a disability.

A disease may run a predictable course and subside—with or without treatment (e.g., pneumonia or influenza), or it may be chronic and controllable but not curable (e.g., asthma, diabetes, human immunodeficiency virus [HIV], acquired immune deficiency syndrome [AIDS]). Other diseases are long term and have symptoms that disappear and recur (i.e., go into a period of remission). This reappearance of symptoms and reactivation of the disease is known as an **exacerbation** of the disease (e.g., as happens with multiple sclerosis).

Remission of a disease can occur spontaneously or be induced by treatment. In the case of multiple sclerosis, for example, the use of immunosuppressive drugs can result in a treatment-related remission. A remission's length varies. The main aim of treatment for leukemia is a complete remission—that is, no signs of the disease from a symptomatic or pathological perspective. If a remission lasts more than five years, some consider the person to be cured. In the case of any kind of cancer, however, the word *cure* is used cautiously; some physicians avoid ever saying a person is cured, regardless of the length of time he or she has been cancer-free.

Exacerbation
A period of time when a disease (usually chronic) is active and the person has symptoms. *Exacerbation* may also refer to an increase in the severity of a disease.

Remission
A period of time during which a chronic disease is neither active nor acute and the person has no obvious symptoms.

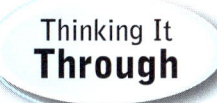 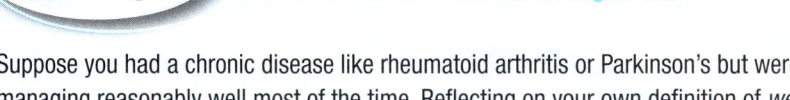

Suppose you had a chronic disease like rheumatoid arthritis or Parkinson's but were managing reasonably well most of the time. Reflecting on your own definition of *wellness*, answer the following:

1. Do you think you would consider yourself to be well?

2. Do you think your outlook would by influenced by periods of remission or of exacerbation of the condition?

Disability

A deviation from normal function, a **disability** can be physical, sensory (e.g., blindness, deafness), cognitive (e.g., Alzheimer's disease), or intellectual (e.g., Down syndrome). A disability can occur in conjunction with or as a result of a disease (e.g., a person with diabetes may undergo amputation of part of a leg because of impaired circulation); be caused by an accident; or be present at birth, either as a result of genetics or due to complications during delivery (e.g., an absence of a limb, cerebral palsy, spina bifida).

Disability
A physical or mental incapacity that differs from what is perceived as normal function. A disability can result from an illness or accident or be genetic in nature.

The language used to describe people with a disability has changed over the years, moving toward more sensitive, less hurtful terminology. For example, today, a person with a cognitive or intellectual disability is most likely to be deemed *mentally handicapped* or *intellectually impaired*. Along with improved terminology has come the recognition that people with disabilities deserve the same rights and opportunities as all other members of society (Box 2.2).

> **Box 2.2 People With Disabilities: Rights Are Formally Recognized**
>
> Historically, people with disabilities have been viewed as individuals who need societal protection, evoking sympathy rather than respect. In an effort to change this perception and to ensure that all people have the opportunity to live life to their fullest potential, in December 2006, the United Nations formally adopted the *Convention on the Rights of Persons With Disabilities*, the first such inclusive human rights treaty of this century. The convention covers a number of key areas, including accessibility, personal mobility, health care, education, employment, rehabilitation, participation in political life, equality, and nondiscrimination. All jurisdictions have acts or other pieces of legislation to protect people with disabilities, and almost all are constantly being improved. For example, an amendment to the *Accessibility for Ontarians With Disabilities Act* will require both public and private organizations to comply with components of the Act by 2025. Timelines for compliance and penalties for noncompliance by individuals and organizations are common concerns.
>
> Source: United Nations. (2006). *Rights of persons with disabilities*. Retrieved from http://www.un.org/disabilities/.

HEALTH MODELS

Health model
A concept of an approach to care, including the development of a treatment plan and involvement and communication with a patient.

A person's health, wellness, illness, disease, or disability—and the resulting interaction with health care providers—usually relates in some capacity to a **health model**. Defined as a design for delivering health care, a health model can influence both a health care provider's practice and his or her delivery of health care, which, in turn, affects treatment, priorities, and outcome measurements. The three most common types of health care models are the medical model, the holistic model, and the wellness model, all of which continue to evolve.

The principles of the wellness model—stressing wellness and illness prevention—are most commonly pursued in our current health care climate. Physicians are embracing evidence-informed decision making and using best practices to deliver patient-focused care in a team-oriented environment.

Medical Model

The medical model was founded on a simple definition: health is the absence of disease. More recently, this model has expanded to consider aspects of functioning, disability, and limitation of activity, thus accepting that a person with physical limitations may nevertheless be healthy.

In the twenty-first century, critics of the medical model argue that the model's scope is too narrow and that the presence or absence of disease alone does not define one's health. This model does not consider social causes of disease that are beyond an individual's control (e.g., disparities in socioeconomic status and education). And, by emphasizing the diagnosis and treatment of disease, the medical model ignores the role of prevention—efforts to stop disease and disability before they occur (Larson, 1991).

Holistic Model

The **holistic** approach to health considers all parts of the person. This approach has been used for some time by alternative practitioners, such as naturopaths; only recently has it been integrated into mainstream medicine.

Focusing on the positive aspects of health—not on the negatives of illness and disease that inform the medical model—the holistic model strives for a state of health that encompasses the entire person, rather than just aiming for a lack of disease and disability. Although similar to the original WHO definition of *health* introduced in 1948 (see Box 2.1), the holistic definition of *health* goes much further by recognizing the impact of factors such as lifestyle, spirituality, economics, and culture on an individual's health.

Although initially described as "utopian" (i.e., impossible to achieve), the holistic model has become widely accepted as a better alternative to the medical model (Larson, 1991).

> **Holistic**
> Whole. In health care, a holistic approach treats the whole person, not an individual part of the person. For example, a holistic approach to treating a person with a heart condition would consider the patient's emotional state, diet, and fitness level, not just his or her heart problem.

Wellness Model

The wellness model builds on the medical and holistic models. It considers health a process that continues to evolve and to progress toward a future state of improved health. Viewing health as a state of feeling, an experience based on an internal process rather than on external symptoms (Larson, 1991), the wellness model encompasses an individual's or a group's ability to cope with health-related challenges.

In the wellness model, people assume responsibility for their own health and make informed choices about such things as lifestyle and **self-imposed risk behaviours**. The wellness model also considers a person with a disability or

> **Self-imposed risk behaviours**
> Actions (such as smoking tobacco) that a person willfully engages in despite knowing they pose a danger to his or her health.

illness to be healthy if that person can function, meet self-imposed goals, and is not incapacitated by pain.

The common thread linking the holistic and wellness health models is the inclusion of a broad spectrum of factors—physical, spiritual, social, emotional, economic, and cultural.

International Classification of Functioning Disability and Health

Introduced in the 1980s by the World Health Organization, the International Classification of Functioning Disability and Health (ICF) is both a classification system and a health model. As a classification system, the ICF measures the health of individuals as well as the health of designated populations. It considers health and health-related issues from the perspectives of the environment, the body's structure and function, and the individual's health-related activities (promoting personal health). As a model, the ICF considers health and disability a little differently. It holds that everyone at some point during the lifespan will experience altered health and may, with that, experience some form of disability. Disabilities then are considered common, experienced by many, not just a few. This model also considers the social components of living with a disability and the effects a disability has on affected individuals and those around them; it emphasizes the effects of a disability rather than the cause. As a model, the ICF is used clinically by health care providers to access patients' social and functional challenges and capacities, set realistic goals, formulate treatment plans, and measure outcomes.

CHANGING PERCEPTIONS OF HEALTH

How a person views health will affect how that person responds to alterations in health. A person who is feeling happy and optimistic may pass off an illness as trivial or as something he or she can cope with. If that same person is feeling down, stressed, or otherwise vulnerable, however, an illness may seem more draining. Consequently, a positive frame of mind can help a person deal more effectively with stress and fight disease.

Until the early 1960s, Canadians, for the most part, held the attitude that if they were sick, they would seek medical care, and the doctor would make them better. Few people recognized the impact of lifestyle on their health. Engaging in self-imposed risk behaviours, such as a sedentary lifestyle, poor nutritional habits, smoking, and alcohol abuse, was rarely directly linked to changes in health status. Canadians functioned very much within the realm of the medical model.

This way of thinking began to change in the 1960s and 1970s. With the help of government initiatives and the establishment of a population health approach to health care, Canadians started to see the value of prevention and to consider what they could do on a personal level to stay healthy—that is, they began to take more responsibility for their own well-being. Slowly, community and group involvement in health promotion and disease prevention emerged.

A federal public initiative, aptly called ParticipACTION, was launched in 1971 to promote a healthy lifestyle through increased physical activity. This initiative resulted from a 1969 study by the National Advisory Council for Fitness and Amateur Sport, which found Canadians to be largely sedentary (i.e., inactive), unfit, and, worse yet, uninterested in the concept of exercise and its health benefits (ParticipACTION, 1969). ParticipACTION has evolved into a network of both public sector and nongovernment organizations (NGOs) whose goal is to promote physical activity, including participation in sports activities. The network sponsors commercials encouraging physical activity as well as a ParticipACTION Web site with the tag line "Let's get moving." The Web site offers information on programs and events, ideas for becoming active, a blog, and more. Individuals can log in to receive email updates.

Other organizations do their bit to encourage a healthy lifestyle. The Heart and Stroke Association, for example, sponsors riveting commercials on lifestyle and related risks. One particularly effective series depicted Canadians spending the last ten years of their lives in illness. Suitably graphic and disturbing, the commercials made a clear impact on viewers.

Today, Canadians have a much broader-based understanding of the link between lifestyle and health. Most people recognize that smoking causes lung cancer and respiratory disease. And many know that being active can lower their chances of developing high blood pressure, osteoporosis, cardiovascular disease, and even some types of cancer.

Still, much work remains to be done. In 2011, the majority of Canadians were considered either active or moderately active, at 54% engaging in physical activity. Almost 72% of Canadians 12 to 19 years old were considered moderately active or active, compared with 44% of those aged 65 years and older (Employment and Social Development Canada, 2014). According to a study done at Queen's University and sanctioned by the Public Health Association of Canada, inactivity in Canadian adults costs taxpayers $6.8 billion per year and accounts for about 3.8% of total health care costs in Canada (Queen's University, 2012).

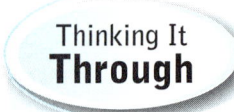

A close friend of yours, a very heavy smoker (two packs of cigarettes daily), is diagnosed with high blood pressure and has a family history of cancer. In spite of this situation, he refuses to stop smoking, stating, "It's my life, and I love to smoke." You believe that he does not comprehend the consequences of his habit and feel very strongly that he should quit. How might you influence his decision—or would you try?

THE PSYCHOLOGY OF HEALTH BEHAVIOUR

Demonstrated by a person's response or reaction to altered health, **health behaviour** has a significant impact on what a person does to maintain good physical and psychological health. Many factors, including what a person believes to be true about health, prevention, treatment, and vulnerability, influence how people act when they are ill or perceive they are ill. Health behaviour also depends on a person's level of health knowledge, personal motivation, cognitive processes, and perceived risk factors. One's culture and ethnicity will invariably affect all of these areas.

To explain human health behaviour, several models have been developed, including the transtheoretical model, the social–ecological model, the protection motivation theory, and the health belief model (developed in the 1950s by the United States Public Health Service). Elements of the health belief model are relevant in one way or another to all of the others, so it is described in the most detail below.

TRANSTHEORETICAL MODEL

The transtheoretical model of health behaviour proposes that people must progress through the following series of steps before their health behaviour completely changes (i.e., improves): precontemplation, contemplation, preparation, action, maintenance, and termination. Integrated into these steps are ten cognitive and behavioural activities that further facilitate change. For example, during the precontemplation stage, although aware that a behaviour modification may improve his or her health, the person has no desire or motivation to make a change and may resist any attempts to help him or her to change. During the next step, the contemplation stage, the person is ready

Health behaviour
The activities a person engages in to acquire and maintain good physical and psychological health.

to think about making changes and may consider the risks and benefits of a behaviour change. The person moves through the remaining steps, ending in the termination stage. At this final stage, the person has established adaptive behaviour and has no desire to return to his or her previous behaviour. In this model, to be successful, a person must be able to make and commit to decisions (Prochaska, 1979).

Social–Ecological Model

The social–ecological model maintains that many levels of influence shape one's health behaviour. Such influences include a person's education, occupation, or profession; the type of social support (personal, community) he or she has; his or her environment (e.g., workplace, availability of health care); and the public policies of various levels of government. The ideal environment is one that promotes good health, health education, and a healthy workplace and welcomes government policies that support and endorse effective health care (Bronfenbrenner, 1979).

Protection Motivation Theory

Building upon the health belief model (discussed below), protection motivation theory asserts that self-preservation is what motivates a person to change his or her health behaviour. The fear of illness, physical decline, or even death can encourage adaptive (or maladaptive) health behaviours. The person's actions depend on how severe he or she perceives a threat to be. For example, if a man fears that he will develop lung cancer, his health behaviours will be altered by how vulnerable he thinks he is (i.e., his likelihood of actually getting lung cancer), what he has to do to avoid this threat (e.g., quit smoking), and his ability (or motivation) to take action (Rogers, 1975).

Health Belief Model

People's health beliefs affect their health behaviour. **Health beliefs** are things people believe to be true about their personal health and susceptibility to illness and about illness, prevention, and treatment in general. Beliefs are acquired largely through social interaction and experience. Around since the mid-1950s, the concept that health beliefs affect health behaviour is widely accepted and is based on a number of assumptions—for example, if people feel that by taking a certain action, they can avoid a negative outcome, they will take that action (Case Example 2.1).

> **Health beliefs**
> Things people believe to be true about their personal health and susceptibility to illness and about illness, prevention, and treatment in general.

Case Example 2.1

Marcy is 17 years old and sexually active. She is convinced that if she takes the birth control pill, she will avoid becoming pregnant.

Many things can stop people from following a recommended course of action to avoid a negative health event—for example, how "at risk" a person feels. Consider Marcy. She may *know* that taking a birth control pill will prevent a pregnancy, but she may also feel that the chances of an unplanned pregnancy happening to her are so slim that she is inclined not to bother taking the pill. She may convince herself that using the withdrawal or rhythm method will be enough to prevent pregnancy. In other words, she does not believe that she is vulnerable.

Another factor that influences people's choices and level of concern is the perceived seriousness of the condition or illness if acquired. Marcy may think that a pregnancy would be devastating, or she may believe that she and her boyfriend would marry and live happily ever after. She may also think that an abortion is a viable option if pregnancy were to occur.

Culture and religion also influence health beliefs and value systems. As a multicultural country, Canada requires health care providers to pay close attention to and to respect cultural and religious traditions. The respect, or lack thereof, shown for such beliefs can affect how the patient feels about seeking health care (e.g., at what point and from whom) and following treatment plans (compliance).

Culture and religion may affect a patient's outlook on mental and physical health, wellness, disease, and disability. These beliefs often include the etiology or origin of the infirmity and how it should be treated. Western medicine is largely scientifically based—for example, we typically believe that an acute infection is caused by a pathogen, whereas some other cultures may believe that spirits, the supernatural, or disharmony with nature is the cause. Specific beliefs as to the origin of an illness will likely dictate what type of treatment the person will accept and comply with.

In Canada, the patient's right to participate in his or her health care is valued. In some other cultures, however, the patient's autonomy to make personal health-related decisions is not considered necessary or important; instead, a family member may assume this responsibility. Often, in these cultures (e.g., Asian and some Aboriginal cultures), the welfare of the whole family is considered in making decisions, possibly without even consulting the patient. Some cultures view doctors and other health care providers as figures of authority, so patients

> **Culture**
> Common elements of a social group, including its beliefs, practices, behaviours, values, and attitudes. Culture can relate to a society or to subgroups within a society.

may find discussing their treatment options difficult because they are accustomed to doing as they are told. People within some cultures may not report cognitive problems or mental illness because of perceptions that such illnesses are spiritually induced (i.e., possession by demons), reveal a lack of self-control, or are a source of shame. Religion, cultural customs, education, and language barriers also influence health behaviours and beliefs and decisions around death and dying. For example, people of Chinese or South Asian descent, Muslims, and Orthodox Jews may question requests for organ donation or the withdrawal of life support even if the patient is deemed brain dead: the belief that life is sacred dominates.

It may be that second- and third-generation Canadians do not hold the same beliefs—or do but not to the same degree—as their parents. Sometimes, within a family, generational differences of opinion may cause conflict when it comes to treatment plans (Euromed Info, n.d.).

THE HEALTH–ILLNESS CONTINUUM

No matter what health beliefs and religious or cultural background a person has, everyone measures his or her health and illness in some manner. A *continuum* is a method of measurement usually represented by a straight line with an opposing state at each end. The **health–illness continuum** measures one's perception of his or her state of health between "optimum health" and "poor health" or "death." In the middle is a section called **compensation** (Figure 2.2). The health–illness continuum includes all of the dimensions of health and wellness, from physiological to spiritual and psychological health, and is, then, congruent with the principles of the wellness model.

Movement on the continuum is constant. An individual may wake up feeling good and then develop a headache two hours later, altering his or her perceived placement on the continuum. Also, one person may have a bad cold but not feel

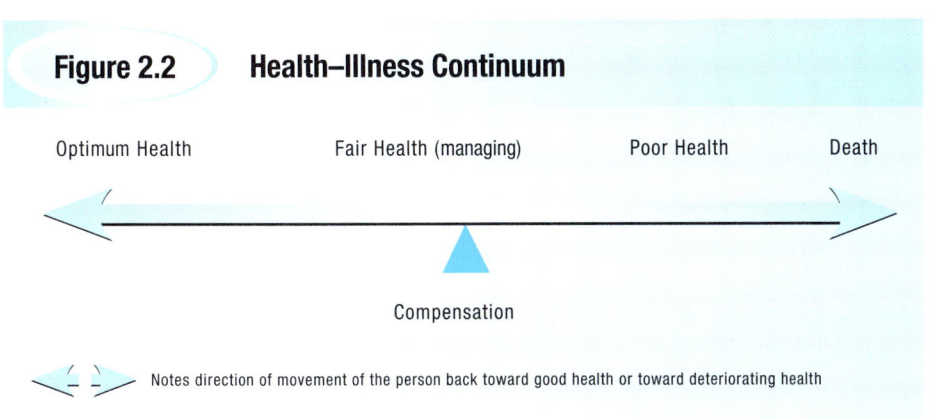

Figure 2.2 Health–Illness Continuum

Health–illness continuum
A method of measuring one's state of health at any given point in time. A person's health state may range from optimum health at one end to death at the other end.

Compensation
That part of the health–illness continuum in which a person is neither in good nor poor health, is able to accommodate a malady, and is continuing on with daily life.

particularly ill so may place him- or herself on the "good health" part of the continuum. Someone else with a similar cold may feel unable to function and place him- or herself in compensation on the continuum (Case Example 2.2).

People with disabilities also place themselves on different places on the continuum. Consider Dr. Stephen Hawking, a world-famous physicist who has had amyotrophic lateral sclerosis (ALS) for many years and, although he is quite disabled, pursues life with a vengeance. Likely he would put himself in the compensation range of the continuum. Others who choose not to face a progressive disability may consider their health to be closer to the negative end of the spectrum and find themselves making some difficult choices. For the competent adult, the right to end one's life with medical assistance, for example, remained illegal in Canada until the statute was changed. (In the News: Landmark Ruling on Physician-Assisted Suicide).

In the News

Landmark Ruling on Physician-Assisted Suicide

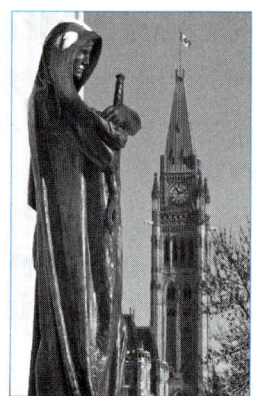

On February 6, 2015, in the case of *Carter vs. Canada*, the Supreme Court of Canada ruled unanimously that the Criminal Code's prohibition against assisting a person in taking his or her own life is an unconstitutional infringement on one's Charter rights to life, liberty, and security of the person.

The Court suspended the effect of its ruling for a year from the date of the judgment to give Canadian lawmakers the opportunity to enact permissive legislation with properly designed and administered safeguards capable of protecting vulnerable people from abuse and error.

Such a permissive scheme would have to permit physician-assisted suicide in the case of a competent adult who clearly consents to the termination of life, and has a grievous and irremediable medical condition (including an illness, disease, or disability) that causes enduring suffering that is intolerable to the individual in the circumstances of his or her condition.

Sources: Courtesy of Ontario Superior Court Justice Douglas Rutherford.
Photo Credit: © Can Stock Photo/michelloiselle

Case Example 2.2

Angela has always enjoyed good health and, for the most part, eats sensibly and exercises regularly. Recently, however, she began to have some epigastric discomfort. She was diagnosed with an ulcer and treated accordingly. Symptoms began to improve within a couple of days. On the health–illness continuum, Angela considers herself to be in compensation but moving toward good health. For Angela, the direction of movement would be noted by an arrow moving toward optimum health (←). Figure 2.3 shows Angela on the continuum near "fair health" and moving toward "optimum health."

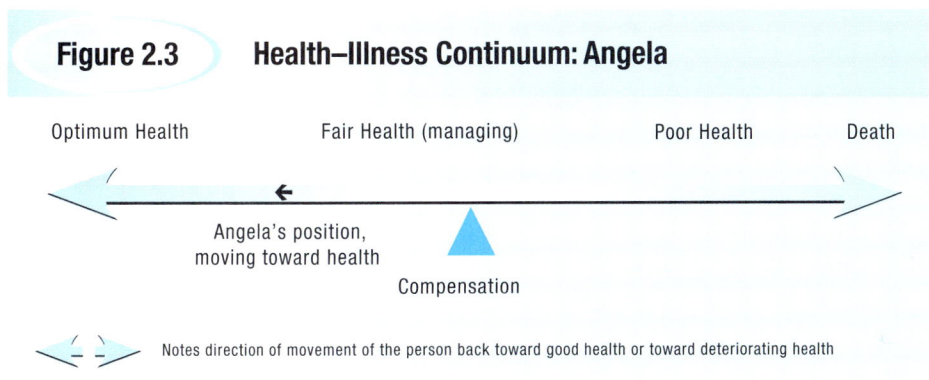

Figure 2.3 Health–Illness Continuum: Angela

SICK ROLE BEHAVIOUR

It is widely accepted that when people are ill, their behaviours, roles, and attitudes change. This response to illness is sometimes referred to as **sick role behaviour** or behavioural illness response (Thompson, 2005). The stress of being ill can alter people's perceptions and the way they interact with others, from those close to them to the health care providers they deal with. Illness can also influence the behaviour of those associating with the unwell person, in large part because these people often have a burden placed on them. They may be required to provide extra support to the ill person or to assume his or her responsibilities, causing both a change in their daily routine and stress.

To better understand sick role behaviour, consider the fact that we all behave differently at different times, with different people, and in different situations. These varying behaviours affect, among other things, the diverse

Sick role behaviour
A person's response to disease or illness. Removed from normal societal expectations and responsibilities, the sick person may respond to situations differently from when he or she is well. Sick role behaviour is usually temporary in nature.

roles and responsibilities we assume throughout our lifetime. Persons who are ill are often relieved from the roles and responsibilities they have in society—which ones and to what extent depend on the nature and severity of their illness.

The majority of patients respond to their illness in an adaptive manner. Other patients, particularly those with a more serious illness or prolonged health problems, will respond by being "more of what they are." For example, people who consistently complain about their health, call frequently, and rely heavily on health care providers will likely become more extreme in these behaviours. On the other hand, components of a person's character not usually seen can emerge: a normally easygoing patient may become inwardly focused and quiet or disagreeable and demanding (Case Example 2.3).

Although pronounced changes in attitude are more apt to be evident when a person suffers a serious illness, the stress of a relatively minor illness or accident (for example, a broken leg or pneumonia) can also be problematic—especially if the illness limits or alters the patient's activities, role functions, or ability to work, even for a short period of time. Such limitations will invariably affect the patient's attitude and outlook, as well as the attitudes of those close to the patient.

Case Example 2.3

Ashma, a student nurse, was looking after a young mother in labour and delivery. The mother was uncommunicative, almost passive, as labour progressed, making it impossible for Ashma to assess her needs accurately. The next day, when she went to see the new mother on the postpartum unit, Ashma was greeted by a big smile and an outgoing, chatty, and cheery demeanour. Ashma could not believe this was the same person.

Health care providers can do their part by maintaining their professional role and respecting the fact that patients will present moods and attitudes that differ from those they display in good health. Family members may also become upset, short-tempered, and demanding. It is important to remember that they, too, are coping with the stress of altered roles and functions and are probably frightened and concerned about their loved one who is ill. Managing patients and family members in such situations requires the ability to remain calm, listen to their concerns, answer questions simply and honestly, and connect them to the appropriate resources as required. A calm, caring, and supportive demeanour most often brings about the most positive responses.

Behaviour in Hospitalized Patients

When hospitalized, patients are more likely to display visible changes in behaviour. Such changes occur, in part, because hospitalization interferes with a person's sense of autonomy and independence. A person must adapt to hospital rules and routines that may seem restrictive or excessive. While in the hospital, patients experience changes in their role function and must relinquish many of their responsibilities. They may worry about their jobs and day-to-day activities in their home and social lives. The resulting stress may cause a person to become passive and dependent or irritable and noncompliant. These changes often become more pronounced the longer the patient is in the hospital.

It is important that all health care providers, regardless of their role in the patient's care or recovery, show sensitivity for the patient's demeanour and recognize his or her need for support and encouragement.

When patients are disagreeable and noncompliant with treatment, consider the nature and the severity of their illness and try to understand their viewpoint. Sometimes just asking why they are upset or refuse treatment can aid a situation. Patients' behaviour may relate to their previous experiences, a lack of knowledge, or some other problem that can be addressed. Importantly, do not mistake their sick role behaviour for their "normal" behaviour. Try to remain patient, good-humoured, and resourceful in creating a supportive environment, and do not take insults or criticism personally.

Take into account the fact that language barriers or cultural or religious beliefs may also affect how a patient responds to hospitalization and medical care. Read the patient's body language and responses. As health care providers, we are taught that touch can be comforting to a patient—even a hand on the arm or shoulder—and that eye contact is important. A male Orthodox Jew, however, may recoil from an attempt at touch by a female health care provider; contact by a member of the opposite sex except when giving direct care is unwelcome. An Aboriginal or Chinese patient may avoid eye contact, thereby appearing disinterested, nervous, or upset. In fact, avoiding eye contact, especially with someone deemed to be in authority, is considered a sign of respect and politeness in some Asian cultures. Modesty, as well, is a concern of people from some cultures (Case Example 2.4) (Thompson, 2013; Chin, 1996; Schwartz, 1991). Sometimes it is necessary for health care providers to seek the help of other team members to ensure optimal care and treatment.

Case Example 2.4

Nishtha, a 65-year-old woman from India, refused to let David, a registered nurse, assist her with her bed bath. She drew the covers up under her chin and waved him away. Confused, David reported that Nishtha had refused care. In Nishtha's culture, modesty is very important, and female caregivers are preferred.

It is important to note that health care providers must avoid stereotyping or generalizing behaviour based on the patient's cultural background. For example, Nishtha's daughter was born in Canada and may not share the same level of modesty.

Signs
Those things related to an illness that a person or examiner can see (e.g., a rash).

Symptoms
Those things that a person feels that may relate to an illness (e.g., fatigue, a headache). Symptoms are sometimes referred to as *clinical signs*.

STAGES OF ILLNESS: INFLUENCE ON PATIENT BEHAVIOUR

A patient's acceptance of a diagnosis and treatment plan normally follows a relatively predictable path through the stages of illness. But a person's response and choice of course of action depend on his or her health beliefs, health behaviours, and other variables (e.g., the seriousness of the health issue) discussed in this chapter. A person may have an illness "brewing" for some time before symptoms appear. How long the illness has been present will affect the nature and severity of the **signs** or **symptoms** of the illness once they do become apparent, as well as the outcome of the illness. The stages of illness and probable responses are summarized in Box 2.3.

Box 2.3 Stages of Illness

Preliminary Phase: Suspecting Symptoms

- Symptoms, possibly subtle, appear; they may progress or abate.
- Person either acknowledges or ignores symptoms.
- Person may seek immediate medical advice or look for information elsewhere (e.g., on the Internet).

Acknowledgement Phase: Sustained Clinical Signs

- Person decides symptoms cannot be ignored.
- Person seeks advice from family or friends, self-treats, or considers making an appointment with the doctor.

Action Phase: Seeking Treatment

- Symptoms become problematic and concerning.
- Person seeks medical advice.

Transitional Phase: Diagnosis and Treatment

- Person receives a diagnosis, a treatment plan, or both.
- Person may seek a second opinion if the diagnosis is serious.
- Person may accept treatment, becoming involved in the treatment plan, or may refuse treatment or even deny the diagnosis (e.g., in the case of a terminal disease).

Resolution Phase: Recovery and Rehabilitation

- Person may recover completely with minimal intervention or may require surgery, ongoing care, or rehabilitation.
- Person may or may not embrace and comply with the rehabilitation plan; if the illness becomes chronic, the person will reposition him- or herself on the health–illness continuum.

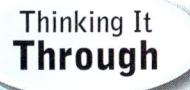
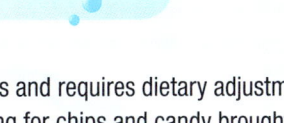

A hospitalized patient has been diagnosed with diabetes and requires dietary adjustments and insulin injections. He refuses to eat his meals, opting for chips and candy brought in by friends. As a dietary assistant, you have been asked to review his meal plan with him. The patient grumbles about the fuss everyone is making and does not understand the need for any changes to his lifestyle. What approach would you take with this patient?

SELF-IMPOSED RISK BEHAVIOURS

Examples of self-imposed risk behaviours include smoking, unhealthy eating habits, inactivity, alcohol or drug abuse, and sexual promiscuity (see page 49). People engage in risk behaviours for a number of reasons, including habit (which often becomes addictive behaviour) and thrill-seeking. A common initiator among young people is peer pressure. For example, if a teen's friends smoke or take drugs, he or she may try it rather than risk not fitting in. Risk behaviour includes indirect activity. For instance, people who choose not to smoke may nevertheless find themselves in danger of inhaling second-hand smoke (they may not realize the implications or find it difficult to remove themselves from the situation), or they may drive sensibly but voluntarily ride in a car with an impaired driver.

Health promotion and illness prevention initiatives undertaken by all levels of government aim to reduce self-imposed risk behaviour for two reasons: to ease the financial burden on our health care system and to promote the health and longevity of Canadians.

THE HEALTH OF CANADIANS TODAY

> **Life expectancy**
> The number of years a population or parts of a population are expected to live as determined by statistics.

Canadians are living longer. The **life expectancy** for both men and women continues to rise and, at birth, is currently estimated to be 81.1 years. On average, women are living 83.3 years, and men are living 78.8 years, although this gap between the sexes is closing (Table 2.1).

Table 2.1 Life Expectancy by Sex and Geography

	Both Sexes (Years)	Males (Years)	Females (Years)
Canada	**80.1**	**78.8**	**83.3**
Newfoundland and Labrador	78.9	76.5	81.2
Prince Edward Island	80.2	77.5	82.8
Nova Scotia	80.1	77.7	82.4
New Brunswick	80.2	77.5	82.8
Quebec	81.2	78.8	83.4
Ontario	81.5	79.2	83.6
Manitoba	79.5	77.0	81.9
Saskatchewan	79.6	77.0	82.1
Alberta	80.7	78.5	83.0
British Columbia	81.7	79.5	83.9
Territories[1]	75.1	72.5	78.2

Notes: Life expectancies are calculated with a method that uses three years of data.
1. Yukon, Northwest Territories, and Nunavut.

Source: Statistics Canada. (2012, May 31). *Life expectancy, at birth and at age 65, by sex and by province and territory* [CANSIM table 102-0512]. Retrieved from http://www.statcan.gc.ca/tables-tableaux/sum-som/l01/cst01/health72a-eng.htm.

It is interesting to note that cancer, for the first time, is the single leading cause of death in every province and territory, emphasizing the need for continued cancer research. The current emphasis on disease prevention and health promotion targets a number of preventable conditions, such as cardiovascular disease.

For infants, the leading cause of death is congenital abnormalities, followed by premature births and low birth weight (Statistics Canada, 2008). Accidents are the leading cause of death for individuals aged 1 to 34, cancer for those aged 35 to 84, and heart disease for those 85 years of age and older. Accidents, suicide, and homicide are the leading causes of death for young adults aged 15 to 24. Suicide and accidental deaths are the leading causes of death among **Aboriginal Canadians**.

The rate of **infant mortality** is often used as a measure of the effectiveness of a country's health care system. Canada's infant mortality rate has declined over the last several decades, but not as fast as the rate in other developed nations. According to the Mundi Index, the mortality rate in 2012 was 4.78, down from 5.08 in 2000 (IndexMundi, 2013). Within the country, infant mortality rates remain higher in areas that are populated predominately by Aboriginal people (discussed in Chapter 10).

Canada still fares poorly on the world stage, ranking sixteenth out of 17 countries for infant mortality rates, according to the Organisation for Economic Co-operation and Development (OECD). The same study showed that Japan had the lowest infant mortality rate (2.4%), followed by Sweden, Finland, Denmark, and Norway. The United States had the highest at 6.5%. Japan, Sweden, and Finland all have infant mortality rates of under three deaths per 1000 live births (Conference Board of Canada, 2012).

It is important to note that countries calculate infant mortality rates differently; Canada and the United States, for example, include in their rates very premature babies whose chances of survival are low, elevating their statistics, and some countries do not register infant deaths occurring within the first 24 weeks of life. According to research, if corrected neonatal mortality rates are applied, Canada ranks twelfth, not sixteenth (CBC News, 2012). Other factors responsible for Canada's poor showing on the world stage include advances in technology that may increase the number of premature births (e.g., more multiple births resulting from fertility treatments).

Leading Causes of Death in Canada

The following is a brief discussion on the three leading causes of death in Canada: cancer, cardiovascular disease, and cerebrovascular disease (Figure 2.4).

Cancer

Cancer results from abnormal cellular growth within the body. Along with familial or genetic causes, many cancers are associated with risk factors. Some risk factors are within our control (i.e., self-imposed risk behaviour); others we have little or no control over (e.g., a genetic propensity). Smoking tobacco, eating an unhealthy diet, abusing alcohol, and being exposed to toxic chemicals (e.g., environmental) are risk factors that increase a person's chances of getting cancer.

Aboriginal Canadians
Individuals indigenous to Canada: First Nations, Inuit, and Métis people.

Infant mortality
The death of an infant (i.e., within the first year of life).

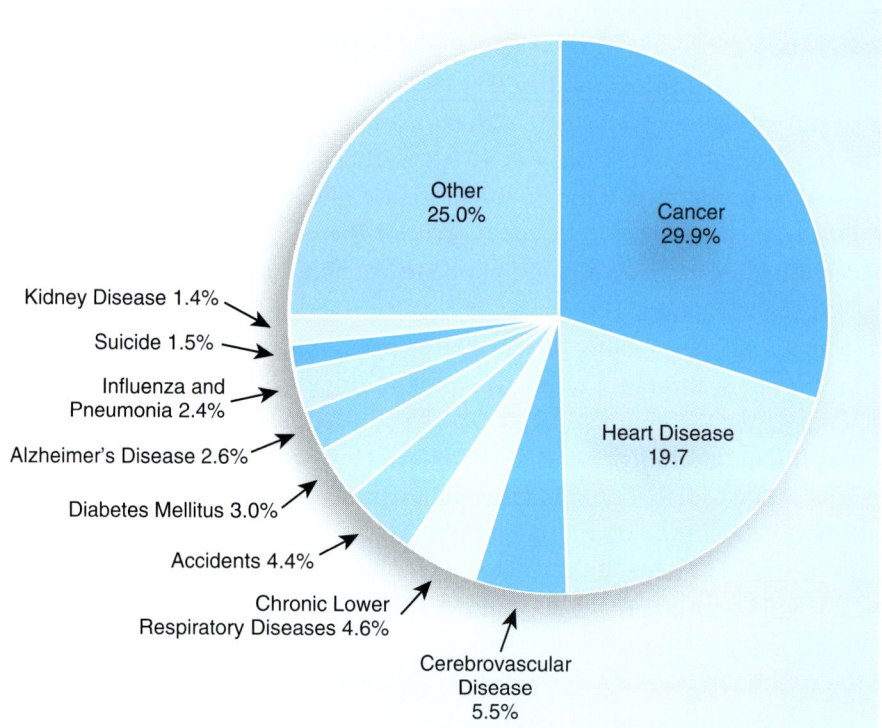

Figure 2.4   Leading Causes of Death in Canada

Source: Data from Statistics Canada. (2014, January 28). *Leading causes of death, by sex* [CANSIM table 102-0561]. Retrieved from http://www.statcan.gc.ca/tables-tableaux/sum-som/l01/cst01/hlth36a-eng.htm.

While the incidence of some types of cancers have decreased (e.g., throat and stomach), others (e.g., breast cancer) have seen a moderate increase, and some (e.g., liver and thyroid) have seen significant increases. The incidence of thyroid cancer is increasing more rapidly than all of the other major types of cancer (Public Health Agency of Canada, 2013).

Women are three times more likely to develop thyroid cancer than men; however, as of 2012, breast cancer remained the most common type of cancer in women over the age of 20. Although mortality rates from breast cancer are declining, breast cancer remains the second leading cause of cancer deaths for women (Canadian Breast Cancer Foundation, 2014).

Prostate cancer is the leading cause of cancer in men. Mortality rates are relatively low because of early diagnosis, treatment when indicated, and the fact that most prostate cancers are slow growing. Because of the low mortality rates, there is controversy over how aggressively to screen for and treat diagnosed cases of prostate cancer. The age of the individual is a factor in treatment. Diagnosing and watching the progress of prostate cancer are achieved through monitoring prostate-specific antigen (PSA) levels. Most provinces will cover the cost of a PSA test, but others have limitations on payment. In British Columbia, for example, the cost of the test is covered by the medical services plan if there is a strong suspicion of prostate cancer or in the course of treatment, but not as part of a routine examination to exclude the presence of prostate cancer. Coverage is similar in Ontario (Associated Press, 2012).

Lung cancer remains the leading cause of all cancer-related deaths in both males and females, with an estimated 25,600 new cases diagnosed in 2012 and 20,100 deaths the same year (Public Health Agency of Canada, 2013). Morbidity and mortality rates from lung cancer in both sexes combined are highest in Nunavut and lowest in Ontario (Canadian Cancer Society, 2014).

Cardiovascular Diseases

Cardiovascular disease (CVD) is one of the main causes of death in Canada, with ischemic heart disease (IHD) accounting for more than 50% of all CVD deaths in 2008. IHD mortality rates have decreased substantially over the past few decades. This overall decrease has been attributed largely to primary prevention (e.g., reductions in risk factors and changes in lifestyle) and better treatment options (Heart and Stroke Foundation, 2014).

According to the Canadian Medical Association (2013), only 1 in 10 Canadians is considered to have excellent cardiovascular health. Cardiovascular diseases include IHD (also called *coronary artery disease*), congestive heart failure (the heart not pumping effectively), arrhythmia (abnormal heartbeat), and peripheral vascular disease (problems with circulation, primarily in the legs). Of these, IHD is the most common.

The mortality rate for cardiovascular disease has dropped significantly over the last ten years, due in part to Canadians' reducing risk factors related to lifestyle (e.g., increasing activity, stopping smoking, eating a healthy diet), prevention (e.g., screening, identification of high-risk individuals, counselling, public education initiatives), and improved treatments (e.g., newer and more effective medications and rehabilitation programs for those who have had a heart attack).

Population health initiatives on the part of Health Canada and provincial and territorial governments have also contributed to lower mortality rates from heart disease. For example, Health Canada funds programs such as ParticipACTION to promote a healthy lifestyle. It has also recently introduced regulations forcing manufacturers to lower the amount of trans fats in prepared foods, launched public campaigns to encourage manufacturers to lower sodium content in foods, and made efforts to reduce the sale of unhealthy foods in schools.

> **Cardiovascular disease**
> Disease that affects the heart and vascular system (i.e., blood vessels).

Cerebrovascular Disease

Cerebrovascular disease includes a number of conditions that affect the flow of blood to the brain, the most serious of which is stroke. Stroke occurs when there is a blockage of oxygen to part of the brain. It is caused by an interruption in the blood flow, most commonly a blood clot. As the third leading cause of death, stroke is responsible for 6% of all deaths in the country and affects more women than men (Statistics Canada, 2012).

Heart disease and stroke are also the leading causes of hospitalization in Canada and, according to the Conference Board of Canada (Heart and Stroke Foundation, 2014), cost the Canadian economy $20.9 billion per year. A 2013 report on the health of Canadians sponsored by the Canadian Heart and Stroke Association claims that, without immediate action, older Canadians (mostly baby boomers) will spend the last ten years of their lives living with illness, disability, and mobility problems (Heart and Stroke Foundation, 2013b). Supporting this, Stats Canada reports that there is a gap "between how long we live, and how long we live in health" (Heart and Stroke Foundation, 2013a). One can only assume from these facts that the message that we Canadians can do much to reduce our risk factors for acquiring a variety of infirmities, including stroke and heart disease, is somehow not getting through, even though access to health information and teaching materials has been greatly enhanced by the Internet. More work is clearly needed to teach Canadians that adopting a healthy lifestyle at an early age will increase the chances of enjoying better health in one's later years.

> **Cerebrovascular disease**
> A number of conditions that affect the flow of blood to the brain, the most serious of which is a stroke.

SUMMARY

2.1 Today, the key concepts of health, wellness, and illness are defined in less black-and-white terms. Definitions of health relate to such things as an individual's own culture, background, and experiences. Wellness goes beyond having good physical and mental health and considers how a person feels about his or her health and quality of life. The many dimensions of wellness include physical, emotional, intellectual, spiritual, social, environmental, and occupational health. *Disease* refers to a condition in which a person's mental or bodily functions are different from normal. The term *illness*, often used to denote the presence of disease, can also refer to how a person feels about his or her health, whether or not a disease is present. A disability can be physical, sensory, cognitive, or intellectual and can occur in conjunction with or as a result of a disease or be caused by an accident.

2.2 How health care is delivered is reflected in a design, a philosophy, and an approach. Three approaches, or models, are most frequently used: the medical, holistic, and wellness models. Some people prefer a natural approach to health care—noninvasive, leaning away from mainstream diagnosis and intervention. Others have more faith in proven treatments. Still others will blend philosophies.

2.3 Several factors influence how people respond when their health is compromised. These include past experiences and one's outlook on life (e.g., optimistic, pessimistic). Over the past several years, Canadians, for the most part, have assumed more responsibility for their own health, assessing their own risk behaviours and focusing on health promotion and disease prevention.

2.4 Health behaviour is how a person responds to all aspects of altered health. How they react affects their relationship with health care providers, family members, and others close to them. A person's response to an altered health situation is unique to each person and influenced by his or her background, social and cultural beliefs, and past experiences with the health care system. Understanding that deviations from a person's normal behaviour are just that—and supporting him or her appropriately—will go a long way to helping a patient recover.

2.5 By some standards, such as the health–illness continuum, a person's health is measurable. How a person feels about his or her health changes frequently and is influenced by the type and severity of an infirmity, personal health beliefs, and the health model the person most closely relates to.

2.6 Overall, the health of Canadians has improved over the past decade, yet challenges remain in providing prompt and effective care, particularly for those with cancer, cardiovascular diseases, and diseases of the respiratory system—the leading causes of morbidity and mortality in the country. Aboriginal peoples are particularly at risk for socioeconomic reasons and, for many, because of the lack of proximity to larger treatment centres.

Review Questions

1. List and describe the dimensions of wellness, and explain how wellness goes beyond having good health.
2. Differentiate between a disease and a disability and provide examples of both.
3. Compare and contrast the medical, holistic, and wellness models of health, identifying the key points of each.
4. What is the International Classification of Functioning Disability and Health (ICF)?
5. Explain how Canadians' attitudes toward their health and well-being have changed since the 1960s.
6. Differentiate between health beliefs and health behaviours.
7. Briefly describe how a person's health behaviour can affect how you as a health care provider treat that person.
8. Explain how sick role behaviour may affect where someone places him- or herself on the health–illness continuum.
9. Describe how the different stages of illness may influence patient behaviour.
10. How and why have the leading causes of death in Canada changed over the past ten years?

References

Associated Press. (2012, March 14). Prostate cancer screening not saving lives. *CBC.* Retrieved from http://www.cbc.ca/news/health/story/2012/03/14/prostate-cancer-screening.html.

Bronfenbrenner, U. (1979). *The ecology of human development: Experiments by nature and design.* Cambridge, MA: Harvard University Press.

Canadian Breast Cancer Foundation. (2014). *Breast cancer in Canada, 2013.* Retrieved from http://www.cbcf.org/central/AboutBreastCancerMain/AboutBreastCancer/Pages/BreastCancerinCanada.aspx.

Canadian Cancer Society. (2014). *Cancer statistics at a glance.* Retrieved from http://www.cancer.ca/en/cancer-information/cancer-101/cancer-statistics-at-a-glance/?region=on.

Canadian Medical Association Journal. (2013). Fewer than 1 in 10 Canadians in ideal cardiovascular health: CANHEART health index measures behaviours and health factors for optimal heart health. *Canadian Medical Association Journal.* . http://dx.doi.org/10.1503/cmaj.131358.

CBC News. (2012, February 17). Canada's rank on infant mortality index called unfair. *CBC.* Retrieved from http://www.cbc.ca/news/health/story/2012/02/17/health-infant-mortality-study.html.

Chin, P. (1996). Chinese Americans. In J. G. Lipson, S. L. Dibble, & P. A. Minarik (Eds.), *Culture and nursing care: A pocket guide* (pp. 74–81). San Francisco, CA: University of California–San Francisco Nursing Press.

Conference Board of Canada. (2012). *Infant mortality.* Retrieved from http://www.conferenceboard.ca/hcp/details/health/infant-mortality-rate.aspx.

Employment and Social Development Canada. (2014). *Indicators of well-being in Canada.* Retrieved from http://www4.hrsdc.gc.ca/.3ndic.1t.4r@-eng.jsp?iid=8.

Euromed Info. (n.d.). *How culture influences health beliefs.* Retrieved from http://www.euromedinfo.eu/how-culture-influences-health-beliefs.html/.

Heart and Stroke Foundation. (2013a). *Canadians face decade of sickness in later years.* Retrieved from http://www.heartandstroke.ab.ca/site/pp.aspx?c=lqIRL1PJJtH&b=8554975&.

Heart and Stroke Foundation. (2013b). *2013 report on the health of Canadians.* Retrieved from http://www.heartandstroke.com/atf/cf/%7B99452D8B-E7F1-4BD6-A57D-B136CE6C95BF%7D/Report-on-Cnd-Health-D17.pdf.

Heart and Stroke Foundation. (2014). *Statistics.* Retrieved from http://www.heartandstroke.com/site/c.ikIQLcMWJtE/b.3483991/k.34A8/Statistics.htm.

IndexMundi. (2013). *Canada infant mortality rate.* Retrieved from http://www.indexmundi.com/canada/infant_mortality_rate.html.

Larson, J. S. (1991). *The measurement of health: Concepts and indicators.* New York: Greenwood Press.

ParticipACTION. (1969). *The ParticipACTION archive project.* Retrieved from http://www.usask.ca:80/archives/participaction/english/impact/index.html.

Prochaska, J. O. (1979). *Systems of psychotherapy: A transtheoretical analysis.* Georgetown, ON: Dorsey Press.

Public Health Agency of Canada. (2013). *Canadian cancer statistics 2012.* Retrieved from http://www.phac-aspc.gc.ca/cd-mc/cancer/ccs-scc-2012-eng.php.

Queen's University. (2012, February 2). *Physical inactivity a $6.8 billion annual burden to Canadians.* Retrieved from http://www.queensu.ca/news/articles/physical-inactivity-68-billion-annual-burden-canadians.

Rogers, R. W. (1975). A protection motivation theory of fear appeals and attitude change. *Journal of Psychology, 91,* 93–114.

Schwartz, E. (1991). Jewish Americans. In J. N. Giger, & R. E. Davidhizar (Eds.), *Transcultural nursing* (pp. 491–520). Chicago: Mosby.

Statistics Canada. (2008, January 14). Deaths. *The daily* (No. 84F0211XWE). Retrieved from http://www.statcan.gc.ca/daily-quotidien/080114/dq080114b-eng.htm.

Statistics Canada. (2012, July 25). Highlights. In *Leading causes of death in Canada, 2009.* Retrieved from http://www.statcan.gc.ca/pub/84-215-x/2012001/hl-fs-eng.htm.

Thompson, V. (2005). *Administrative and clinical procedures for the health office professional.* Toronto: Pearson Prentice Hall.

Thompson, V. (2013). *Administrative and clinical procedures for the Canadian health professional.* Toronto: Pearson Education.

CHAPTER THREE

Population Health: Introduction and Principles

Learning Outcomes

3.1 Explain the concept of population health.
3.2 Describe the key determinants of health.
3.3 Discuss the major events leading to the use of a population health approach in Canada.
3.4 List the partners instrumental in implementing population health in Canada.
3.5 Demonstrate an understanding of the Public Health Agency of Canada's template for implementing a population health approach.
3.6 Debate how the key determinants of health are used as indicators in the population health promotion model.
3.7 Review the current status of the population health approach in Canada.

KEY TERMS

Determinants of health, p. 71
Disease prevention, p. 71
Epidemiology, p. 92
Health indicators, p. 90
Health promotion, p. 71
Inequities in health, p. 81
Intersectoral cooperation, p. 86
Population-based surveillance, p. 92
Population health, p. 70
Primary care, p. 79
Primary health care, p. 81
Public health, p. 71
Qualitative research, p. 93
Quantitative research, p. 97
Socioeconomic gradient (SES gradient), p. 73
Upstream investments, p. 94

How healthy are Canadians? What is most affecting their health? What do they need to do to prevent illness in themselves and their children? What can they do now to improve their health? The answers are found in a population health approach to health care—collaborative efforts by various government departments, community groups, and individuals to promote health strategies, health, and well-being—and the development of public health strategies. This chapter teaches learners about population health—what it is, how it was introduced in Canada, and the impact it continues to have on the health of Canadians. Students will become familiar with the determinants of health and will better understand Canadians' current health status, where their health ought to be, and what Canadians need to do to raise their level of health. They will also see that, although many strategies for health promotion and disease prevention exist at a national level, each province and territory has its own agenda and timeline.

POPULATION HEALTH APPROACH

A **population health** approach looks at health in broad terms—that is, it aims to improve the health status of the population, rather than that of the individual. It is a framework for gathering and analyzing data about the factors that affect a population's health and the causes behind some groups' being healthier than others. The population health approach also looks for ways to improve health and to reduce inequities in health status through reductions in material and social imbalance. The benefits of a population health approach, therefore, extend beyond improving population health to building a sustainable and integrated

> **Population health**
> A framework for gathering and analyzing information about conditions that affect the health of a population. The aim is to both maintain and improve the health of the entire population and to reduce inequities in health status among population groups.

health care system, increasing national growth and productivity, and strengthening social cohesion and citizen involvement in health care.

Population health embraces the newer, broader definitions of health and wellness discussed in Chapter 2. It also moves away from the medical model of health and illness toward holistic concepts like the wellness model (also discussed in Chapter 2). Population health incorporates **public health** initiatives, **health promotion, disease prevention**, and the concept of wellness. Public health strategies are funded and implemented primarily by government, although health care providers, industry, community agencies, and individuals play a role as well. Such strategies are frequently based on population health outcomes.

The terms *population health* and *public health* are often used interchangeably but are different entities with a common denominator—health information. Population health is a scientific, organized approach to health promotion and disease prevention that is both social and political in nature. It looks at how lifestyles and living conditions affect the health of individuals and population groups. Often using data from population health studies, public health focuses on the practice of promoting health and preventing disease. See Box 3.1 for a description of the difference between population health and public health.

> **Public health**
> The use of health information from a variety of resources (e.g., Statistics Canada, the WHO, provincial, territorial, and regional sources) to improve the health of communities. Public health programs often carry out recommendations made by population health studies.
>
> **Health promotion**
> Initiatives that inform people about things they can do to remain healthy and to prevent disease and illness.
>
> **Disease prevention**
> Used in conjunction with health promotion. Information initiatives aimed at encouraging individuals, especially those in high-risk population groups (e.g., with a family history of diabetes or heart disease), to adopt strategies to prevent diseases.

Box 3.1   Population Health Versus Public Health

Population Health
- Studies the health of a population using scientific approaches to prevent disease and promote good health (e.g., using health indicators and the determinants of health—see below)
- Analyzes the information gathered
- Makes recommendations to improve the health of a population or population group

Public Health
- Uses health information to prevent disease and promote good health for groups of people or an entire country
- Applies strategies to improve health rather than analyzing and researching strategies
- Carries out recommendations derived from population health studies

KEY DETERMINANTS OF HEALTH

Since the Canadian Institute for Advanced Research (CIFAR) introduced the concept of population health in 1989, the Public Health Agency of Canada (PHAC) has identified a number of factors known to influence the health of individuals, population groups, and communities, called **determinants of health**

> **Determinants of health**
> The conditions (economic, social, environmental, etc.) in which people live that affect their current and future health.

(see Figure 3.1). Health is influenced not by one determinant in isolation but rather by the interaction of multiple determinants. How these determinants work together to affect the health of a population is not clearly understood.

Determinants of health are always changing. Every stage of life poses different challenges. For example, we strive to ensure proper conditions for healthy child development, to find ways to reduce rising trends in obesity in our population, and also to keep Canada's aging population as healthy as possible. The 12 determinants put forth by the PHAC as most instrumental in influencing the health of Canadians are discussed below.

Figure 3.1 Key Determinants of Health

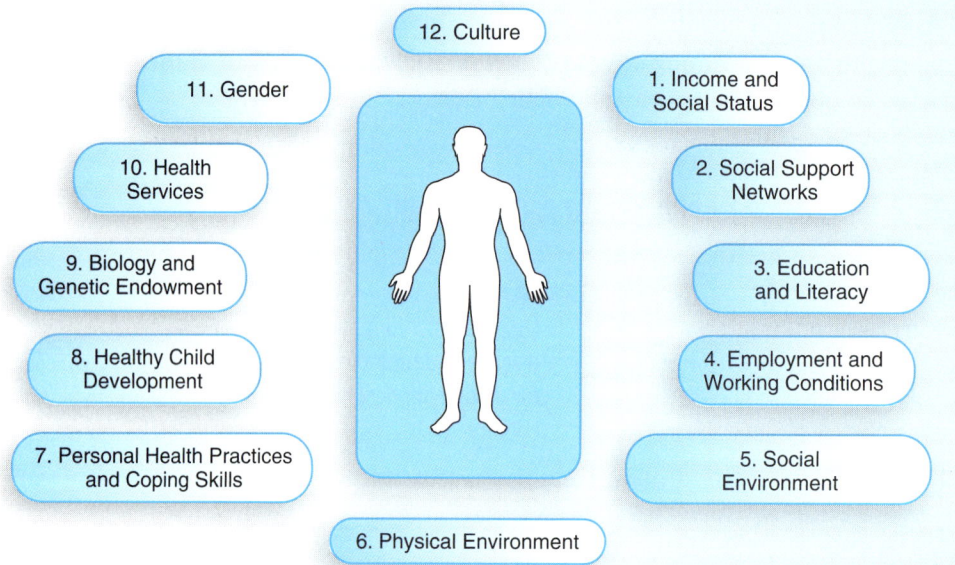

Source: Based on Public Health Agency of Canada. (2001). *Determinants of health: What makes Canadians healthy or unhealthy?* Retrieved May 29, 2009, from http://www.phac-aspc.gc.ca/ph-sp/determinants/index-eng.php#determinants.

1. Income and Social Status

Income and social status appear to be the most important determinants of health. Extensive research demonstrates the link between income, social status, and health (Public Health Agency of Canada, 2011). A lower socioeconomic status appears to be associated with poorer health and an earlier death, and a higher socioeconomic

> **Box 3.2** **The SES Gradient**
>
> The **socioeconomic gradient (SES gradient)** is a measurement of health or health inequalities as they relate to a person's or population's socioeconomic circumstances. *SES gradient* is a term widely used in population health studies today. At the bottom of the gradient are people who are below the poverty line, perhaps unemployed, living in a poor socioeconomic environment, and, therefore, at risk for poor health. As an individual's or group's socioeconomic status improves, so does the individual's or group's health. For example, those living in what we might consider a middle-class environment tend to be healthier than those in a lower-class group. Those living in the highest socioeconomic bracket, according to the SES gradient, enjoy the highest level of health. We also know, however, that people who are born into a lower socioeconomic environment can enjoy good health and be happy, productive individuals. So the theory is not absolute, and variables within and relationships among the determinants are not clearly understood.
>
> Source: Keating, D. P., & Hertzman, C. (Eds.). (1999). *Developmental health and the wealth of nations: Social, biological, and educational dynamics.* New York: Guilford Press.

Socioeconomic gradient (SES gradient)
A measurement of health or health inequalities as they relate to a person's or population's socioeconomic circumstances.

status, with better health; in other words, an individual's health tends to be proportional to his or her position on the socioeconomic gradient, or SES gradient (Box 3.2).

Poor living conditions, such as substandard housing and food, can, of course, negatively influence people's health. However, research indicates that the degree of control that people have over their lives and their ability to act also significantly affect their health status. Higher income and social status generally allow for more control. Lower income and social status are often accompanied by poor self-confidence and self-esteem, which diminish an individual's ability to make choices and exercise control and, ultimately, increase his or her risk for poor health (Public Health Agency of Canada, 2013; World Health Organization, n.d.; Mikkonen & Raphael, 2010).

Thinking It Through

In many cases, individuals faced with continuing challenges, such as a limited income, alcoholism, or drug addiction, overcome these adversities. They are able to find opportunities, graduate from high school and postsecondary facilities, find rewarding employment, become financially secure, and be well adapted socially.

1. Is there something about an individual's character that carries that person through adversity to achieve goals beyond what would be expected for him or her?

2. Is there another common denominator that is responsible for some people moving up the socioeconomic scale?

2. Social Support Networks

The opportunity to share feelings, discuss problems, and receive the clear support of others relieves stress and enhances a sense of well-being. It promotes the feeling of being wanted, supported, and valued and improves a person's physical and emotional health. Social support can come from family members, friends, or a community (e.g., a support group). The type and level of support a person has or seeks are influenced by many factors, including sex, gender, and culture. Typically, men are less likely to form supportive networks and share feelings. Similarly, in some more reserved cultures, sharing personal feelings with others is discouraged. Consider Case Examples 3.1 and 3.2.

Case Example 3.1

Mary is 35 years old and has been married for five years. Her husband, Eric, is an alcoholic. They have two children. Mary is under great stress trying to cope with the effects of Eric's alcoholism on both herself and her family. She joins Al-Anon, a support group for friends and families of alcoholics. There she sees that she is not alone and learns coping mechanisms for dealing with her husband's drinking.

Case Example 3.2

Kumar is 50 years old and has been married to Reena for 15 years. They have been having marital problems for some time. Kumar is uncomfortable voicing personal problems and does not have a close friend with whom he could discuss such issues. He bottles up his feelings and, as a result, is bad tempered most of the time. His mood affects his family, friends, and colleagues. He has trouble sleeping, and his blood pressure is rising. Reena, on the other hand, is able to reach out for support and is learning to deal with her problems in a proactive way.

Kumar's behaviour is not unusual for many men. Statistically, men die at a younger age than women. This may be due, in part, to men's inability to access a social network for support and advice. In fact, recent reports show a link between the social environment and the risks of morbidity and mortality, exclusive of the effects of other health determinants. Findings also indicate that social environment can influence the course of a disease. For example, a person with cancer or cardiovascular disease will survive much longer if he or she accesses supportive social networks. This may relate, in part, to a reduction in stress and a positive, even optimistic, outlook generated by a loving and caring environment (Haydon, Roerecke, Giesbrecht, et al., 2006; Mikkonen & Raphael, 2010; Koven, 2013; Holt-Lunstad, Smith, & Layton, 2010; Institute of Medicine (US) Committee on Health and Behavior, 2001).

3. EDUCATION AND LITERACY

Literacy and access to education often encourage a higher level of education, which, in turn, usually leads to jobs with higher social status and an established, steady income. Financial security increases opportunities for a person and his or her family on a number of different fronts. For example, children may benefit from participating in organized sports or taking lessons.

A higher level of education also widens people's knowledge base and their ability to think logically and to problem-solve. Higher education can develop right-brain activities such as enjoyment of the arts, creativity, philosophy, and politics, and it can motivate people to engage in meaningful relationships, become involved in the community, and, in general, be more satisfied.

4. EMPLOYMENT AND WORKING CONDITIONS

Individuals who are unemployed or work at menial jobs in which satisfaction is low and stress is high tend to have poorer health (Box 3.3). These people have a higher mortality rate at a younger age (e.g., from suicide—particularly among Canada's Aboriginal people living in isolated communities) and higher morbidity rates from chronic diseases (e.g., cardio-respiratory disease). Families of unemployed or underemployed individuals can also have poorer health, probably because of resulting high stress levels, related emotional problems, and a lower socioeconomic environment. Unemployment is cited as one of the largest stressors that a person or family can face. One study found that those who are unemployed experience significantly more psychological distress, anxiety, depressive symptoms, health problems, and hospitalizations, as well as take more disability days and face more activity limitations than do those who are employed (D'Arcy, 1986).

Box 3.3 Landmark Studies Support the Link Between Employment and Health Status

The Whitehall I Study, a classic study conducted at the British Civil Service from 1967 to 1977, demonstrated the link between health outcomes and levels of employment in the civil service. The study found that those at the lowest level of the employment scale (i.e., those with jobs that were menial and offered little job satisfaction and little control, such as messengers or doorkeepers), had a mortality rate three times higher than those in the highest employment bracket (e.g., supervisors and administrators). Furthermore, those at the lower end of the employment scale engaged in more risk behaviours (e.g., smoking, stress and unhealthy diet leading to obesity, inactivity) that

Continued on next page

contributed to the higher mortality rate. Interestingly, none of the individuals involved in the study was poor in the strict sense of the word. They each had a steady income and equal access to health care.

A follow-up study, Whitehall II, showed that individuals in high-status jobs in the British Civil Service did not have a higher risk of heart disease. Whitehall II supported previous findings that employment status relates to health status but went further to suggest that the way a work environment is organized and the work atmosphere itself (e.g., how individuals are treated, relationships among employees, how much control individuals have over their work environment), along with other social influences, contribute to the SES gradient (see Box 3.2).

Sources: Marmot, M., Rose, G., Shipley, M. J., et al. (1978). Employment grade and coronary heart disease in British civil servants. *Journal of Epidemiology and Community Health, 32*, 244–249; Ferrie, J. E. (2004). *Work, stress and health: The Whitehall II study*. London: Public and Commercial Services Union on behalf of Council of Civil Service Unions/Cabinet Office. Retrieved from http://www.ucl.ac.uk/whitehallII/pdf/Whitehallbooklet_1_.pdf.

5. Social Environment

The social environment is constructed by how individuals behave; their relationships with others and their community; their gender, culture, and ethnic group; their education and roles in the workforce; the conditions and communities in which they live; and how they feel about themselves. These elements overlap with other determinants to influence health and life expectancy. Individuals in the same or similar social environments have been shown to demonstrate similar values, outlook on life, and ways of thinking.

The tighter knit and more organized a community is, and the more involved the population is with activities within the community, the greater the health of that community is. Volunteerism, for example, improves the well-being of the social environment, apparently increasing a community's level of compassion, harmony, and cohesiveness. Volunteers themselves generally live longer and suffer less from depression and heart disease (Public Health Agency of Canada, n.d.).

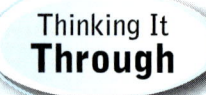

You have an opportunity to volunteer at your community health centre. You know it is a good cause but wonder if you can find the time with all your other commitments at school and home.

1. Do you believe that being a volunteer can contribute to your physical and social well-being?

2. Would volunteering in your chosen field add value to your résumé?

A well-organized community has agencies and resources that support community residents—for example, community- or government-sponsored child care. This affects the entire family positively by reducing stress and financial burden. Social stability fosters positive relationships, recognition and acceptance of cultural diversity, and unified communities that inspire confidence, a sense of being valued, and assurances of support—all of which have a powerful effect on reducing health risks.

6. Physical Environment

The physical environment consists of the "natural" environment and the "manufactured" environment. The "natural" environment includes the food people eat, the water they drink, the air they breathe, and the places they live—the outside or physical world. The "manufactured" environment refers to the homes people live in, the buildings they attend school or work in, the roads they travel, and the recreational areas such as parks and community structures they use. How this built environment is structured and constructed affects health status. For example, the phrase *sick building syndrome* describes nonspecific illnesses that are attributed to time spent in a specific building. This syndrome appears to be a growing concern. In 1984, the World Health Organization (WHO) reported that up to 30% of buildings, particularly newer and remodelled structures that are airtight and well insulated, were associated with health-related complaints. The assumption is that these health issues are linked to poor air quality, although this is not an established fact in many cases (United States Environmental Protection Agency, 1991).

Currently, environmental issues are top of mind, with widespread concern over drinking water and related infrastructure, air pollution, environmental warming, pollution of agricultural land, and depletion of natural resources.

7. Personal Health Practices and Coping Skills

Personal health practices relate to self-imposed risk behaviours, health beliefs, and health behaviours (as discussed in Chapter 1). Personal health practices are often linked to a person's level of self-esteem, sense of control, and level of confidence. Coping skills help an individual deal with situations and problems and are, in part, a component of his or her genetic makeup. Some people are better able to deal with problems, stress, and daily challenges than others. Most health problems that are associated with this particular determinant of health relate to risk behaviour such as smoking, alcohol abuse, drug use, and poor dietary habits (e.g., eating when depressed, smoking when stressed, drinking alcohol when not wanting to face a problem) (Public Health Agency of Canada, 2003).

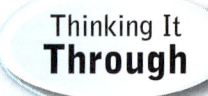

As a student, you are likely faced with new challenges such as living away from home, meeting new people, and dealing with academic responsibilities.

1. How do you respond to these stressors?

2. Are you likely to approach a professor, friend, or family member for support?

3. Are you aware of the resources at your university or college that can offer you support?

8. Healthy Child Development

Many determinants of health affect the growth and development of a child, even before conception. The mother's nutritional intake, whether or not she engages in risk behaviours, and the quality and amount of her prenatal care all affect the baby during pregnancy and have lasting effects after birth. The formative years are influential in terms of the child's current and future health. Other influential determinants include socioeconomic status, biology and genetic endowment, and the physical environment. For example, babies born to mothers who have a lower position on the income scale are more likely to have a low birth weight (Mikkonen & Raphael, 2010), which, in itself, is associated with a variety of health problems; to eat a poor diet; and to experience both health and social problems throughout their lives.

9. Biology and Genetic Endowment

The phrase *biology and genetic endowment* refers to all the attributes that people inherit from their parents. These inherited attributes can make a person vulnerable to developing specific diseases and other health problems. Individuals can have genetic studies done that will help them to understand their risk of developing certain diseases (e.g., Huntington's disease, cystic fibrosis, certain forms of cancer—such as breast cancer—and, more recently, Alzheimer's disease). Such information may also be used to help individuals understand the risk of passing certain conditions on to their children. How individuals use this information varies, and some may choose not to know. In 2013, actress Angelina Jolie discovered she had a gene that increased her chances of developing breast cancer, and made a difficult decision to address her newfound knowledge (In the News: Angelina Jolie's Medical Choice).

In the News: Angelina Jolie's Medical Choice

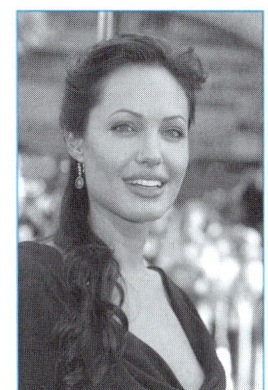

In May 2013, Angelina Jolie announced that she underwent an elective double mastectomy to reduce her chances of developing breast cancer. Along with her having a strong family history of breast cancer, genetic studies revealed she carried the BRCA1 gene, exponentially increasing her risk of developing the disease. She clearly stated it was her "medical choice" to have her breasts surgically removed. She has been both praised and criticized for her decision.

Following the release of this story, centres for genetic testing in Canada had a large increase in calls from women requesting the testing. The cost of the test ranges from $3000 to $4000 and is covered in Canada only for women who meet certain criteria, which vary among jurisdictions (the common qualifier is that the woman has two or more blood relatives who have had breast or ovarian cancer). Anyone can go to a private clinic in the United States to have the testing done.

Sources: Associated Press. (2013, May 14). Angelina Jolie has double mastectomy due to breast cancer risk. *CBC News*. Retrieved from http://www.cbc.ca/m/touch/arts/story/1.1348853; Mayer, A. (2013, May 18). Should genetic testing for cancer be available to all Canadians? *CBC News*. Retrieved from http://www.cbc.ca/m/touch/news/story/1.1314320.

Photo source: © Pictorial Press Ltd/Alamy.

10. HEALTH SERVICES

Health services include diagnosis, treatment, disease prevention, and health promotion. The type of health care services offered and their method of delivery affect the health of a population. Greater availability of **primary care** services and of health promotion and disease prevention programs (e.g., immunizations, preventive care such as breast screening, prenatal care, and well-baby initiatives) can lead to a healthier population.

Under the *Canada Health Act*, all Canadians are entitled to equal access to any and all medically necessary services. However, researchers are convinced that availability of health care plays only a small part in ensuring that a population's health is maximized, believing that the accessibility of the best health care services in the world would not guarantee a population overall good health.

Primary care
Front-line care, direction, and advice provided by multidisciplinary health care teams. Primary care also involves initiatives that seek to improve access to, quality of, and continuity of care; patient and health care provider satisfaction; and cost-effectiveness of health care services (Health Canada, 2006).

11. GENDER

The word *gender* is often used interchangeably with *sex*, the latter of which indicates whether a person is male or female. However, *gender*, by definition, refers to social, not biological, differences. For example, gender identity is how a person perceives himself or herself socially (i.e., as a male or female). According to WHO, "Gender refers to the socially constructed roles and responsibilities assigned to women and men in a given culture. Thus, gender is distinct from sex, which is biologically determined" (Zaman & Underwood, 2003).

As a determinant of health, gender considers factors that produce inequities between men and women that affect their health, such as employment opportunities (e.g., men tend to have more opportunities, including greater opportunities for advancement) and income inequities (e.g., women tend to make less money). Gender also includes roles determined by society (e.g., until the late twentieth century, females were directed into such professions as teaching and nursing), attitudes, values, and personality traits.

12. Culture

Culture can be described as a way of life (e.g., behaviours, values, attitudes, geographic and political factors) that is attributed to a group of people. *Ethnicity* refers more to race, origin or ancestry, identity, language, and religion. Culture and ethnicity are often linked—and both affect health, particularly in terms of health beliefs, health behaviours, and lifestyle choices.

Those with different social, religious, value, and belief systems than others in their community are more likely to face inequities, marginalization, socioeconomic problems, and isolation.

Minorities are especially at risk because the larger group's socioeconomic and cultural environments tend to dominate the community, and the needs of minorities can be overshadowed. Risk factors for minorities include health beliefs and health behaviours—for example, how and at what point they will approach the health care system. Barriers to seeking care may include fear, language struggles, and noninvolvement of family members. (Family members often contribute significantly by contacting a physician, providing transportation to the physician's office or hospital, explaining the rationale for treatments, and translating information when required.)

INTRODUCTION OF POPULATION HEALTH TO CANADA

The reports and conferences discussed in this section were instrumental in the introduction and development of population health in Canada. The Lalonde Report, written in 1974, was the first that had Canadians looking at health differently, recognizing it as a resource that is influenced by a broad range of factors rather than by biology alone.

THE LALONDE REPORT, 1974

In 1974, Marc Lalonde, then the minister of National Health and Welfare (which became Health Canada in 1993), created a landmark document instrumental in introducing the concept of population health to Canada. This document, entitled *A New Perspective on the Health of Canadians* and informally called the Lalonde Report, is considered to be the first document acknowledged by a major industrialized nation to state that health is determined by more than just biology and that improved health could be achieved through changes in the environment, lifestyle, and health care organizations. (The full report can be found on the Evolve Web site.)

ALMA-ATA CONFERENCE, 1978

In September 1978, the World Health Organization convened the international Alma-Ata conference in Kazakhstan to address the need for global cooperation on health issues and in health care reform. A slogan that emerged from that conference was "Health for All—2000," which reflected the shared goal to reduce **inequities in health** across the globe through an emphasis on primary health care initiatives. **Primary health care**, as defined by the conference (Box 3.4), encompassed a broad range of concerns that paralleled those of the population health approach.

The conference's ten-point declaration (see Appendix, p. 397) claimed health as a fundamental right and stated that attaining an optimum level of health should be given the highest priority by all nations. The declaration called for the right of people and communities to be involved in planning their own health care and challenged governments to develop strategies to improve primary health care (In the News: The World Health Organization: In Support of Primary Health Care).

Inequities in health
Unfair and unequal distribution of health resources in relation to resources available and the population involved.

Primary health care
Health care with an emphasis on individuals and their communities. It includes essential medical and curative care received at the primary, secondary, or tertiary levels and involves health care providers, as well as community members, delivering, within the community, care that is cost-effective, comprehensive, and collaborative (i.e., uses a team approach).

Box 3.4   Alma-Ata Definition of *Primary Health Care*

Primary health care is essential health care based on practical, scientifically sound and socially acceptable methods and technology made universally accessible to individuals and families in the community through their full participation and at a cost that the community and country can afford to maintain at every stage of their development in the spirit of self-reliance and self-determination.

Reproduced, with the permission of the publisher, from *Declaration of Alma-Ata: International conference on primary health care*, Alma-Ata, USSR, 6–12 September 1978. World Health Organization. (1978). Retrieved from http://www.who.int/publications/almaata_declaration_en.pdf.

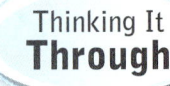
Thinking It Through

The *Declaration of Alma-Ata* identified primary health care as the key strategy for attaining universal health by the year 2000. "Health for All" was universally accepted as the main social goal (i.e., not merely a health goal) by the world health community. Today, efforts to improve the delivery of primary health care are under way in most regions across Canada, yet thousands of individuals remain without family doctors.

1. What improvements (if any) to health care have you seen in your own community?

2. If it were up to you, what changes to health care would you implement?

In the News

The World Health Organization: In Support of Primary Health Care

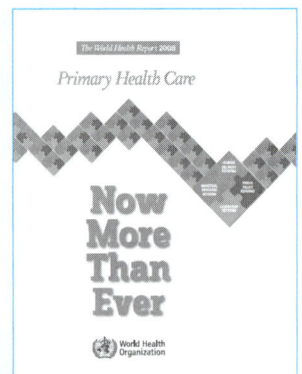

To commemorate the thirtieth anniversary of the Alma-Ata conference, WHO issued a new report in October 2008 entitled *Primary Health Care—Now More Than Ever*. This report documents the many failures that have left the health status of different populations, both within and among countries, dangerously out of balance. The inequities revealed by this report, listed below, are striking:

- Differences in life expectancy between the richest and poorest countries now exceed 40 years.
- Across the world, government spending on health ranges from as little as $20 US per person to well over $6000 US per person.
- Personal spending on health now pushes more than 100 million people below the poverty line each year.

To improve the performance of health systems globally, this recent report calls for a renewal of the focus on primary health care that was originally launched at the Alma-Ata conference:

> Primary health care brings balance back to health care and puts families and communities at the hub of the health system. With an emphasis on local ownership, it honours the resilience and ingenuity of the human spirit and makes space for solutions created by communities, owned by them, and sustained by them.

Reproduced, with the permission of the publisher, from *World health report calls for return to primary health care approach* [News release]. World Health Organization. (2008). Retrieved from http://www.who.int/mediacentre/news/releases/2008/pr38/en/.

Reproduced, with the permission of the publisher, *The world health report 2008: Primary health care—Now more than ever*. The World Health Organization. (2008).

OTTAWA CHARTER FOR HEALTH PROMOTION, 1986

The 1986 WHO conference in Ottawa was convened to review and expand on the proposals put forward at the Alma-Ata conference and to determine what progress had been made toward assuring health for all by the year 2000.

At the Ottawa conference, the original factors affecting health, outlined in the Lalonde Report, were broadened and termed "health prerequisites" and the need for a collaborative approach to address health-related problems was reinforced. Five principles emerged from the conference, including the need for all levels of government to become involved in health promotion and for individuals to assume responsibility for their own health (not just seeing the doctor when sick and expecting him or her to make them well). The charter also looked at strategies at the community level that would enhance health; for example, government-funded day care was cited as a strategy that would ultimately benefit the health and well-being of both the child and the parent.

Thinking It Through

Some people believe government-funded day care should be available to everyone. Others feel that child care should be the responsibility of the family and that government involvement only adds to the taxpayer's burden.

1. Should day care for your children be universally funded? Why or why not?"

2. Do you think that day care facilities would be better regulated thus safer if universal funding was implemented?

THE EPP REPORT, 1986

The Epp Report, *Achieving Health for All: A Framework for Health Promotion* by Jake Epp, minister of health and welfare, was released at the 1986 Ottawa conference. Its focus was proposals to reduce inequities for disadvantaged groups, to better manage chronic diseases, and to prevent disease, and it recommended that these initiatives have financial support from all levels of government (Epp, 1986).

THE PUBLIC HEALTH PROGRAM INITIATIVE

Designed by the Canadian Institute for Advanced Research—discussed on page 87—the Public Health Program Initiative reviewed the determinants of health;

analyzed their impact on the health of the Canadian population; and assessed the efficiency and effectiveness of the health care system. Recommendations made upon completion of the project in 2003 supported extending the idea that the determinants of health identified at previous conferences were linked—that is, that health outcomes were tied to multiple factors. For example, low income alone did not contribute to ill health, nor did a low position on the socioeconomic scale. Consider the potential outcomes in the life of Hinze (Case Example 3.3).

Case Example 3.3

If Hinze is in a low income bracket, chances are he will also be in a lower socioeconomic group or subject to less desirable living conditions, or both. As a result, Hinze may have less opportunity or motivation to advance his education or to obtain meaningful and satisfying employment. Perhaps he smokes or drinks alcohol to relieve stress. Cumulatively, he may then feel socially isolated or have low self-esteem and little confidence. He may also have poor nutritional habits perhaps because of a lack of knowledge about nutrition or because he cannot afford nutritious food. Combine these factors, and Hinze is at risk for multiple health problems ranging from depression to cancer or heart disease.

Remember the SES gradient in Box 3.2? While Hinze may develop a serious health problem, his friend Gus, who lives an almost identical lifestyle, is the picture of good health. This disparity has frequently been observed among groups of people living in similar conditions. Why are some groups affected and some not, given common denominators? Research in this field continues today. One area under close scrutiny is the inequity in the health of Canadians despite universal access to health care.

TOWARD A HEALTHY FUTURE: THE FIRST REPORT ON THE HEALTH OF CANADIANS, 1996

The first *Report on the Health of Canadians* was released in September 1996 by federal health minister David Dingwall and Ontario health minister Jim Wilson. Its recommendations carried forward the proposals made by CIFAR in 1989. This report was the first to officially recognize and incorporate the determinants of health into its findings and recommendations.

The report concluded that Canadians were among the healthiest populations in the world and emphasized that collaboration among all levels of government, industry, and the private sector must be intensified to improve the health of Canadians (Federal, Provincial and Territory Advisory Committee on Population Health, 1996). Box 3.5 lists strategies specified by the report to improve or maintain the health of Canadians, a further endorsement of the principles of the population health approach.

Box 3.5   Strategies for Improving the Health of Canadians

- Create a thriving and sustainable economy, with meaningful work for all.
- Ensure an adequate income for all Canadians.
- Reduce the number of families living in poverty in Canada.
- Achieve an equitable distribution of income.
- Ensure healthy working conditions.
- Encourage lifelong learning.
- Foster friendships and social support networks among families and communities.
- Create a healthy and sustainable environment for all.
- Ensure suitable, adequate, and affordable housing.
- Develop safe and well-designed communities.
- Foster healthy child development.
- Encourage healthy life-choice decisions.
- Provide appropriate and affordable health services, accessible to all.
- Reduce preventable illness, injury, and death.

Source: Health Canada. (1996). *Report on the health of Canadians.* Retrieved from http://publications.gc.ca/collections/Collection/H39-385-1996-1E.pdf.

NATIONAL FORUM ON HEALTH, 1994–1997

The National Forum on Health was the blueprint for current Health Canada initiatives. The forum was launched by the Right Honourable Jean Chrétien in 1994 and wrapped up in 1997. An integral part of this forum was public input—the beliefs and values of people across the country were sought through public discussion groups, conferences, meetings with experts, commissioned papers, letters, and briefs.

In February 1997, the forum published two final reports: *Canada Health Action: Building on the Legacy, Vol. I: Final Report* and *Canada Health Action: Building on the Legacy, Vol. II: Synthesis Reports and Issue Papers.* One of the key recommendations emerging from this forum was the need for more analysis and concrete evidence (i.e., an evidence-informed approach) to support initiatives for improving health.

All of these reports, beginning with the Lalonde Report, were significant in initiating a united population health approach to achieving better health for

Canadians. Recent reports—including *Toward a Healthy Future: The Second Report on the Health of Canadians, 1999; Building a Healthy Future, 2000; Final Report on the Health of Canadians, 2002* (also known as the Kirby Report); and *Building on Values: The Future of Health Care in Canada, 2002* (more commonly known as the Romanow Report) (see Chapter 1)—have analyzed the health of Canadians using a population health approach and offered recommendations for action.

PARTNERS IN POPULATION HEALTH ACTION

> **Intersectoral cooperation**
> Joint action among the public, the government, and nongovernment or community-based organizations.

The implementation of population health requires a formal plan, which ensures that steps are executed in a coordinated manner, that critical elements are identified, and that the role of agencies or individuals is clearly defined. Outlining a mission statement, goals, objectives, and methodology will help to ensure that all stakeholders understand the direction the approach will take. A clear plan is also necessary for the success and sustainability of **intersectoral cooperation**, a critical element of a population health approach. Planning should be transparent and flexible and should invite input from everyone involved.

Thinking It Through

In Canada, it is widely recommended (with a few exceptions) that everyone over the age of 6 months get an annual flu shot. Targeted or high-risk groups (e.g., older adults and people working in health care) are especially encouraged to get their vaccinations early. Since the H1N1 pandemic, the H1N1 virus has been included as one of the strains in the annual flu vaccine. Yet, in 2013–2014, a significant number of cases of H1N1 flu developed across Canada. People who had not gotten the flu shot then lined up to be immunized.

1. What is your opinion about getting the flu shot?

2. How would you feel if you (or a family member) were in hospital and being cared for by an unvaccinated health care provider who thus had a higher potential of transmitting the flu virus?

Source: Public Health Agency of Canada. (2014). FluWatch. Retrieved from http://www.phac-aspc.gc.ca/fluwatch/index-eng.php.

A number of departments, agencies, and organizations are instrumental in researching, gathering information, planning, and recommending strategies for Canada's population health approach. Various agencies, particularly at the community level, act as valuable resources for ideas related to the population health approach. The population health approach also energizes community members to be proactive, involved, and accepting of initiatives because they have been part of the planning process.

Discussed below are the roles that Health Canada, the Public Health Agency of Canada (PHAC), the Canadian Institutes of Health Research (CIHR), the Canadian Institute for Advanced Research (CIFAR), Canadian Policy Research Networks (CPRN), Statistics Canada, and the Canadian Institute for Health Information (CIHI) play in the formulation of Canada's population health approach.

HEALTH CANADA

Health Canada is the federal department ultimately responsible for helping Canadians maintain and improve their health. The department is "committed to improving the lives of all of Canada's people and to making this country's population among the healthiest in the world as measured by longevity, lifestyle and effective use of the public health care system" (Health Canada, 2011).

Health Canada's philosophy stresses that disease prevention and health promotion strategies will lead to better health for Canadians and will ultimately control the soaring costs of health care in the country. Health Canada partners with numerous other agencies and health care organizations to ensure its efforts meet the needs of all Canadians (see also Chapter 6).

PUBLIC HEALTH AGENCY OF CANADA

The Public Health Agency of Canada (PHAC) is a centralized agency under the umbrella of Health Canada. The PHAC's role is to respond to national emergencies and to implement health promotion and disease and injury prevention initiatives (see also Chapter 6).

To increase the public profile of population health, the Public Health Agency of Canada developed a symbol for use on all materials pertaining to population health. The design features a flower, which signifies growth and renewal and suggests the complexity of health and health care in Canada as well as the efforts to encourage a healthier population.

THE CANADIAN INSTITUTES OF HEALTH RESEARCH

Established by the federal government, the Canadian Institutes of Health Research is an organization responsible for funding health research in Canada. The mandate of this agency is to apply new research it has produced to the improvement of health and health care delivery in Canada. It is composed of a number of "institutes" that collaborate on and provide funding for research initiatives, including those concerning social, cultural, and environmental factors that affect population health. One of these institutes is the Institute of Population and Public Health, whose focus is almost exclusively on public and population health.

A recent research project by the CIHR involved working with Aboriginal people to integrate traditional and Western health practices in an attempt to provide more culturally sensitive, effective health care for that population (In the News: Health Research Model).

In the News — Health Research Model

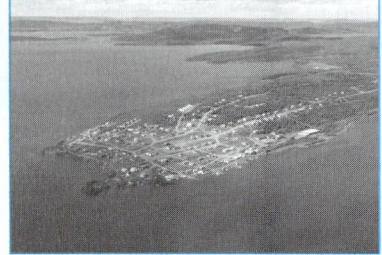

In 2012, the CIHR launched an operating grant for research into Aboriginal health, a project called Two-Eyed Seeing developed by the University of Cape Breton. The idea was to promote the integration of Aboriginal health–related customs and scientific (Western) methodologies to establish a best practices formula. This formula is to be applied to research aimed at improving the health of Aboriginal communities. With researchers and Aboriginal communities across Canada working together on this initiative, Aboriginal people are being given a say in the type of research carried out within their communities and are providing input on health care issues while also ensuring that their cultural beliefs and practices are considered.

Sources: Canadian Institutes of Health Research. (2013, May 15). *About PPH*. Retrieved from http://www.cihr-irsc.gc.ca/e/13787.html; Canadian Institutes of Health Research. (2011, July 26). *IPPH strategic research priorities*. Retrieved from http://www.cihr-irsc.gc.ca/e/27322.html; Canadian Institutes of Health Research. (2013, May 1). *Research profiles: Two-eyed seeing: Bringing Aboriginal perspectives to health research*. Retrieved from http://www.cihr-irsc.gc.ca/e/46646.html; Cape Breton University. (2013, January 18). *Two-eyed seeing model developed in Cape Breton drives new national grant for Aboriginal health research*. Retrieved from http://www.cbu.ca/news/two-eyed-seeing-model-developed-cape-breton-drives-new-national-grant-aboriginal-health-researc.

Photo source: Jason Pineau/All Canada Photos.

CANADIAN INSTITUTE FOR ADVANCED RESEARCH

A nonprofit organization relying on both public and private funds to sustain its research initiatives, the Canadian Institute for Advanced Research (CIFAR) brings together researchers from around the world to share ideas, thoughts, and theories concerning a wide variety of subjects. CIFAR specializes in advanced research, much of which is important to designing and implementing strategies used in population health. This agency remains a vital resource for both research and insight into health issues on national and international fronts.

Canadian Policy Research Networks

Founded in 1994, Canadian Policy Research Networks (CPRN) is a think tank whose main objective is to generate knowledge and discussion about socioeconomic issues in Canada. CPRN, which functions collaboratively with a variety of organizations, including all levels of government, and with industry, unions, educational institutions, and volunteer organizations, currently has the following four networks: family, health, public involvement, and work. The think tank conducts workshops, dialogues, and advisory committee meetings to generate information and debate in an impartial arena in which knowledge can be freely shared.

Statistics Canada

Statistics Canada is a branch of the federal government whose primary purpose is to gather information from every province and territory and to publish accurate statistics on almost every aspect of life imaginable. Statistics Canada is used extensively by government and agencies involved in public health and population health initiatives (e.g., for gathering data regarding births, deaths, and causes of morbidity and mortality).

Every five years, in the first and sixth years of every decade, Statistics Canada conducts a national census, which every household by law must participate in. The last national census was in 2011. For the first time, only the short-form questionnaire (with two questions on language added) was mandatory. The National Household Survey (NHS) replaced the previous long-form questionnaire and was voluntary. In 2010, amid much controversy, the federal government did away with the mandatory long-form census.

The Canadian Institute for Health Information

An independent organization, the Canadian Institute for Health Information (CIHI) works closely with CIHR and Statistics Canada to gather and assimilate information from numerous sources, including surveys, hospitals, clinics, and other health care centres. Funded by the federal, provincial, and territorial governments, CIHI reports to an independent board of directors that represents government health departments, regional health authorities, hospitals, and health-sector leaders across the country.

The data collected, organized, and distributed by this agency provide valuable, comprehensive information for organizations and individuals within and outside of Health Canada—the general public, government bodies, hospitals, professional organizations, educational facilities, researchers, and organizations at the municipal level (e.g., regional health authorities). The information helps in planning, organizing, and implementing policies and strategies.

CIHI maps the pattern of health care in Canada by working with 20 national and provincial information systems to gather data about the costing and delivery of health care services and the supply and distribution of health care providers. The organization produces an annual report of general information as well as a number of specific reports, such as *Women's Health*; *Supply, Distribution and Migration of Canadian Physicians*; and *Health Indicators*.

THE PUBLIC HEALTH AGENCY OF CANADA TEMPLATE

A template is much like a design or plan an architect would use to build a house. The Public Health Agency of Canada (PHAC) template has eight key elements, which appear in the shaded boxes in Figure 3.2. The white boxes in the figure indicate the basic steps necessary to link the key elements and to facilitate the entire population health process. In this process, the determinants of health are used as a means of analyzing the health of Canadians.

The PHAC template can act as a guide for policymakers, program planners, health educators, evaluators, researchers, and academics.

MEASURE THE POPULATION HEALTH STATUS

Measuring the health status of the population can answer the following key questions (Public Health Agency of Canada, 2012):

- How healthy is a population, and is its health improving?
- What can be learned about current trends in health status to help plan for future initiatives?
- What are the most important health issues?

> **Health indicators**
> Measurements that help to gauge the state of health and wellness of a population.

The first step in measuring population health is to select indicators for gauging the health status of that population. **Health indicators** are standardized measures that assist in assessing the health issues in a population and identifying any change in health status. A framework for health indicators was developed in 1999 by the CIHI and Stats Canada. These indicators were categorized as health status (how healthy and able a person is), nonmedical indicators (e.g., nutrition, risk behaviour, socioeconomic status), equity, and components related to the efficiency and effectiveness of health care and health care delivery (Canadian Institute for Health Information, 2013). Traditional health indicators also used include mortality (e.g., infant death, life expectancy, death due to cancer and

Figure 3.2 Template for Implementing a Population Health Approach in Canada

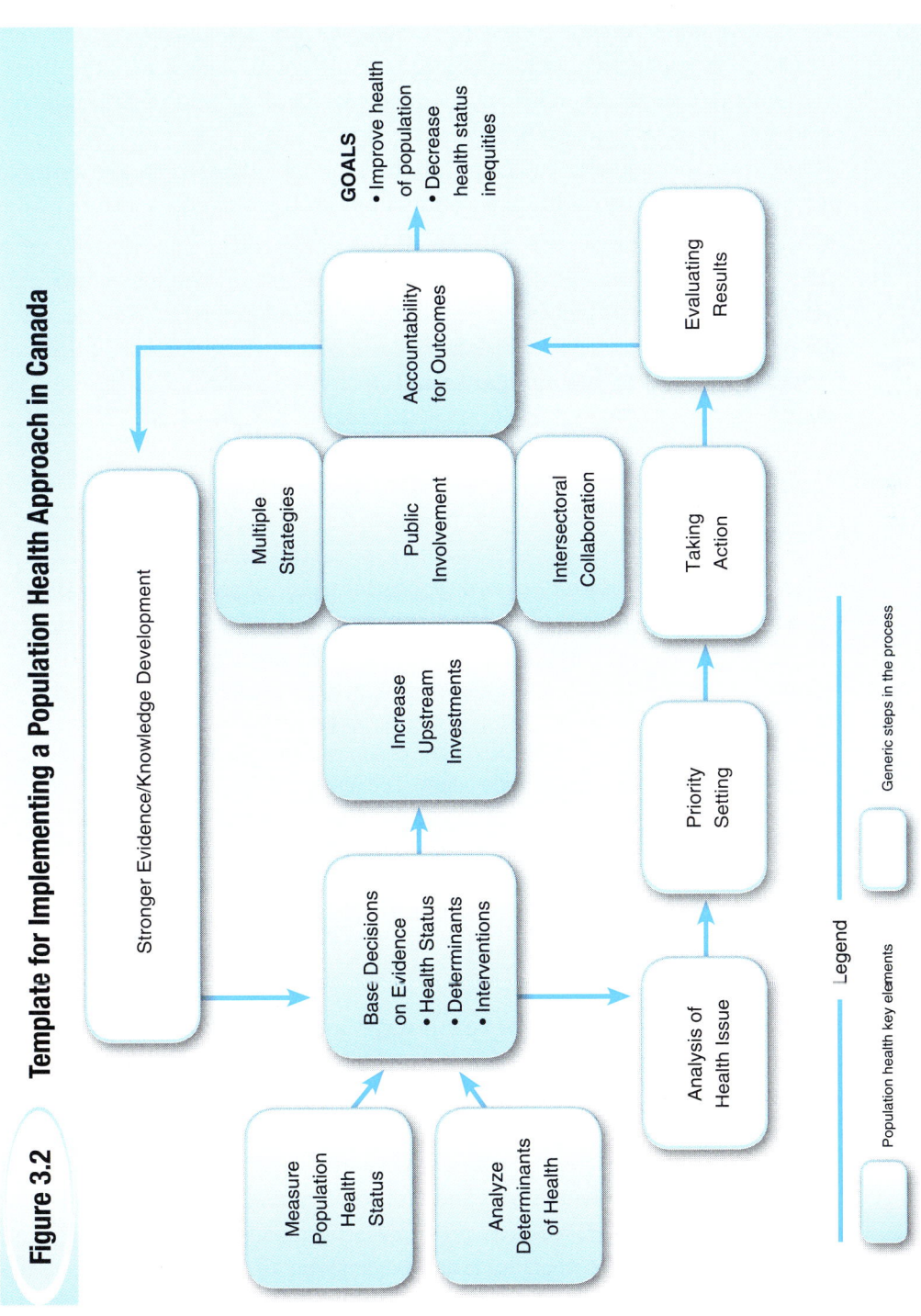

Source: © All rights reserved. The *Population Health Template Working Tool*. Public Health Agency of Canada, 2001. Reproduced with permission from the Minister of Health, 2014.

heart disease) and hospitalization rates. While important, these indicators do not provide the whole picture where population health status is concerned; they need to be supplemented with enhanced measures of morbidity, with the effects of chronic disease or disability on the quality of life, and with measures of the positive factors that improve health.

Based on these health indicators, information is gathered in the form of **population-based surveillance**. Information for this surveillance comes from a range of sources, including **epidemiology** (Box 3.6), socioeconomic data, health indicators (e.g., cancer rates, life expectancy, morbidity and mortality related to hospital infection rates), and data on the use of health services.

Population-based surveillance
The collection and analysis of data that are needed to plan, implement, and evaluate population health initiatives.

Epidemiology
The study of diseases in populations.

Box 3.6 Epidemiology Explained

Translated literally from Greek, *epidemiology* means "the study of people"; however, the term is used more specifically to denote the study of such entities as disease, injury, and death.

Epidemiology describes disease patterns in different groups of people, including how often they occur; identifies the causes of diseases; and then provides the information needed to plan, implement, and evaluate services to prevent, treat, and control diseases. Professionals who work in the field of epidemiology are known as *epidemiologists*.

In epidemiology studies, various assessment tools are used. For example, the incidence rate looks at the number of new cases of disease in a specified period of time; morbidity rates account for how many people are affected by a disease or an accident; and mortality rates provide information about deaths (Chapter 2).

Epidemiology remains the most important method of studying and understanding population health. In recent years, it has played a key role in the study of epidemics and in identifying emerging health issues in populations, from infectious diseases like acquired immune deficiency syndrome (AIDS) and influenza outbreaks to occupational hazards like asbestos.

Age is a social determinant of health regardless of immigration status. However, immigrant seniors, especially those who came to Canada in their later years, are more prone to poor health in the long run than are Canadian-born seniors because of their limited social networks, inadequate knowledge of official languages, and relatively low income, particularly if they live alone. More data on immigrant seniors' health status and more analyses of currently available data are needed to improve policies and practices (see Box 3.7).

Ongoing population surveillance is an excellent way to identify inequities in the health care system. For example, consider the inequities that exist between Canada's Aboriginal people living in the north and those Aboriginals living in urban areas.

> **Box 3.7** **An Aging Population: An Example of Population-Based Surveillance.**
>
> Canada's aging population is already stressing the health care system and the economy. Reasons for a proportionately larger older population include the post–World War II baby boom (1946–1965), increased longevity, and a lower birth rate. Statistics Canada (2008) predicts that by 2056, older-adult Canadians will account for 25% to 30% of the population. In terms of demographics, this population mix has both social and economic consequences. As older Canadians retire, fewer young people are moving into the workforce. As well as affecting the economy in general, this demographic shift will mean that fewer people are working to support Canada's social safety net, including seniors' pensions and health care benefits. Possible solutions that the government may consider include efforts to raise the birth rate and increase immigration. Continued monitoring of Canada's aging population, the birth rate, and immigration patterns, combined with other information, will provide data for strategies to improve the general well-being and health of Canadians.
>
> Source: Health Council of Canada. (2011, January). *A citizen's guide to health indicators: A reference guide for Canadians.* Retrieved from http://www.healthcouncilcanada.ca/rpt_det.php?id=130.

ANALYZE THE DETERMINANTS OF HEALTH

Population health considers all of the factors (determinants) that affect health status. As outlined in Figure 3.1, determinants of health include social, economic, and physical environments; early childhood development; gender; personal health practices and coping skills; culture; and biology and genetic endowment.

These determinants are scrutinized in terms of how they interact with one another and how they affect health status; this information then forms the basis for developing and implementing population health interventions.

USE EVIDENCE-INFORMED DECISION MAKING

All stages of a population health approach—selecting issues to be worked on, choosing interventions, deciding to implement and continue these interventions—are supported by decisions based on the most current best evidence available, a process called *evidence-informed decision making*.

An evidence-informed approach uses the full range of data, both qualitative and quantitative in nature. **Qualitative research** examines the way a population group thinks, how it acts, and its health beliefs and health behaviours. Qualitative research is conducted in a number of ways, including the administration of surveys and holding of open forums. **Quantitative research** deals primarily

Qualitative research
A method of research that examines the way a population group thinks and behaves. The analysis is largely subjective in nature.

Quantitative research
A method of objective research that deals with the measurement of data, such as the number of deaths from cancer.

with numbers, which are interpreted most frequently as statistics. Data can be generated through epidemiological studies, databases, and surveys, such as the census mentioned earlier in the chapter.

Employ Upstream Investments

> **Upstream investments**
> Actions that can be taken to improve the health of a population or to prevent illness when the potential for a problem is first recognized.

The term **upstream investments** refers to the process of making decisions that will benefit the health of a population group *before* a problem occurs. Being proactive regarding prevention saves money and gives a population a healthier future. Short-term and long-term goals are set and prioritized, and strategies are implemented using evidence-informed decision making. For example, encouraging Canadians to undergo periodic health exams, which are supported by most provinces, is a strategy to identify health problems at an early stage; similarly, immunizations prevent an array of diseases, such as diphtheria, polio, measles, mumps, and hepatitis, ensuring outbreaks of these illnesses do not put a strain on the system.

In 2012, in its annual report, the Mental Health Commission of Canada addressed Canadians' concerns about the state of mental health services (see Chapter 10). If the recommendations in the report are implemented, the result would be an upstream investment in mental health in Canada to improve diagnosis, treatment, and support for those with mental health problems.

Use Multiple Strategies

Once a population health goal is set, the next step is to introduce interventions to achieve the goal. No one action is likely to accomplish this, so a multifaceted approach must be taken. Actions must relate directly to the situation; suit the age range, health status, and environment of the target population; and be implemented over a chosen time frame. Such interventions must also address all of the health determinants involved, recognizing that they are interrelated.

Those involved in implementing a population health strategy must accept both the goal and the plan of action. Collaboration is essential. It is up to the government, then, to work with all sectors deemed to have an influence on the success of the interventions (e.g., the individual, the community, industry, related agencies, and local, provincial, and territorial governments).

Consider the introduction of the Gardasil vaccine. This upstream investment aimed to vaccinate all females at risk. The question was how to conduct the vaccination effectively and efficiently so that parents would allow their children to be vaccinated and so that those old enough to make their own decisions would understand and accept the rationale behind the vaccination program.

The government launched a massive public relations campaign, primarily through radio and television advertising, and engaged schools, public health units, and family doctors as champions of the program.

Engage the Public

Without public support, most health-care-related implementations will fail, in part because it is the public's health at issue and its tax dollars that fund implementation. Public involvement increases the likelihood that citizens will embrace a plan in a meaningful way. The key is to capture the public's interest early and in a positive manner. Plans to achieve positive public interest must be carefully considered and executed so as not to turn public opinion against the plan, especially because attempting to reverse public opinion can be difficult, if not impossible. For example, publicized concerns over the safety and adverse effects of Gardasil illustrate how public opinion can dissuade a significant number of people within a population or community from participating in an immunization campaign (Consumer Reports, 2009). Engaging the public requires the establishment of trust and an open process of decision making and implementation. Questions must be addressed promptly, properly, and persuasively.

Think Intersectoral Collaboration

Intersectoral collaboration involves developing partnerships between different segments of society—private citizens, community groups, industry, health and educational agencies, and various levels of government—to improve health. Each group comes to the table with its own values, outlook, opinions, and agenda. Harmonizing these variables is a challenge, but the benefits are profound: a commitment to common goals and an assurance that plans are implemented to meet these goals.

Efforts of the World Health Organization to control the AIDS epidemic, particularly in developing countries, are illustrative of this collaborative approach. Initially, most of the responsibility for treating and controlling the spread of the human immunodeficiency virus (HIV) rested with health care authorities. Subsequently, the involvement of other sectors was initiated through advertising campaigns on a number of fronts (e.g., educating populations on how HIV is contracted; involving schools and community agencies in the promotion of safer sex). Furthermore, a strategy to ensure a safe blood supply targeted all groups within the population and educated the public about behaviours that could reduce HIV transmission.

Demonstrate Accountability for Health Outcomes

A population health approach emphasizes the accountability for health outcomes—that is, the ability to determine if any changes in health outcomes can actually be attributed to specific policies or programs. The concept of accountability has an impact on planning and goal setting since it encourages the selection of interventions or strategies that produce the greatest health results.

Important steps in establishing accountability, therefore, include determining baseline measures (i.e., a standard against which to gauge progress), setting targets, and monitoring progress so that a thorough evaluation can be done. Evaluation tools provide criteria for determining the impact of policies or programs on population health. Finally, making evaluation results public is critical for gaining widespread support for successful population health initiatives.

Population Health Promotion Model

The population health promotion model (Figure 3.3) is an approach for promoting health on a population-wide basis. The model organizes population health into three areas:

1. What—looking to the health determinants to measure the health of populations
2. How—creating and implementing prioritized strategies to improve health
3. Who—engaging multiple stakeholders to participate in health improvement strategies

The population health promotion model demonstrates the complexity of health promotion. The model emulates the population health approach by using the determinants of health as indicators to measure health and to gather information for health promotion initiatives.

Decisions about health promotion policies are made using three sources of evidence:

1. Research studies on health issues (i.e., the underlying factors, the interventions, and their impact)
2. Knowledge gained through experience
3. Evaluation of current programs to anticipate strategies needed in the future—in other words, upstream investments in health promotion

Figure 3.3 Population Health Promotion Model

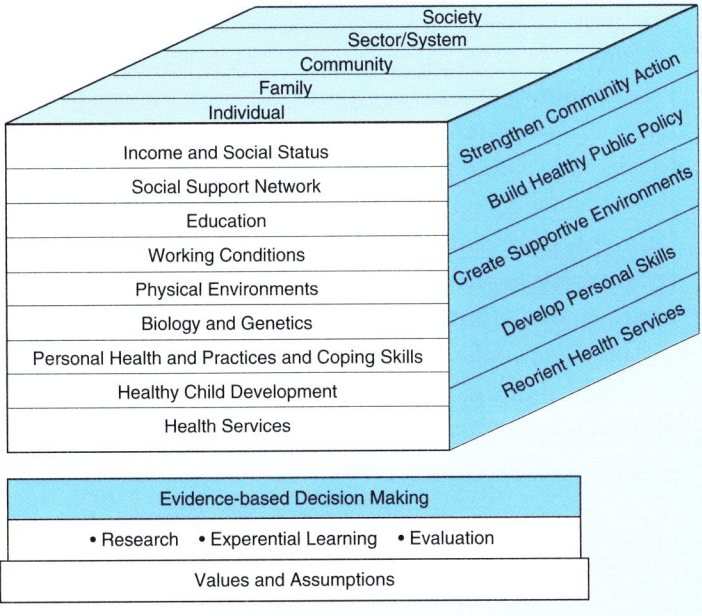

Source: © All rights reserved. *Population Health Promotion: An Integrated Model of Population Health and Health Promotion.* Public Health Agency of Canada, 2001. Reproduced with permission from the Minister of Health, 2014.

Collectively, stakeholders should address the full range of health determinants when adopting a population health promotion approach. Particular organizations, however, may wish to focus on specific determinants.

The population health promotion model can be used by any level of government, community agency, or group and can be accessed from any point of entry, depending on the health issue. Consider an industry wanting to improve working conditions. It would conduct research, draw information from other industries in which similar working conditions exist, evaluate identified strategies, and recommend action.

POPULATION HEALTH IN CANADA AND ABROAD

The general consensus among Canadians seems to be that the population health approach has been relatively successful but that it requires ongoing funding and commitment by all levels of government to have a truly positive impact on the health of Canadians. All provinces and territories have agencies within their own ministries that are responsible for their unique population health initiatives.

Information gathered by the PHAC and other departments at the federal level may have similar implications for all jurisdictions, but how each province or territory deals with any given issue may differ (e.g., planning for more hospital and long-term care beds as their population ages). Likewise, strategies and goals set may have different priorities and timelines. Consider Alberta's Vision 2020, which outlines five goals—from improving the delivery of health care across the board to strengthening public health services—to improve the health of Albertans by the year 2020 (Alberta Health and Wellness, 2008). British Columbia has also developed a guiding framework for public health. Its identifies seven goals, including strategies to enhance methods of preventing communicable diseases, and supports a population health approach and a public health role to ensure health equity (British Columbia Ministry of Health, 2013).

Although population health initiatives are used in most developed countries, they are almost nonexistent in developing nations. Data such as births, deaths, and causes of death are not usually recorded. Consequently, the health profile of these developing nations (many of which have the highest burden of disease) is virtually absent.

SUMMARY

3.1 Population health is a framework for measuring the health status of groups of people. The framework has been around for many years but has only recently been applied in an organized manner in Canada.

3.2 Since the late 1980s, the concept of health promotion has emphasized that adopting a healthy lifestyle is an important step toward achieving and maintaining good health and preventing diseases. As a result, definitions of health have been expanded, and more emphasis is given to the impact that elements in our social and physical environments have on our health status. These variables are called *determinants of health* and are now the foundation on which to gather data, analyze them, and propose solutions for health problems at national, provincial, territorial, and community levels. That the determinants interrelate to influence health issues is well known; how they do so, however, is not clearly understood.

3.3 Several reports issued by the federal government were instrumental in launching the population health initiative, beginning with the Lalonde Report in 1974. Following this report, Canadians began thinking about health in terms of prevention, with campaigns at both the federal and provincial levels of government urging the population to look at lifestyle and risk behaviours.

3.4 A number of government agencies work together to gather data and develop strategies. These include the Public Health Agency of Canada, the Canadian Institute for Health Information, the Canadian Institutes of Health Research, the Canadian Institute for Advanced Research, the Canadian Policy Research Networks, and Statistics Canada.

3.5 The Public Health Agency of Canada has developed a template and a logo for population health. The agency uses the template as a tool for the ongoing measurement of the health of Canadians and for the subsequent development of strategies to improve health.

3.6 The population health promotion model arranges population health into three segments: what, how, and who, through which it identifies *what* the problem is, *how* it can best be dealt with, and *whom* it affects. Evidence-informed decision making is a critical component for making strategies effective.

3.7 Information gathered by various organizations at the federal level is available to all provinces and territories across Canada. Each jurisdiction may use the information differently, tailoring it to the specific needs of its population.

Review Questions

1. Compare and contrast the principal elements of population health, health promotion, and public health.
2. What role did the *Declaration of Alma-Ata* play in developing population health initiatives?
3. Explain the purpose of the Public Health Agency of Canada's population health template.
4. What is the relationship between health care services and the health of a population?
5. What are inequities in health?
6. State the advantages of engaging the public in developing population health initiatives.
7. How does the population health promotion model differ from population health itself?
8. What might make the population health needs of one province or territory different from those of another?

References

Alberta Health and Wellness. (2008). *Vision 2020*. Retrieved from http://www.health.alberta.ca/documents/Vision-2020-Phase-1-2008.pdf.

British Columbia Ministry of Health. (2013). *Promote, protect, prevent: Our health starts here*. Retrieved from http://www.health.gov.bc.ca/library/publications/year/2013/BC-guiding-framework-for-public-health.pdf.

Canadian Institute for Health Information. (2012). *Health indicators 2012*. Retrieved from https://secure.cihi.ca/free_products/health_indicators_2012_en.pdf.

Canadian Institute for Health Information. (2013). *Health indicators 2013*. Retrieved from https://secure.cihi.ca/free_products/HI2013_EN.pdf.

Consumer Reports. (2009). Gardasil: Safety concerns persist, but may be unfounded. *Consumerreports.org*. Retrieved from http://www.consumerreports.org/cro/2012/04/gardasil-safety-concerns-persist-but-may-be-unfounded/index.htm.

D'Arcy, C. (1986). Unemployment and health: Data and implications. *Canadian Journal of Public Health*, 77(Suppl. 1), 124–131.

References

Epp, J. (1986). *Achieving health for all: A framework for health promotion*. Ottawa: Health and Welfare Canada. Retrieved from http://www.hc-sc.gc.ca/hcs-sss/pubs/system-regime/1986-frame-plan-promotion/index-eng.php.

Federal, Provincial and Territory Advisory Committee on Population Health. (1996). *Report on the health of Canadians*. Retrieved from http://publications.gc.ca/collections/Collection/H39-385-1996-1E.pdf.

Haydon, E., Roerecke, M., Giesbrecht, N., et al. (2006). Chronic disease in Ontario and Canada: Determinants, risk factors and prevention priorities. *Ontario Chronic Disease Prevention Alliance and the Ontario Public Health Association*. Retrieved from http://ocdpa.echidnadev.ca/sites/default/files/publications/CDP-FullReport-Mar06.pdf.

Health Canada. (2006). *Health care system: About primary health care*. Retrieved from http://www.hc-sc.gc.ca/hcs-sss/prim/about-apropos-eng.php.

Health Canada. (2011). *Health Canada Privacy Act annual report 2010–2011*. Retrieved from http://www.hc-sc.gc.ca/ahc-asc/pubs/_atip-aiprp/2011priv-prot/index-eng.php.

Holt-Lunstad, J., Smith, T. B., & Layton, J. B. (2010). Social relationships and mortality risk: A meta-analytic review. *PLOS Medicine*. Retrieved from http://dx.doi.org/10.1371/journal.pmed.1000316.

Institute of Medicine (US) Committee on Health and Behavior: Research, Practice, and Policy. (2001). Social risk factors. In *Health and behavior: The interplay of biological, behavioral, and societal influences*. Washington, DC: National Academies Press (US). Retrieved from http://www.ncbi.nlm.nih.gov/books/NBK43750/.

Koven, S. (2013). Social support matters in cancer survival. *KevinMD.com* Retrieved from http://www.kevinmd.com/blog/2013/10/social-support-matters-cancer-survival.html.

Mikkonen, J., & Raphael, D. (2010). *Social determinants of health: The Canadian facts*. Toronto: York University School of Health Policy and Management. Retrieved from http://www.thecanadianfacts.org/The_Canadian_Facts.pdf.

Public Health Agency of Canada. (n.d.). *Volunteering as a vehicle for social support and life satisfaction*, Factsheet, p. 1.

Public Health Agency of Canada. (2003). *What makes Canadians healthy or unhealthy?*. Retrieved from http://www.phac-aspc.gc.ca/ph-sp/determinants/determinants-eng.php.

Public Health Agency of Canada. (2011). *What determines health?*. Retrieved from http://www.phac-aspc.gc.ca/ph-sp/determinants/determinants-eng.php#income.

Public Health Agency of Canada. (2012). *What is the population health approach?*. Retrieved from http://www.phac-aspc.gc.ca/ph-sp/approach-approche/index-eng.php.

Public Health Agency of Canada. (2013). *What makes Canadians healthy or unhealthy?*. Retrieved from http://www.phac-aspc.gc.ca/ph-sp/determinants/determinants-eng.php.

Statistics Canada. (2008). *Some facts about the demographic and ethnocultural composition of the population*. Retrieved from http://www.statcan.gc.ca/pub/91-003-x/2007001/4129904-eng.htm.

United States Environmental Protection Agency. (1991). *Indoor air facts no. 4 (revised): Sick building syndrome (SBS)*. Retrieved from http://www.epa.gov/iaq/pdfs/sick_building_factsheet.pdf.

World Health Organization. (n.d.) *Health impact assessment: The determinants of health*. Retrieved from http://www.who.int/hia/evidence/doh/en/.

Zaman, F., & Underwood, C. (2003). *The gender guide for health communication programs*. Baltimore: Center Publication No. 102. Johns Hopkins Bloomberg School of Public Health/Center for Communication Programs.

Chapter Four

The Law and Health Care

 Learning Outcomes

4.1 Describe the laws used in health care legislation and their classifications.
4.2 Explain the federal and provincial jurisdictional framework in Canada.
4.3 Outline the concerns about and the issues related to health care's being a right.
4.4 Discuss the legality of offering private services in Canada.
4.5 Understand the basic principles of consent to treatment.
4.6 Discuss the health record and issues surrounding the privacy of health information.
4.7 Describe the role of self-governing health care professions in legal matters.
4.8 Identify some other important legal issues in Canadian health care.

Key Terms

Act, p. 104
Age of majority, p. 135
Assisted suicide, p. 123
Circle of care, p. 130
Civil law, p. 105
Code of ethics, p. 141
Common law, p. 105
Confidentiality, p. 136
Conflict of interest, p. 126
Constitutional law, p. 103
Contract law, p. 108
Controlled Drugs and Substances Act, p. 112
Criminal law, p. 109
Drug-seeking behaviour, p. 113
Duty of care, p. 108
Electronic health record (EHR), p. 139
Electronic medical record (EMR), p. 139
Fiduciary duty, p. 126
Good Samaritan law, p. 143
Implied consent, p. 130
Incident report, p. 110
Informed consent, p. 127
Inpatient, p. 143
Jurisdiction, p. 111
Legislation, p. 103
Malpractice, p. 107
Minor, p. 131
Negligence, p. 107
Oral consent, p. 130
Personal Information Protection and Electronic Documents Act (PIPEDA), p. 135
Power of attorney, p. 131
Privacy, p. 137
Professional misconduct, p. 107
Proxy consent, p. 132
Quarantine Act, p. 118
Regulation, p. 104
Regulatory law, p. 104
Statutory law, p. 104
Tort, p. 106
Whistleblower, p. 144
Workplace Hazardous Materials Information System (WHMIS) legislation, p. 112

This chapter provides a practical overview of the relationship between the law and health care in Canada. It concentrates on basic elements of health care and the application of related legal issues, rather than on specific laws and legislation. Because laws vary among the provinces and territories, it is more meaningful for students to research those within their own jurisdiction to access specific information.

Most health care providers, hospitals, regional health authorities, and regulated professions are governed by legislation, regulations, or guidelines, which affect how they function. This chapter begins by examining the division of legislative powers between the federal government and the provincial and territorial governments where health care is concerned. It also discusses the legal responsibilities of the federal government with respect to safety legislation and sections within criminal law that affect health care.

The chapter also addresses the legal right of Canadians to health care and discusses court challenges that have been launched (some successfully, some not) regarding the right of Canadians to timely medical intervention under the Canadian Charter of Rights and Freedoms.

Legislation regarding private enterprise in health care varies across Canada's jurisdictions. This chapter looks at restrictions imposed on Canadians with regard to seeking health care from private clinics and the right of Canadians to purchase private insurance for medically necessary services that the provinces or territories cannot provide within reasonable time frames.

The chapter also examines the legal guidelines and responsibilities of health care providers regarding consent to treatment. The effects of the law on health care providers, as well as on their moral and legal obligations to patients, are also highlighted. Finally, this chapter addresses health information management, confidentiality, and current privacy legislation—and the challenges presented by electronic health records.

LAWS USED IN HEALTH CARE LEGISLATION

Law in Canada includes both statutory law (i.e., derived from acts) and common law (i.e., made by judges in deciding cases). Various levels of government are authorized to create laws. Some types of law apply to the health care industry more than others, including constitutional, statutory, regulatory, and common (or case) law, all of which are described in the sections that follow.

Constitutional Law

Constitutional law addresses the relationship between the people and their government, and establishes, allocates, and limits public power. In Canada, cases

Legislation
Laws made by a provincial or territorial legislature or by Parliament. To become law, a bill (i.e., proposed legislation) that has been introduced to Parliament requires the agreement of the House of Commons, the Senate, and the Crown (i.e., the Governor General, the representative of the British monarch in Canada).

Constitutional law
The area of law dealing with legislation derived from or related to Canada's Constitution.

challenging a person's right to health care have been based on the Canadian Charter of Rights and Freedoms, part of the Canadian Constitution. Under the Constitution, everyone has the following fundamental freedoms (Canadian Charter of Rights and Freedoms, 1982):

- Freedom of conscience and religion
- Freedom of thought, belief, opinion, and expression, including freedom of the press and other media of communication
- Freedom of peaceful assembly
- Freedom of association

A Canadian citizen denied any of these rights can challenge the person, persons, or organization denying him or her such rights based on the related section of the Charter. Challenges regarding the right to health care often occur under sections 7 and 15 (see page 115).

STATUTORY LAW

A *statute* is a law or an **act**. **Statutory laws** are the laws passed in Parliament (i.e., at the federal level) or in the provincial or territorial legislatures. Statutory laws under federal authority include those dealing with immigration, taxation, and divorce. Statutory laws under provincial or territorial jurisdiction include those related to education, family, and health care.

REGULATORY LAW

Regulatory law possesses the legally binding feature of an act; however, regulatory law is not made by Parliament (i.e., at the federal level) or by provincial or territorial legislatures but rather by delegated persons or organizations, such as an administrative agency or a tribunal (e.g., the National Energy Board, the Public Utilities Board of Yukon and the Northwest Territories). The authority to implement **regulations**, however, must be specifically outlined in a federal, provincial, or territorial act—for example, in Manitoba, the *Regional Health Authorities Act* gives regional health authorities the power to make, implement, and enforce regulations. Federally, the *Food and Drugs Act* enables Health Canada's *Food and Drug Regulations*.

In health care, regulatory law affects hospital boards, health care institutions, and bodies governing health care providers. Under provincial and territorial health care professions acts (e.g., Ontario's *Regulated Health Professions Act*), the minister of health oversees the manner in which health care professions operate and govern themselves and also retains the power to request a council make, amend, or revoke a particular regulation.

Act
A usually comprehensive body of laws passed by Parliament or a provincial or territorial legislature.

Statutory law
Written law, formally created or established by the legislature.

Regulatory law
Laws made not by Parliament or by a legislature but by authorized persons or organizations to govern a particular group; these laws are ultimately subject to the provincial, territorial, or federal act that governs the administrative body, organization, or tribunal.

Regulation
A form of law, made by persons or organizations (e.g., an administrative agency) awarded such authority within an act (whether federal or provincial or territorial), that has the binding legal power of an act.

Common (Case) Law and Civil Law in Canada

In Canada, law in all provinces and territories except Quebec is based on **common law**. Quebec, however, operates under **civil law**, based on the French *Code Napoléon* or *Civil Code*.

Common law is not established within legislature or formally written like statutory law. Also called *case law*, it results from the decisions of judges. These decisions are based on precedents—rulings other judges made in previous similar cases. Although Quebec's civil law system relies heavily on written laws, judges in Quebec courts often seek guidance from precedents set in earlier cases, as is done in common law systems. As well, common law may govern litigation conducted before the Federal Court of Canada, which sits in both Montreal and Quebec City.

Common law may serve to define obligations and legal rights or to further explain an element of, for example, the Charter or the *Privacy Act* or a regulation under the *Occupational Health and Safety Act*. (See Box 4.4, which details a Charter case.)

Classifications of Law: Public and Private Law

Laws are classified as public or private. Public law pertains to matters between an individual and society as a whole and, therefore, includes criminal, tax, constitutional, administrative, and human rights laws. For example, when an individual breaks a criminal law, his or her breach is considered a wrong against society, not just a wrong against another person or a select group of people. Public law is the same across Canada.

Private law governs matters concerning relationships between people and includes contract and property law, matters relating to inheritance, family law, tort law (e.g., negligence), and corporate law. As mentioned above, two systems deal with private law issues: civil law in Quebec and common law throughout the rest of Canada.

To illustrate the difference between public law and private law, if a nurse believed a patient was better off dead and actively helped that person to die (active euthanasia), the police, acting on behalf of the state, would arrest the nurse and charge him or her under the Criminal Code, part of public law. If found guilty, the nurse could be sentenced to jail or be ordered to pay a fine (i.e., to the state). The victim's family could also launch a civil suit against the nurse under private law. If the family were awarded damages, the nurse would have to pay these directly to the family.

Some provinces and territories have specialized agencies called Criminal Injury Compensation Boards (see Web Resources on Evolve) to which a victim (or the family of a victim) can apply for damages, bypassing the necessity of launching a civil suit, once an individual has been convicted in a criminal court. The government assesses the damages, which are awarded from public funds.

> **Common law**
> Laws established over time by judges based on decisions made on similar cases; sometimes referred to as *case law*.
>
> **Civil law**
> A legal system in which laws governing civil rights and relationships within society, between people and property, and within families are written rather than being determined by judges.

In British Columbia, a landmark civil case fundamentally changed access to health care for hearing impaired persons across Canada and had implications for others with disabilities (Box 4.1).

> **Box 4.1 Equality of Care for Hearing Impaired People**
>
> Linda and John Warren and John Eldridge were born deaf. For many years, a private, nonprofit organization provided sign interpreters to help them communicate with health care providers during doctors' appointments, hospital visits, medical tests, and the like. Sign language was their preferred method of communication.
>
> In 1990, because of funding shortfalls, the organization that had provided the interpreter discontinued this service. Several appeals for financing proved futile, and the trio was left with no support to hire an interpreter. They claimed that the absence of a sign interpreter interfered with their ability to effectively communicate with health care providers, increasing the opportunity for errors in diagnosis and treatment and impeding their ability to understand treatment options and to make informed decisions. Requests to the provincial and federal governments for support were repeatedly denied.
>
> After a long legal battle ending at the Supreme Court of Canada, the Court ruled that the *Hospital Services Act* and the *Medical and Health Care Services Act* contravened section 15(1) of the Charter (equality rights) by failing to address the need for services for individuals to communicate effectively with health care providers. The Supreme Court directed that both acts—as well as those of other provinces and territories—be changed to accommodate these rights.
>
> Source: *Eldridge v. British Columbia* (Attorney General), 1997, 3 SCR 624.

A person can sue a business, a dentist, a doctor, a hospital, a primary health care organization, or any individual for damages under private law, which includes the torts of libel and slander, breaches in privacy and confidentiality, and negligence suits.

Tort Law

Tort
A civil wrong committed against a person or his or her property.

A **tort** occurs when one person or that person's property is wronged or harmed by another, either intentionally (deliberately) or unintentionally. Tort law cases can be complicated—what might initially be seen as an unintentional act, perhaps attributed to human error, may well end up as a case of negligence.

Intentional Tort

An intentional tort occurs when the harmful act is deliberate. In health care, it usually involves physical aggression or forcing unwanted medical treatment on a patient. An intentional tort could result if, for example, a health care aide was proven to have treated a patient roughly, resulting in injury to that patient or if a health care provider successfully performed cardiopulmonary resuscitation (CPR) on an individual who had a known do-not-resuscitate order.

Unintentional Tort

An unintentional tort occurs when the act caused physical or emotional injury or property damage but was not deliberate or calculated. Unintentional torts usually result from acts of human error, misjudgement, or negligence. For example, human error might be considered the cause if a respiratory therapist gave an inhalation treatment to a child and mistakenly used the wrong drug (although in some cases negligence might be proven). A physiotherapist might misjudge a patient's ability to ambulate, resulting in a fall the first time he or she tried to get up independently. Negligence is one of the most common torts, and cases are often complicated.

Negligence

Negligence as part of tort law is sometimes referred to as **malpractice** or, depending on the case, **professional misconduct**. **Negligence** occurs when a health care provider fails, whether intentionally or unintentionally, to meet the standards of care required of his or her profession. Negligence can result from forgetting to perform an action, not caring or confirming whether a particular action is performed, providing improper or substandard care, providing a patient with unclear instructions, or failing to successfully instruct a patient in how to follow a treatment plan (Case Example 4.1).

Health care providers may find themselves accused of a tort if a patient experiences physical or emotional injury resulting from something the health care provider did, whether intentionally or unintentionally. In Canada, an injured party who cannot prove negligence would rarely receive compensation.

Malpractice
Illegal, negligent, or substandard treatment (failing to meet the treatment standards of one's profession) by a medical practitioner. Malpractice may be intentional or unintentional wrongdoing that may or may not result in injury to a patient.

Professional misconduct
Behaviour or some act or omission that falls short of what would be proper in the circumstances. Examples include deviating from a profession's standards of practice or violating the boundaries of a professional–patient relationship.

Negligence
The failure of a health care provider, whether intentional or unintentional, to meet the standards of care required of his or her profession; also sometimes referred to as *malpractice*, especially when resulting in harm or injury to the patient.

Case Example 4.1

Andrea, a physiotherapy assistant, has been asked to get 85-year-old Edgar (who has advanced Alzheimer's disease) up for a short walk and then help him back to bed. After leaving the floor, Andrea remembers that she failed to put up Edgar's side rail. Running late, she thinks, "Someone will have done it by now," and leaves the hospital. Edgar falls out of bed, breaking both legs. His family sues the hospital and Andrea, the assistant.

Duty plays a significant role in both medical ethics and medical law. Held more accountable in terms of their duty to their patients than people in many other professions, health care providers will face litigation if it is proven that they failed to fulfill their duty to the patient. Duty becomes part of the patient–health care provider relationship as soon as the professional relationship begins. For example, Jeremy has made an appointment with a new doctor. Their professional relationship begins once the doctor has seen Jeremy, assessed him, and recommended a treatment plan. Before the appointment, Jeremy could not claim that the doctor was negligent in a health-related matter and bring legal action against him or her. The doctor is responsible for Jeremy's care until the doctor–patient relationship ends and Jeremy has transferred his care to another practitioner. Facilities likewise can be held responsible for incidents when substandard care is proven (e.g., inadequate staffing levels in a nursing home resulting in harm to a resident) because the facility itself is responsible for setting and maintaining standards of care.

Results from a negligent incident may not be immediately apparent to anyone involved. For example, cases of adverse effects due to saline breast implants have often come to light several years after being implanted.

Litigation and the Duty of Care

> **Duty of care**
> The obligation to act in a competent manner according to the standards of practice.

Almost all health care providers are bound by a **duty of care** that is in keeping with their profession's standards of care. Litigation in such cases considers the standard of competency that a "reasonable person" (i.e., a person with similar training in a similar situation) is expected to meet. This standard generally remains constant within a profession but varies among professions (e.g., a registered nurse would be held to a higher standard of care than a personal support worker, or a nurse practitioner may be held to a higher standard of care than a registered nurse, depending, of course, on the situation).

Contract Law

> **Contract law**
> The branch of law dealing with agreements between parties, including the interpretation or enforcement of agreements when there is a dispute.

Contract law concerns legally binding contracts—voluntary agreements between two or more parties. Contracts can exist between, for example, an employer and an employee or a health care provider and a patient. They also may be either expressed (i.e., openly spoken or written) or implied (i.e., unspoken but considered understood).

A breach of contract occurs when one of the parties fails to meet the terms of the agreement. A plastic surgeon, for example, can agree to perform a facelift on a patient for a given price. If, for some reason, the physician fails to complete the procedure or if the patient refuses to pay the agreed-upon price, one can sue the other for breach of contract. Another example: A private health care organization hires a dentist on a one-year contract. After two months, the dentist finds a higher-paying position and leaves. The health care organization can sue the dentist for breach of contract.

Criminal Law

The field of **criminal law** deals with crimes against the state or crimes deemed intolerable within society, such as murder, racism, and theft (In the News: Nondisclosure: A Criminal Offence?). In the health care field, examples of crimes punishable under criminal law include someone using another person's health card fraudulently, a surgeon practising without a licence, a person trafficking narcotics, and someone assisting a person or patient to commit suicide. Box 4.2 suggests ways for those in clinical practice to avoid legal problems in the health care environment.

A person charged with a criminal offence may be found not guilty in a criminal court but later be found guilty in a civil court (Case Example 4.2).

> **Criminal law**
> The field of law dealing with crimes against the state or against society. Criminal law defines offences and controls the regulations concerning the apprehension, charging, and trying of those believed to have committed a criminal offence.

In the News: Nondisclosure: A Criminal Offence?

In April 2009, Johnson Aziga, a Hamilton, Ontario, man, was found guilty in a criminal court of two counts of first-degree murder after causing the human immunodeficiency virus (HIV)–related deaths of two women by having unprotected sex with them and not divulging that he was HIV positive. This case is unprecedented in Canada, according to Crown Attorney Karen Shea.

Source: Canadian Press. (2009, April 5). Man spreading HIV convicted of murders. *CNews*. Retrieved from http://cnews.canoe.ca/CNEWS/Canada/2009/04/04/9006741-cp.html.

Photo credit: Hamilton Spectator-Gary Yokoyama/The Canadian Press.

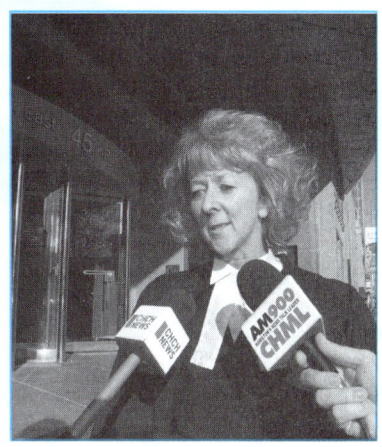

Box 4.2 Strategies for Avoiding Legal Problems

- Most health care facilities require criminal checks both for potential employees and for students who apply to complete a work or co-op placement. Complete any such checks as requested and, if criminal activity exists in your background, tell your potential employer. Trying to hide something and having it surface later causes more harm. In most areas, criminal checks can be attained for a fee by contacting the nearest police station. The check may take several days or several weeks.

Continued on next page

Incident report
A legal document outlining all relevant information concerning any negative occurrence in the workplace.

- Work only within your scope of practice. If asked to do something outside of your scope of practice or something you are not licensed to do, say no. If you feel unsure about how to perform a specific task within your scope of practice, ask for help. It is not a crime to seek assistance; it could be a crime if you do not.
- Complete, concise, and accurate documentation protects everyone—you, the organization you work for, and your patient. Keep required charting current and accurate. Record all events, even those that seem trivial. In the event of litigation, the medical record may be the most important document in determining the outcome of a case.
- Most facilities maintain a formal process for the reporting of adverse events. These procedures usually involve completing a form called an **incident report**. Information on this form must be concise and accurate. In most cases, if the incident involves a patient in the hospital setting, the information recorded on the incident report appears on the patient's medical chart only if it relates directly to the patient's health. The incident report itself is sent to the risk manager, who uses it to assess the occurrence and to implement measures to prevent similar future occurrences.
- Adhere to privacy and confidentiality laws. Think before you speak about work or information relating to work. Never access anyone's files (electronic or written) unless you have a legal right to do so. Being a friend or relative does not give you legal access to another's private health information. Remember, good news related to health information also must remain confidential.
- Always do your best. Never provide substandard care or treatment. Take the extra time to complete a task properly. An ounce of prevention goes a long way.
- Be an advocate for your patients. If you suspect that something is wrong, use the appropriate chain of command and talk to someone, rather than ignoring the incident. Your patient may be afraid to address the situation personally or may feel that he or she will simply be ignored.
- Do not ignore unethical or illegal activities.
- Ensure that you have some type of liability insurance through your place of employment or your professional college or organization that will cover you for mishaps or wrongdoing.

Case Example 4.2

Jessica, a respiratory therapist, was charged with criminal negligence after she administered the wrong inhalation treatment to Hanna, a patient. Hanna suffered a cardiac arrest because of an allergy to the medication administered. Jessica was found not guilty of criminal negligence, but when Hanna brought a civil charge against Jessica, the civil court upheld the charge and awarded Hanna $200,000 in damages.

FEDERAL AND PROVINCIAL JURISDICTIONAL FRAMEWORK

The law has played a role in health care since the *British North America Act* (now the *Constitution Act*) was passed in 1867, granting jurisdiction over some areas of health care to the federal government and jurisdiction over other areas to the provincial and territorial governments. A government's having **jurisdiction** means that it has authority over specific designated geographic and legislative areas and also possesses the right to draft, pass, and enact laws within its region.

Initially, the provinces assumed responsibility for "the establishment, maintenance, and management of hospitals, asylums, charities in and for the province, other than for marine hospitals" (*Constitution Act*, 1982). The federal government retained authority over health care for certain population groups, including members of the Royal Canadian Mounted Police (RCMP), inmates of federal penitentiaries, and Aboriginal peoples.

In addition to its fiscal influence over health care (see Chapter 6), the federal government controls certain components of health care activity covered by the Criminal Code of Canada. For example, the vague phrase "peace, order, and good government" (*Constitution Act*, 1982) allows the federal government to pass legislation on matters that would normally fall under provincial or territorial jurisdiction—in particular, the enactment of emergency powers, such as quarantine.

The next section examines federal authority in key areas of health care as it applies to the safety and protection of physicians, other health care providers, and the general public.

> **Jurisdiction**
> Authority or power over a designated region or geographic area.

WORKPLACE SAFETY

Several Canadian organizations—including the Canadian Centre for Occupational Health and Safety (CCOHS), the Workers' Compensation Board (WCB, or equivalent), and the Workplace Hazardous Materials Information System (WHMIS)—strive to maintain the health of working Canadians by ensuring that they have a safe and healthy workplace.

Health care providers may have to interact with CCOHS and WCB in some manner, possibly by helping a patient regain health and mobility in order to return to his or her current workplace or to transfer to a new career.

Occupational Health and Safety: Jurisdictions

In Canada, occupational health and safety legislation is divided among 14 jurisdictions: ten provincial, three territorial, and one federal. The federal government manages labour affairs for certain sectors, including employees of the federal government and of federal corporations. The federal government also has jurisdiction over individuals working in occupations that cross provincial and territorial lines (e.g., transportation and communication) and in the federal public service sector.

Each province and territory hosts an occupational health and safety agency, which enacts its own legislation, generally called the *Occupational Health and Safety Act* or something similar.

Occupational Health and Safety Legislation: Objectives

Aiming to ensure a safe workplace for all Canadians and to support the rights of workers to a safe environment, occupational health and safety legislation sets guidelines, provides for legal enforcement of these guidelines, and outlines the rights of employees, including the following:

- The right to be aware of potential safety and health hazards
- The right to take part in activities (e.g., by serving on committees or acting as a health and safety representative) aimed at preventing occupational accidents and diseases
- The right to refuse to engage in dangerous work without jeopardizing his or her job

Workers' Compensation Boards work hand-in-hand with the CCOHS but concentrate specifically on assisting injured employees by providing wages, rehabilitation, and training. Legislation related to these boards or commissions, drafted and administered by each province and territory, is typically named the *Workers' Compensation Act*. The Northwest Territories and Nunavut share a Workers' Compensation Board.

Workplace Hazardous Materials Information System

The CCOHS oversees the **Workplace Hazardous Materials Information System (WHMIS) legislation**, which became law through complementary federal, provincial, and territorial legislation in October 1988.

The national standards for WHMIS legislation were established by the federal *Hazardous Products Act* and the Controlled Products Regulations. Enforced by the federal, provincial, and territorial governments, this legislation applies to all Canadian workplaces in which identified hazardous materials are used. The national office for WHMIS operates as a division within Health Canada.

Some may think that WHMIS legislation would apply only to industrial settings, but hazardous materials are present in many areas of the health care industry. Hospitals, for example, house hazardous substances used in diagnostic testing (e.g., radioactive products), chemotherapeutic agents, combustible agents (e.g., oxygen), infectious material, and medical waste.

DRUGS AND THE LAW

Canada's drug laws are covered primarily by federal legislation called the **Controlled Drugs and Substances Act**. This Act replaced the *Narcotic Control Act* and the *Food and*

Workplace Hazardous Materials Information Systems (WHMIS) legislation
A group of laws, rules, or statutes enacted by a government (federal, provincial, territorial, or municipal).

Controlled Drugs and Substances Act
Federal legislation addressing Canada's drug laws, including a classification system for drugs.

Drugs Act, Parts III and IV, in May 1997. The new Act established different categories of drugs, called *schedules*. The classification system addresses the properties of drugs and their potential for harm. Schedule I, for example, includes cocaine, heroin, opium, oxycodone, morphine, and codeine; Schedule II addresses cannabis.

Controlled Drugs and Prescriptions

The *Controlled Drugs and Substances Act* outlines who can prescribe controlled drugs (e.g., doctors, dentists) and the conditions and terms of use for prescription narcotics. The prescribing of controlled substances occurs under combined federal, provincial, and territorial legislation. There has been much controversy over the drug oxycodone, with provincial and territorial governments disagreeing about how to effectively deal with abuse issues (In the News: A Significant Drug Problem: Who Should Assume Responsibility?).

Dispensing Controlled Drugs in Facilities

Most hospitals and other health care facilities maintain a closely monitored supply of restricted drugs (e.g., hydromorphine). These drugs must be prescribed by a physician and carefully dispensed by the pharmacy. Most jurisdictions require that health care facilities that stock such drugs keep them under double lock at all times. In many hospitals, even controlled drugs are electronically dispensed (with appropriate protocols), reducing the margin of error and misuse. Each dose is carefully recorded.

In the past, only a registered nurse was allowed to handle or dispense controlled drugs in acute care settings. Increasingly, however, registered or licensed practical nurses (RPNs or LPNs) are assuming this responsibility as well. In almost all nursing homes, LPNs (RPNs in Ontario) may dispense and sign for narcotics.

Prescribing Controlled Drugs

Under federal legislation, it is illegal for any medical practitioner to administer, prescribe, or provide a person with narcotics except for legal, therapeutic purposes. The legislation states that physicians must remain alert for behaviours that suggest patients are seeking drugs for unlawful purposes.

Among the prescription drugs that are commonly abused are tranquillizers or benzodiazepines (e.g., diazepam, lorazepam) and opioids (e.g., oxycodone, codeine) (Canadian Centre on Substance Abuse, n.d.). These powerful drugs have addictive properties and are targets for illegal use and trafficking. Misused, the effects can be tragic, ranging from addiction to death. Despite strict monitoring of the acquisition, storing, prescribing, and use of these drugs, misuse does occur. Individuals looking for controlled medication will often offer a variety of explanations as to why they want prescriptions renewed. Some explanations may be entirely legitimate; however, repeat requests from the same person may indicate **drug-seeking behaviour**

> **Drug-seeking behaviour**
> A behaviour or activity focused on obtaining access to addictive controlled substances.

and should be regarded with a degree of concern. Health care providers may also find themselves approached by unfamiliar patients with atypical stories that cannot be verified. Case Example 4.3 illustrates a situation in which a patient presents with a suspicious explanation.

In the News: A Significant Drug Problem: Who Should Assume Responsibility?

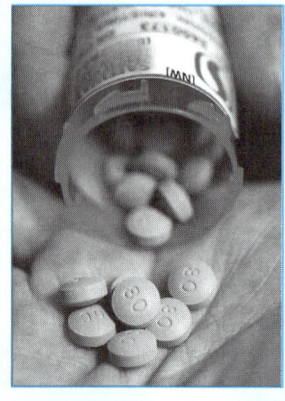

The drug OxyContin was brought to market by Perdu Pharmaceuticals in early 2000. OxyContin is a narcotic analgesic that contains a highly addictive opioid agonist called oxycodone. In 2012, Perdu voluntarily withdrew OxyContin from the market several months before the drug's patent expired. The company replaced the drug with another, supposedly safer drug called OxyNeo. All jurisdictions urged Health Canada to limit the use of OxyNeo and to refuse to grant companies permission to produce generic forms of OxyContin after Perdu's patent expired in 2012. The federal minister of health refused, stating that federal laws prohibit banning drugs because of abuse issues.

Effective in 2013, however, the federal government did tighten licensing rules for companies dispensing oxycodone in any form, requiring that companies producing the drug track sales more diligently, report sharp increases in sales, and monitor distribution patterns.

Source: Eban, K. (2011, November 9). OxyContin: Purdue Pharma's painful medicine. *Fortune*. Retrieved from http://fortune.com/2011/11/09/oxycontin-purdue-pharmas-painful-medicine/.

Photo credit: © Norma Jean Gargasz/Alamy.

Case Example 4.3

Manny comes to the office to try to have his prescription for diazepam (Valium) renewed before his current prescription runs out. He says, "I dropped my bottle in the sink, and the pills went down the drain."

Practitioners eligible to prescribe drugs are legally and morally bound to prescribe properly (i.e., to meet the patient's health care needs while also adhering to the law) and to identify any circumstances that raise suspicions about drug abuse. A prescriber suspecting drug abuse should take action—for example, by treating the patient with another drug if the patient overuses a prescribed narcotic or by reporting suspected criminal action (e.g., selling of drugs) to the police.

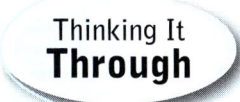

Thinking It Through

You work as an office manager for a family doctor. Genève, a patient, tells you that her cousin Jason, another patient, is selling oxycodone that the doctor prescribed for him for pain. Jason does have a slightly suspicious history of losing his pills or forgetting them when he goes on vacation and has presented with numerous excuses to have more oxycodone prescribed. But he has somehow managed to stay off the radar. Genève tells you not to say anything to the doctor because she would get into trouble if Jason found out. She "just thought you should know." What would you do?

Regardless of the care prescribers take to avoid such situations, some patients will inevitably obtain prescription drugs for their own use or to sell. A province's or territory's college of physicians and surgeons can prevent physicians who prescribe too liberally from prescribing narcotics at all while still allowing them to practise medicine and prescribe other medications. Some physicians have knowingly prescribed drugs for illegal purposes, and some are addicted to drugs themselves.

Under federal legislation, prescribing practitioners must keep detailed records of all controlled substances prescribed and provide authorized inspectors access to these records upon request. In order to dispense controlled drugs, pharmacies must have an original signed prescription.

Health Canada routinely inspects pharmacies selling prescription drugs over the Internet or by mail order to ensure they comply with the *Food and Drugs Act* and *Food and Drug Regulations*. Such pharmacies must maintain an established licence to act as a wholesaler, and, under federal legislation, only certain categories of drugs may be sold in this manner.

Permission to Use Illegal Drugs

Some highly restricted drugs, such as marijuana, can be prescribed for medical purposes. Medical marijuana may be prescribed for individuals with conditions such as cancer; HIV or acquired immune deficiency syndrome (AIDS), which incur symptoms such as severe nausea and pain; severe muscle spasms related to multiple sclerosis or spinal cord injury; epilepsy; and intractable pain caused by severe arthritis. Marijuana for medical use is controlled under both the *Controlled Drugs and Substances Act* and the *Food and Drugs Act*.

Health Canada has made changes to how Canadians can access medical marijuana under the *Marihuana for Medical Purposes Regulations*, which came into effect on April 1, 2014. Under these regulations, the federal government is no longer responsible for producing and distributing medical marijuana. As well, the government no longer issues a personal-use production licence, which authorized individuals using the drug to produce marijuana at home. Instead, the government has approved independent companies (legal "grow ops") to produce the product, but they must meet strict regulation standards. Physicians must fill in a form similar to a prescription for patients requiring the drug. Patients present this completed form directly to the grower or distributor and get the designated amount of marijuana. This process replaces the previous complicated and drawn-out process of both the patient and the doctor filling out forms and declarations. In addition, the newer system is better able to control the quality of the marijuana produced and its distribution. It is estimated that over 30% of approved home grow ops were involved in the illegal distribution of marijuana.

The use of other controlled substances available by prescription—including amphetamines, methamphetamines (which contain caffeine, cocaine, and nicotine), and testosterone—is legislated under the *Food and Drugs Act*. Strict regulations apply to these prescriptions; for example, under most circumstances, they must be written or faxed by the doctor directly to the pharmacist, and automatic refills are not permitted.

Synthetic Marijuana

An area of growing concern in Canada is the production and use of herbal incense, which is widely available across the country with instructions that it is not for human consumption. However, it is often marked as "smokable herbal incense" or "exotic smokable incense" as, when inhaled, it gives a high similar to that of marijuana. Drug effects include hallucinations, psychotic episodes, and seizures. The product is sold under such names as Happy Shaman and Project 420. Products claiming to be marijuana alternatives appear to be in a legal grey area or in legal limbo in Canada, despite the fact that Health Canada considers any product that causes the same effects as marijuana illegal.

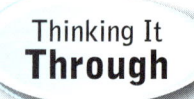 

A large number of people claim that marijuana use provides pain relief and symptom control for a variety of complaints.

1. Should the government control the distributors of medicinal marijuana so tightly?

2. Should the use of marijuana be legalized in Canada?

At times, the provinces and territories challenge federal legislation, illustrating that, in many cases, the margins of law are not as clearly defined as they appear, as demonstrated by the case in Box 4.3.

Box 4.3 Supervised Use of Controlled Drugs

If someone told you that a place existed in Canada where you could use heroin and other prohibited drugs legally, what would you think? And not only that such a place existed but also that someone would provide you with sterile needles and a clean, supervised place to rest and "shoot up." Would you believe that person?

In 2003, a project called Insite was launched in Vancouver (initially under a special exemption from the federal government) with government support and funding, making it the first legalized injection site in North America. Insite, an initiative of Vancouver Coastal Health Authorities, provides impartial access to health care for individuals with addictions, mental illness, and related diseases. Controversially, it also gives people who use injection drugs clean needles and other supplies needed for their habit. Nurses supervise the injection process and offer support, counselling, and, when possible, referrals for medical help. The project aims to provide drug users with support and direction while also reducing the incidence of diseases such as hepatitis and HIV.

Insite was threatened with closure and withdrawal of government support several times over the next few years. After a series of legal battles, in September 2011, the Supreme Court of Canada ruled that Insite could remain open because the overwhelming success of the project had set a precedent. The trial judge found that "the application of ss. 4(1) and 5(1) of the *Controlled Drug and Substance Act* violated the claimants' rights under s. 7 of the Charter." Insite was granted the right to remain open, and free from federal drug laws, under a constitutional exemption.

Other cities across Canada have plans to open similar facilities, so the federal government is working on legislation to govern its decisions regarding future applications for safe injection clinics.

Sources: Mahoney, K. (2012, April 24). The safe injection site precedent: Parliamentary supremacy vs. democratic values?; *ABlawg.ca*. Retrieved from http://ablawg.ca/2012/04/24/the-safe-injection-site-precedent-parliamentary-supremacy-vs-democratic-values/; *Canada (Attorney General) v PHS Community Services Society*, 2011 SCC 44, McLachlin CJC. Retrieved from http://scc.lexum.org/decisia-scc-csc/scc-csc/scc-csc/en/item/7960/index.do; Vancouver Coastal Health Supervised Injection Site. (n.d.). *Insite—Supervised injection site*. Retrieved from http://supervisedinjection.vch.ca/; *PHS Community Services Society v. Attorney General of Canada*, 2008 BCSC 661. Retrieved from http://www.courts.gov.bc.ca/Jdb-txt/SC/08/06/2008BCSC0661err1.htm.

Thinking It Through

The decision by the Supreme Court of Canada to grant Insite a constitutional exemption opens the door for other facilities across the country to operate safe injection clinics.

1. Do you agree that people who suffer alcoholism and drug addiction should be treated the same as people battling any other illness?

2. Given the success of Vancouver's Insite clinic, how would you feel if a similar clinic opened close to where you work or live?

Advertising Prescription Drugs

In Canada, direct-to-consumer advertising of prescription drugs is strictly controlled and must meet certain criteria. Under the *Food and Drugs Act*, advertising a prescription drug is defined as "any representation by any means whatever for the purpose of promoting directly or indirectly the sale or disposal of any food, drug, cosmetic or device." Some drugs can be advertised in Canada under the following two conditions (Health Canada, 2005):

1. "Reminder advertisements": Manufacturers can advertise drugs, using their brand names but not directly mentioning their uses. For example, television ads for "Celebrex" or "Viagra" merely hint at the drug's intended use and end by suggesting that viewers ask their doctor.

2. "Disease-oriented ads": Rather than mentioning a brand name, these commercials discuss a condition, suggesting that the consumer consult his or her physician for available medication.

HEALTH CANADA'S EMERGENCY POWERS

The Constitution states that the federal government has an interest in "peace, order, and good government." As a result, the federal government retains the power to enact laws to manage health-related emergencies of national concern, such as the 2003 SARS epidemic, West Nile virus, and avian influenza. The speed at which these infectious diseases spread has taken many countries by surprise, including Canada, prompting the federal government to renew the severely outdated **Quarantine Act**. Even 10 years ago, immigration, air travel, and the import and export of food and other products did not pose the same level of threat as they do today in terms of furthering the spread of disease. As a result of today's global village, many people believe it is only a matter of time before a worldwide pandemic of some description occurs. The 2009 outbreak of the H1N1 virus fuelled fears of a full-blown pandemic. The World Health Organization (WHO) put the world on alert, adjusting the phase of pandemic alert accordingly (see Chapter 6).

Quarantine Act
Updated in 2005, this legislation gives the federal government powers to assess individuals and detain those who may pose a health risk to Canadians.

The Quarantine Act

A new *Quarantine Act* (Bill C-12) received royal assent and became law in May 2005. Previous legislation had remained unchanged since 1872! Administered by the federal minister of health, the *Quarantine Act* complements the International Health Regulations (discussed next) by allowing Canadian authorities to respond more rapidly to health threats at Canadian borders and better preparing authorities to deal with threats and risks to global public health. The Act is also designed to complement existing provincial and territorial public health legislation.

Provisions under the Act address concerns and threats in society today. The federal government now can:

- Divert aircraft or cruise ships to alternative landing or docking sites
- Designate quarantine facilities anywhere in Canada
- Restrict or even prohibit travellers who represent a serious public health risk from entering Canada (Public Health Agency of Canada, 2004)

The Act also created two new occupational categories: environmental health officers and screening officers. These officers have the authority to assess, screen, and detain individuals who pose a health risk; to investigate and detain ships; and to examine goods and cargo crossing into or out of Canadian borders. Importantly, however, this Act does not restrict the movement of Canadians from one province or territory to another.

International Health Regulations

The International Health Regulations outline strategies to prevent the global spread of infectious diseases and to minimize any resulting disruption to the world economy.

In 1951, the first International Sanitary Conference was held in Paris, France, to develop protective guidelines against the spread of disease. That same year, the member states of the World Health Organization adopted these guidelines; in 1969, they were revised and renamed the International Health Regulations. The regulations have since undergone numerous modifications, the last in 2005, to address evolving concerns, including the reappearance of infectious diseases thought to have been eliminated.

The regulations initially monitored six serious infectious diseases: cholera, plague, yellow fever, smallpox, relapsing fever, and typhus. By 1969, only three diseases remained reportable: cholera, plague, and yellow fever. But by the 1990s, others had resurfaced—cholera outbreaks occurred in South America, plague in India—and new diseases, such as Ebola and hemorrhagic fever, were added to the watch list. All of these diseases are considered global threats because of the ease of transmission in today's world.

International regulations offer many benefits in monitoring and containing risks. Under the WHO's constitution, all member states are bound by law to adhere to the International Health Regulations, which provide ways to identify a global public health emergency and outline measures for quickly gathering and distributing information and global warnings, including travel warnings. Some countries, however, remain resistant to the idea of reporting outbreaks for fear of any negative effects on their economy.

HEALTH CARE AS A RIGHT

Because Canada has a publicly funded health care system and legislation at various levels of government to manage health care, Canadians believe that access to public health care is their right. Certainly, under the *Canada Health Act*, access to health care is a *legal* right. This right, however, remains limited by the principles and conditions of the Act. Notably, the *Canada Health Act* does not guarantee health care as such. It states that qualified Canadians are eligible for prepaid health care for medically necessary services—that is not a guarantee. The Act is federal legislation, and the provinces and territories are not bound by law to adhere to its principles, although the federal government can impose financial penalties on uncooperative jurisdictions. Application of the Act, therefore, varies among jurisdictions, depending on interpretation, resources, finances, and so on.

MEDICALLY NECESSARY: WHAT DOES IT MEAN?

The term *medically necessary* appears throughout the *Canada Health Act* because the principles of the Act developed from the legal right of Canadians to "medically necessary" procedures. At first glance, the term seems straightforward: when one is sick, the services needed to make one well; when one is well, the services needed to maintain that health. However, *medically necessary* is a subjective term at best, in large part because services vary not only among provinces and territories but also *within* provinces and territories. A resident of northern Saskatchewan, for example, does not have access to the same type of health care services as a resident of Saskatoon.

In recent years, decreasing financial and human resources have increased limitations regarding who should receive what medical care (medically necessary or not) and when. As a result, services previously deemed medically necessary have been removed from public insurance plans (i.e., deregulated), resulting in such services being offered privately, a matter discussed later in this chapter.

More recently, with strained resources resulting in long waits for just about every aspect of health care, people have turned to the Charter for legal means to gain improved access to health care services. Canadians want the right to buy insurance for services covered under the public plan and the right to seek services outside of Canada using public insurance. Interestingly, Canada remains one of the few industrial nations that does not offer its citizens a choice between public and private health care. In Canada, it is still illegal to purchase insurance to cover medically necessary procedures.

THE CANADIAN CHARTER OF RIGHTS AND FREEDOMS

The Canadian Charter of Rights and Freedoms, embedded in the Canadian Constitution, was passed into law in 1982 and amended by the Constitutional Amendment in 1983. The Charter guarantees Canadians certain rights and freedoms but is tempered by the phrase "subject only to such reasonable limits prescribed by law as can be demonstrably justified in a free and democratic society" (Canadian Charter of Rights and Freedoms, 1982). The Charter does not specifically identify health care, nor does it guarantee in specific terms that Canadians have a right to health care. The Charter does, however, demand that health care be provided to all persons *equally* and *fairly*.

The following sections within the Charter have met more legal challenges than others relating to the right of Canadians to health care:

- Section 7—life, liberty, and security of person. To determine whether a person's rights have been violated, the court must consider three things: (1) the medical resources available at the time of the person's illness, (2) the demands made on those resources, and (3) the urgency of the individual's medical needs. Under the law, everyone has the right to fair assessment, but this right does not guarantee access to specific services.

- Section 15—equality. Section 15(1) states, "Every individual is equal before and under the law and has the right to equal protection and equal benefit of the law without discrimination and, in particular, without discrimination based on race, national or ethnic origin, colour, religion, sex, age or mental or physical disability." A defendant must prove discrimination (i.e., that he or she has been treated unequally) on the basis of one or more of the criteria outlined in this section.

Several notable challenges regarding people's right to health care have been prompted by long waits for access to surgical services. Probably the most significant is the case of *Chaoulli v. Quebec* (Box 4.4).

Box 4.4 Landmark Court Challenge: *Chaoulli v. Quebec*

In *Chaoulli v. Quebec (Attorney General)*, the Supreme Court of Canada ruled that Quebec's ban on private insurance in the face of long wait times violated the Quebec Charter of Human Rights and Freedoms. The courts held that, when the public system is unable to deliver care within a reasonable time frame, alternatives must

Continued on next page

be considered. Although binding only in Quebec, the landmark decision has had implications for private versus public health care across the country.

George Zeliotis, who required hip surgery, argued that his long wait time for the surgery caused him to suffer from increasing immobility and pain. He claimed this pain interfered with his sleep and compromised almost every aspect of his quality of life. He stated that he should have the right to govern his life, including the right to make decisions that would enhance his quality of life. In his case, that meant he should have access to timely health care.

Mr. Zeliotis's physician, Dr. Jacques Chaoulli (who had opted out of the provincial medical plan), also challenged that he should have the right to treat his patient in either his private facility or a public hospital. The duo demanded that two sections of the province's *Healthcare and Hospital Insurance Act* be struck down, clearing the way for Quebec residents to buy private insurance as well as allowing physicians opted out of the Quebec plan to provide private medical care within both clinics and a public hospital.

The Supreme Court essentially removed restrictions prohibiting individuals from using private insurance to pay for services offered by the public system. The Court held that removing this restriction would guarantee freedom of choice for individuals and improve accessibility of care.

Although it was predicted that this ruling would result in widespread and significant changes to health care services across Canada, this outcome has not happened. Changes have occurred, but slowly. For example, jurisdictions have set benchmark waiting times for procedures and created options in some provinces. Despite the changes, in the years that followed, numerous lawsuits were initiated across the country by individuals claiming they were forced to suffer irreversible harm because of long waits and restrictions preventing them from buying private health insurance to cover a myriad of procedures.

As a result of this court decision, the Quebec government revised the law to allow hospitals to sign contracts with private clinics to perform three types of elective surgeries paid for by the province (hip and knee replacements and cataract surgery). In 2012, a new ruling increased the types of surgeries allowed to be contracted out from three to 56 (Picard, 2009). As well, whereas previously, a physician could work in a public clinic or a private clinic, but not both, the new regulations allowed doctors the freedom to work in either type of clinic or even both. A physician can, therefore, offer a patient the option of having a procedure done in a public hospital in three months, for example, or in a private clinic the next day (but at a cost). Other provinces have since followed suit.

Quebec residents are also now free to purchase private insurance for some surgical procedures, including knee and hip replacements.

Sources: *Chaoulli v. Quebec (Attorney General)*, 2005 SCC 35, McLachlin CJC. Retrieved from http://scc-csc.lexum.com/scc-csc/scc-csc/en/item/2237/index.do; Picard, A. (2009, July 16). Private health care slips under radar. *The Globe and Mail*. Retrieved from http://www.theglobeandmail.com/life/health-and-fitness/private-health-care-slips-under-radar/article788120/.

Many Canadians now know that opportunities to access private health care are available, albeit marginally, and believe that privatization of health care will grow, creating a parallel system to publicly funded health care. Private health care has existed in various forms for some time, particularly in Quebec, Alberta, and British Columbia. As well, the Quebec ruling in the *Chaoulli* case has opened the door for other such cases challenging provincial and territorial governments for the right to private insurance coverage for medically necessary procedures.

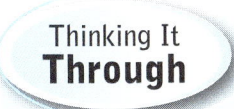

Canadians from coast to coast to coast must endure long waits for access to medical care and treatment.

1. Should the provincial and territorial governments have to pay for treatment elsewhere (even out of country) if it cannot be provided within a designated time frame?
2. What criteria should be used to define a "reasonable wait," given that every case differs?

THE LAW, THE CONSTITUTION, AND END-OF-LIFE ISSUES

Assisted suicide occurs when a person aids another to end his or her life. Until the statute was changed, Canadian law held that assisted suicide or assisted death was illegal under section 241 of the Criminal Code of Canada and carried a penalty of up to 14 years in prison. Those who request assistance to end their life usually have been diagnosed with a degenerative, incurable disease that will lead to a prolonged or painful death.

Several high-profile cases in Canada challenged this law on the basis of the rights of an individual to liberty and autonomy under the Charter of Rights and Freedoms. These Canadians sought the right to end their lives at a time of their choosing. Sue Rodriguez, who suffered from amyotrophic lateral sclerosis (ALS), lost her 1993 case by a ruling of 5 to 4. The ruling held that society's obligation to serve and protect life outweighed her rights to what she claimed was to die with dignity (Fenton, 2013). In 2012, the Supreme Court of British Columbia gave Gloria Taylor, a B.C. resident who also suffered from ALS, the first constitutional exemption to receive physician-assisted suicide. Ms. Taylor died of complications of her illness before she could use her exemption. The Supreme Court of Canada nevertheless appealed this ruling. Even after Ms. Taylor's death, her family continued her quest to change the law (Fong, 2013).

Assisted suicide
A person assists another who wishes to end his or her life but is unable to do so independently.

In June 2014, the Quebec government tabled a controversial bill on medical aid to die. The law allows that if a doctor receives repeated consent from an individual, the doctor can administer a lethal dose of a medication (CBC News, 2013). Already legal in Quebec is palliative sedation, meaning that a person who is near death can be put into a medically induced coma and have life-sustaining measures (e.g., intravenous [IV] medication, feeding tube, respirator) removed. It is legal anywhere in Canada to withdraw feeding tubes and IVs and to render comfort measures only, if in accordance with the patient's wishes. The decision to remove a ventilator is sometimes more complicated and often pits physicians against the family—even when the patient has previously requested this be done (CBC News, 2012).

The Netherlands, Belgium, Colombia, and Switzerland have legalized physician-assisted death (or suicide). On February 6, 2015, the Supreme Court of Canada also legalized physician-assisted suicide (see In The News: Landmark Ruling on Physician-Assisted Suicide, in Chapter 2, page 56). In the United States, Vermont, Montana, and Washington have enacted laws allowing a doctor to write a prescription for a lethal dose of a medication; the patient can then take it at a time of his or her choosing.

THE LEGALITY OF PRIVATE SERVICES IN CANADA

As mentioned, Canada remains one of only very few countries prohibiting private insurance for medically necessary procedures. However, the Supreme Court's ruling on *Chaoulli v. Quebec* (see Box 4.4) may have opened the door for consumers to purchase insurance for core publicly funded health care services.

Those in favour of a purely public health care system worry about the impact of private insurance on the publicly funded system, fearing that it would result in a two-tier health care system in which those with less money would receive inferior care and have to endure longer wait times than would people who can afford to purchase private insurance. Consequently, controversy continues over whether there's a place for expanded private health care beyond complementary and supplementary services in Canada, although it already exists in various forms across the nation. For example, Workers' Compensation Boards, the RCMP, Indian and Northern Affairs Canada, and the Correctional Service of Canada pay for medical services in private surgical clinics for their population groups. Considered justifiable in the case of Workers' Compensation Boards, private health care is deemed essential to ensure workers are treated and returned to their occupations as soon as possible to keep compensation payments down.

All provincial and territorial governments fund certain types of medical care—for example, cataract surgery, hernia repairs, and knee surgery—in private clinics under specified conditions. Governments also pay for other services, such as diagnostics, in private clinics with which they hold contracts. And Canadians everywhere can purchase private insurance for non–medically necessary health care.

Physicians' Opting Out of the Public Plan

It is common belief among Canadians that doctors *legally* must take part in socialized medicine, adhering to the practice of charging the provincial or territorial plan for their services. However, doctors may work in either a public or a private system or in both. Operating entirely outside the public system, though, is not a practical option. Opting out means deregistering themselves from the public plan and billing patients directly for services. In Manitoba, Ontario, and Nova Scotia, opted-out doctors cannot charge the patient more than the public plan would pay for services rendered, which effectively removes any incentive for opting out. Alberta, British Columbia, New Brunswick, Quebec, and Saskatchewan will not reimburse people who use the services of an opted-out physician, making it even more unattractive for a doctor to opt out. Opted-out New Brunswick doctors can ask patients to sign waivers stating that they will pay doctors' fees that are above what the provincial plan pays. Prince Edward Island will not provide funding for physicians (opted-in or -out) who charge more than what the provincial health insurance plan pays for a specific service (Flood & Archibald, 2001).

Independent Health Care Facilities

Hundreds of independent health care facilities across Canada (e.g., diagnostic centres, laboratories, physiotherapy clinics, surgical clinics) offer diagnostic and therapeutic medical services. These private facilities depend on referrals from doctors and, theoretically, can compensate doctors for referring patients to them, which causes legal concern. Doctors may also own such a private facility and refer his or her own patients to the clinic. The question raised is both legal and ethical in nature: Would self-interests influence a physician's clinical judgement (see Case Example 4.4)?

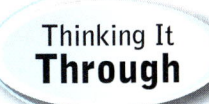 

Thinking It Through

You receive a brochure advertising a comprehensive medical workup, including a physical exam, dietary counselling, routine blood work, and some diagnostic tests, and promising an appointment within a week. The cost is $1000. You could have these assessments done by your family doctor, and the services would be covered by your provincial or territorial health plan—but you would have to wait several months for an appointment. What would you do?

> ### Case Example 4.4
>
> If Dr. Harper owns a clinic that operates magnetic resonance imaging (MRI) and other diagnostic equipment, would he refer patients to that clinic more liberally than he would if he did not possess a financial interest in it? Would unnecessary procedures be done at a public expense? Similarly, if Ribera Medical owned a string of physiotherapy clinics and offered Dr. Harper $25 for each patient he referred, would Dr. Harper suddenly find a large number of patients needing physiotherapy? When such a personal interest exists, a doctor may be influenced by the fact that by referring more patients to the facility, he or she makes more money, creating a conflict of interest.

Conflict of interest
The possible clash of two or more concerns. For example, a personal financial interest in a business may influence one's professional decisions.

Fiduciary duty
A duty binding professionals to act with honesty and integrity, and in the best interests of their patients, with regard to their professional practice.

In Canada, common law governs **conflict of interest** concerns. The law binds physicians to behave with honesty and integrity (i.e., to act according to a **fiduciary duty**) with regard to their medical practice. That is not to say that Dr. Harper in Case Example 4.4. cannot refer patients to his own clinic, but by law, he must disclose to patients his interest in the clinic. However, tracking violations of this law is difficult. Medical organizations, such as the Canadian Medical Association or the provincial and territorial physicians' regulatory bodies, probably carry more weight than other officials in terms of creating and enforcing regulations and guidelines that address these issues.

As is the case with most aspects of health care, provincial or territorial legislation directs the operation of private health care facilities in Canada. In Ontario, for example, the Independent Health Facilities Program (implemented under the *Independent Health Facilities Act*) licenses—in some cases, funds—and coordinates quality-assurance assessments for private facilities. As well, these facilities are subject to routine inspection, often by the provincial or territorial college of physicians and surgeons.

In Alberta, the *Health Care Protection Act* oversees surgical services provided outside of hospitals. Private surgical facilities must have the approval of both Alberta Health and Wellness and the College of Physicians and Surgeons of Alberta; must secure a contract with a regional health authority to provide insured services; must comply with the principles of the *Canada Health Act*; must be a required service within their geographic location; and must not negatively affect the public health system.

Private clinics, such as the False Creek Healthcare Centre locations in Vancouver, British Columbia, and Winnipeg, Manitoba, provide services such as several types of surgery, family practice, urgent care, and sophisticated diagnostics. Another site in Winnipeg is a state-of-the-art facility with three operating rooms, six recovery beds, and five overnight-stay rooms. This centre legally provides services for Workers' Compensation Boards and other designated groups as well as for private citizens (False Creek Surgical Centre, 2014).

Organizations such as Timely Medical Alternatives assist Canadians in accessing any type of health care services—some of which can be obtained within Canada, while others are outsourced to the United States. In most cases, patients pay for these services themselves.

Ottawa-based La Vie Health Centre, Calgary-based Foothills Health Consultants, and Toronto-based Medcan Health Management are just a few of the clinics across Canada that offer services aimed at the prevention and early detection of health problems. For a price, a person can enroll for a one-day comprehensive assessment that includes a three- to four-hour block of time dedicated to testing, screening, and receiving advice, health education, and planning (e.g., working out a diet or exercise plan) from health care providers. Because this service does not involve medically necessary procedures, it does not contravene the *Canada Health Act*. All of the services offered by these organizations are available at publicly funded doctors' offices through the provincial and territorial health plans but will entail waits and multiple visits to different health care providers.

INFORMED CONSENT TO TREATMENT

Throughout Canada, before a health care provider may treat a patient, he or she requires the **informed consent** of the patient. In order to provide informed consent, a patient must understand, consent to, and accept the treatment and its foreseeable risks. When doubt exists about a person's capacity to understand the information provided, in most cases, the health care provider must determine whether the person is capable of giving consent to treatment. Importantly, an individual's capacity to give consent can change. Persons quite capable on one day may be incapable on another day, depending on their mental and physical state. If a previously capable patient becomes unable to understand the nature of an intervention, the issue of consent must be readdressed.

Consent must be both informed and voluntary:

- Informed: Patients must understand the treatment or procedure—the nature and purpose of the proposed treatment, the risks, side effects, benefits, and expected outcomes. Patients must also understand the implications of refusing the recommended treatment and be made aware of alternatives, if any, to the proposed treatment so that they have choices. The health care provider has an obligation to use language that is at an appropriate level and to discuss the information when the patient is not stressed or unhappy (this may require a second explanation of the intervention when the patient is in a calm frame of mind).

Informed consent
A formal agreement signed by a patient consenting to a treatment, procedure, or test administered by a health care provider after the patient has been fully informed of all related risks and benefits.

- Voluntary: Patients must not feel compelled to make a decision for fear of criticism, nor must they feel pressured toward any particular decision by the information provider or anyone else. Sometimes in health care, only a fine line exists between coercing (i.e., bullying) and making a recommendation, especially when the health care provider feels strongly that the patient should consent to a treatment, and the patient is leaning toward refusing it (Case Example 4.5).

Case Example 4.5

Jennifer has terminal cancer. She asks the doctor, "What is really best for me? You have more knowledge and experience than I do, so let's go with what you think is best." In this case, Jennifer is clearly looking for the physician's expertise to help her make a decision.

Alternatively, Jennifer might say, "Dr. Li, I am not sure I want the chemotherapy. You sound almost angry with my decision. I know you think I should have it. I'm confused." Is Dr. Li pushing Jennifer to accept chemotherapy? Jennifer's decision to refuse the treatment could be based on wanting to enjoy a better quality of life during the time she has left rather than living longer but enduring the side effects of chemotherapy. In such cases, Jennifer may want to seek a second opinion or ask her doctor to list the reasons he thinks she should embark on a treatment regime.

The Supreme Court of Canada supports the basic right of every capable person to decide which medical interventions he or she will accept or refuse (*Ciarlariello v. Schacter*, 1993). Involving patients in their health care should be a fundamental policy of all health care providers. Not only does it show respect for the patient and his or her right to autonomy; it also improves patient compliance with treatment regimes.

Each province and territory has enacted its own legislation addressing informed consent. Policies, therefore, vary somewhat among the jurisdictions. Relevant legislation may include the *Adult Guardianship Act*, the *Mental Health Act*, and the *Health Care Consent Act*. Increasingly, physicians and other health care providers are advised to obtain written consent for even minor medical services such as immunizations.

All health care providers in a position to provide care to a patient (e.g., physiotherapists, respiratory therapists, laboratory technicians, nurses, doctors) have both legal and ethical obligations regarding that patient's consent to proposed care. The ethical components of consent are discussed in Chapter 5.

TYPES OF CONSENT

Express Consent

Express consent can be written or oral and indicates a clear choice on the part of the patient. Express consent usually requires that the individual be fully informed as to the benefits, risks, and consequences of any treatment options.

Written Consent

All major medical interventions require signed, written consent as confirmation that the appropriate process for obtaining consent was followed and that the patient has agreed to the proposed intervention. Ideally, the person signing the consent form understands what the intervention is, including its risks and benefits. In reality, however, how much the patient has been told is hard to prove, and how much he or she understands is hard to determine. Although written consent provides health care providers with evidence of consent, a signed consent form may be weighed against any conflicting evidence and, therefore, may not provide a solid defence in the case of legal action.

Most consent forms have to be signed by the patient, dated, and witnessed. People qualifying as a witness to consent vary among jurisdictions and health care organizations. For medical procedures, including minor or major surgery, a physician or registered nurse will usually witness the consent. The witness must ensure the patient understands what he or she is signing. If any doubt remains, the appropriate person (e.g., usually the physician, nurse, or technologist doing the procedure) should speak to the patient and provide clarification. Reviewing the nature of the procedure is important, as medical terms can sometimes be confusing or misleading; the witness must be certain that what the patient has been told agrees with the nature of the procedure he or she is consenting to (Case Example 4.6).

Case Example 4.6

Prepared to sign a consent form for a straightforward hysterectomy, Pia reads through the form the nurse has brought her. The type of surgery named on the form is a *pan-hysterectomy*, which Pia may not understand. If she does not ask for clarification, she will sign consent for removal of her uterus, fallopian tubes, and ovaries.

Note that a multicultural environment may present challenges surrounding consent because of religious, cultural, gender, or social concerns, as well as language barriers. Most hospitals maintain a list of volunteer interpreters should the need arise; however, interpreters capable of delivering health-related information clearly and accurately are not always available. Often, medical staff must rely on a family member to translate for the patient. As a result, what is presumed to be "informed consent" may not be.

Oral Consent

Equally binding as written consent, **oral consent** is given by spoken word over the phone or in person. At times, someone other than the patient offers consent to surgery; however, two people (usually health care providers) must validate that consent has been given. For example, if a husband gives telephone consent for a procedure for his wife, assuming she is unable to give consent, two health care providers must be on the telephone to validate the husband's consent—that consent was given, that he has had all of his questions answered, and that he fully understands the circumstances under and for which consent is being provided. Protocol may vary among facilities and jurisdictions.

When a health care provider receives oral consent, he or she should carefully document it in the patient's chart, describing the intervention discussed, stating that the patient has acknowledged understanding of the intervention, and noting that the patient has agreed to it orally. Written consent remains the preferred alternative, however, for complex treatments.

Implied Consent

Implied consent occurs by virtue of the fact that an individual seeks the care of a physician or other health care provider (i.e., a patient's **circle of care**). For example, may people have received an immunization or another treatment from a family doctor without having signed a consent form; the immunization or treatment has been provided under the umbrella of implied consent. As previously mentioned, however, more and more health care providers are requesting written consent, even for immunizations.

By allowing themselves to be admitted to hospital, patients imply their consent to certain interventions (e.g., allowing the nurse to give them a bath or to take their vital signs). However, when possible, oral consent should be obtained (e.g., "Roger, I am going to begin your exercises now. Is that okay?"; "Emiko, I would like to change your dressing in about an hour. Are you okay with that?"). Patients may provide or deny consent through their actions, such as by nodding ("yes") or shaking their head ("no"). A patient's refusal to treatment should be documented in detail on his or her medical record, along with any reasons provided.

Oral consent
Verbal agreement from a patient to undergo a treatment, procedure, or test performed by a health care provider.

Implied consent
Consent assumed by the patient's actions, such as his or her seeking out the care of a health care provider or his or her failure to resist or protest.

Circle of care
The individuals and health care providers legitimately involved in rendering a patient's care.

Who Can Give Consent

A capable person receiving the intervention most often gives consent for the treatment. If the individual proves incapable of providing consent (e.g., is not mentally competent or is unconscious), the person's legal representative or next of kin (subject to provincial and territorial law) assumes the responsibility. In most jurisdictions, the person who legally has **power of attorney** for personal care (see page 132), the person who is named as proxy for health care decisions for the patient, or a person related to the patient usually takes on this duty.

In the absence of a legally assigned person, most provinces and territories will allow a spouse (whether legal or common law) or another family member to legally provide consent. Some jurisdictions outline a designated order, depending on the availability of particular relatives—for example, a spouse will have such control before a father or mother, who would have control before a sibling, who would have control before an aunt or uncle, and so on.

In Alberta, when a person is deemed unable to give consent (unless mentally incompetent), the only person who can legally provide it is a guardian under the *Dependent Adults Act* or someone named under the *Personal Directives Act*. Under Alberta's *Mental Health Act*, however, a family member can make a decision on behalf of a mentally incompetent individual. In urgent situations, when no legal alternative exists, nor is there time to appoint one, two consenting physicians can sign certificates indicating the need for treatment—ideally, after consultation with the next of kin or other appropriate persons.

Contrary to popular belief, in most jurisdictions, no specific age defines a **minor** when it comes to providing independent consent to treatment or to requesting treatment without a parent's knowledge. As long as the minor fully understands the treatment and its risks and benefits, he or she can make an informed decision about accepting or rejecting the treatment, and health care providers must respect his or her wishes. When a minor's consent is accepted, the minor is referred to as a *mature minor*. Frequently, a minor's consent to treatment is made in conjunction with the parents. *Emancipated minors*—those married, living on their own, or showing independence from their parents in some way—may also validly consent to medical care.

When required, either parent who has legal custody of the minor (or a legally appointed guardian) can provide consent for treatment. If children are travelling, the legal guardian or parent can provide written permission to another adult travelling with the minor to consent to medical treatment in case of an emergency.

In extraordinary circumstances, a province or territory can seek temporary guardianship and order that treatment be implemented. Although the Charter

> **Power of attorney**
> A legal document naming a specific person or persons to act on behalf of another in matters concerning personal care, personal estate, or both.

> **Minor**
> A person under the age of majority in a particular province or territory.

holds that Canadians have the right to freedom of religion, when children are, in the view of the courts, too young to hold and express beliefs or to understand the consequences of receiving treatment or not receiving treatment, courts usually uphold requests made to intervene on the children's behalf.

Even in emergency situations, if at all possible, health care providers should obtain consent from a patient before providing treatment. Under some circumstances (e.g., the individual cannot communicate because of a language barrier or because he or she is unconscious), a health care provider can administer emergency treatment without the patient's permission if, in the professional's opinion, delay in treating the person will result in serious harm or injury. In such circumstances, however, the health care provider must provide clear, detailed, and concise written documentation explaining the decision to give treatment in the patient's medical record.

Finally, a power of attorney, an important legal document, provides a person the legal power to act on behalf of another in matters of estate, personal care, or both. A power of attorney for personal care or a **proxy consent** specifically grants a person (usually a loved one) the right to make health care decisions for another if the second is deemed incapable. Such a document can be, and often is, separate from a power of attorney for matters of finance or estate. See Web Resources on Evolve for samples of various legal forms, including power of attorney packages.

Proxy consent
Consent given by a person authorized by a health care patient to give consent on his or her behalf.

THE HEALTH RECORD

Any person who has received health care in Canada at any time possesses a health record, an accumulation of information relating to his or her interactions with health care services. People who work in the health care industry and deal directly with patients are often in a position to access and record health information relating to services provided for the patient. Most information today is electronically recorded and stored.

Depending on the nature of the facility and those involved in the patient's circle of care, a health record may consist of information gathered from many sources. A health record in the hospital setting will have more components than one in a dentist's office, a chiropractic clinic, or a physiotherapy clinic. In the hospital setting, records (manual or electronic) will contain numerous and varied reports including an admission sheet, patient history, medication records, diagnostic reports, medical or surgical records, flow sheets, and interdisciplinary notes. Interdisciplinary notes are recordings of patient care entered by any health care providers (e.g., nurse, respiratory therapist, social worker, dietician) who render that care or carry out any intervention for the patient.

Clinics or offices may also maintain a variety of reports: diagnostic reports, consultation reports, history sheets (sometimes called a *cumulative profile*), and a record of what happened at each encounter (e.g., details of visits to the family doctor, including the reason for the visit and the treatment received).

THE IMPORTANCE OF ACCURATE RECORDING

In most disciplines, health care providers must, by law, record information clearly, concisely, and accurately. Possibly one of the most important tasks in the field of health care, careful recording provides valuable information that can ensure continuity of patient care. All entries must be dated and signed or initialled (according to agency protocol), either manually or electronically.

What is recorded and how an entry is worded are also important. A person not in a position to diagnose must use words such as *appears to have* instead of *has* and must never record suppositions or inadvertently label someone (e.g., Mr. Smith is a schizophrenic). Each discipline provides related guidelines for appropriate charting. In nursing, several charting methods may be used. For example, if *charting by exception*, nurses will chart only abnormal data, thereby saving time. That means that Mr. Smith's having had a good day would not be recorded, but anything unusual occurring during Mr. Smith's day would. *Narrative charting*, on the other hand, affords more detail.

Health care providers must regard anything that they enter into a health record as information potentially required in any type of litigation. Health records may prove pivotal in a legal proceeding.

OWNERSHIP OF HEALTH INFORMATION

It is important to note that all jurisdictions have legislation that balances the right of access to personal information with appropriate protection of that information. Privacy legislation is discussed later in the chapter.

The health care facility or doctor's office that collects the information and creates the health record owns the patient's physical chart. Physicians, dentists, other health care providers, and health care facilities that maintain such records act as custodians of that information.

The health information itself, however, belongs to the patient. Patients retain the right to request a copy of their information, including consultation reports and copies of reports generated by other physicians at the request of third parties, such as insurance companies. However, patients may not physically remove the record from the facility or alter its data. Office staff should supervise patients viewing their charts to avoid any unauthorized making of changes that may pose legal problems for the health care provider or the facility. Changes, including additions, may be made, but only if the health care provider agrees. Such revisions to data in the chart must be dated and initialled.

When a third party requests a patient's health information, the patient must provide written consent for its release, or a court of law may order the release of such information.

Often, patients who are moving or changing physicians will request a copy of their chart, which may be given to the patient or sent directly to the new physician by registered mail or courier, usually for a fee based on the amount of photocopying required (accounting for both time and paper). Patients should be advised in advance of the cost to receive a copy of their chart. Because of security and privacy issues, patients' health information should never be sent via e-mail.

Under some circumstances, usually to avoid serious negative effects on the patient's mental, emotional, or physical health, a physician may deny a person access to his or her medical information or may selectively remove information from a patient's chart before providing the patient with a copy of it. Although existing provincial or territorial legislation aimed at safeguarding health information usually supports denying a patient access, the physician must be able to justify any such decision. A patient can usually appeal a denial.

STORAGE AND DISPOSAL OF HEALTH INFORMATION

If a physician moves, ceases to practise for some reason, or retires, the medical information he or she accumulated must be retained and stored in such a manner that patients and other health care providers providing care for that patient can access them (with the patient's permission) as needed. If another health care provider assumes responsibility for the practice at the same location, the patients' charts often remain at that location. Patients must receive notification of the change of provider.

When physicians or other health care providers form a group, they should immediately clarify ownership of the charts—for example, does each own the charts of the patients he or she regularly sees, or do all of the records belong to the organization?

When a health care provider leaves a practice and no one assumes direct responsibility for the records (e.g., no one takes over the practice), a custodian—a person or business legally allowed to store or otherwise keep medical records—may take over the charts. Medical file storage companies can charge patients several hundreds of dollars for photocopies of their files. Provincial and territorial governments and regulatory bodies specify guidelines for the storage of records, including how long they must be maintained.

The Canadian Medical Protective Association advises that physicians retain medical records for at least ten years from the date of the last entry or, in the case of minors, for at least ten years from when the **age of majority** is reached. Each jurisdiction sets its own policies on health records' retention; for example, in British Columbia, physicians are required to keep their records for 16 years from the date of last entry or of a patient's age of majority (College of Physicians and Surgeons of British Columbia, n.d.), and Alberta physicians are advised to keep records for a minimum of ten years after the patient was last seen or, in the case of a minor, the greater of ten years or two years beyond the patient's age of majority (College of Physicians and Surgeons of Alberta, 2010). The Canadian Medical Association encourages all physicians across Canada to retain records for a longer period if at all possible (Canadian Medical Protective Association, 2008).

The ultimate destruction of medical records must be accomplished in a manner that will ensure the information can never again be accessed. For example, a health care provider cannot just delete medical information from his or her computer; rather, the hard drive on which the information is stored must be professionally wiped clean.

Age of majority
The age at which a person is considered an adult; depending on the province or territory, age 18 or 19.

FEDERAL LEGISLATION AND PRIVACY LAWS

Each of Canada's provinces and territories implements its own privacy legislation. Some provinces, including Alberta, Manitoba, Saskatchewan, and Ontario, have privacy legislation specific to health care service providers. (See Web Resources on Evolve for a link to privacy legislation for each of the provinces and territories.)

Two related federal acts—the *Privacy Act* (1983) and the **Personal Information Protection and Electronic Documents Act** (2004), known as *PIPEDA*—contribute to this protection.

Personal Information Protection and Electronic Documents Act (PIPEDA)
A federal act ensuring the protection of personal information in the private sector.

Privacy Act

Enacted in July 1983, the *Privacy Act* requires federal government departments and agencies to limit the private information they collect from individuals. As well, the Act restricts the use and sharing of any collected information. The *Privacy Act* also allows individuals to access any information federal government organizations have about them.

Personal Information Protection and Electronic Documents Act

PIPEDA protects personal information preserved in the private sector. The Act supports and promotes both online and traditional commercial activities by protecting personal information that is collected, used, or disclosed under certain circumstances. It defines personal information as "information about an identifiable individual" and includes any factual or subjective information, recorded or not, in any form. For example, the following would be considered personal information:

- Name, address, telephone number, gender
- Identification numbers, income, or blood type
- Credit records, loan records, existence of a dispute between a consumer and a merchant, and intentions to acquire goods or services

Known as consent-based legislation, *PIPEDA* requires any organization collecting and using personal information to present patients with consent forms that fully disclose how their personal information will be collected and managed, and to have these forms signed. For example, a dentist's office collecting information for research purposes for commercial gain must reveal to the patient all personal information gathered and seek permission before using it.

Since January 2004, all Canadian businesses have had to comply with the privacy principles set out by *PIPEDA*, except those businesses in provinces with privacy legislation similar to *PIPEDA* (e.g., British Columbia, Alberta, Quebec). *PIPEDA* protects information throughout Nunavut, the Northwest Territories, and Yukon because most organizations, other than hospitals and schools, remain under federal jurisdiction there.

PIPEDA does not usually affect hospitals and other health care facilities since most are not overtly involved with commercial activities. The legality of exempting some publicly funded organizations from *PIPEDA* legislation has been questioned, however, because some functions within health care facilities (e.g., a privately owned diagnostic clinic operating within the hospital) mimic those of a private organization.

In most jurisdictions, personal information collected by health care facilities remains under the protection of province- or territory-generated, public-sector legislation (e.g., in Ontario, the *Personal Health Information Protection Act* [*PHIPA*]; in British Columbia, both the *Freedom of Information and Protection of Privacy Act* [*FIPPA*] and *Personal Information Protection Act* [*PIPA*]). FIPPA, for example, gives individuals the right to access their own records as well as the right to insist that any errors found are corrected. At the same time, the Act outlines limited exceptions to the right to access.

Some jurisdictions, such as New Brunswick, Newfoundland and Labrador, Nova Scotia, and Prince Edward Island, lack specific privacy legislation for private-sector organizations and use *PIPEDA* instead.

CONFIDENTIALITY

All health care providers must legally and ethically keep all health information confidential. The concept of **confidentiality** refers to the health care provider's moral obligation to keep a patient's health information private.

Confidential
Kept private or shared only with authorized individuals (e.g., in health care, shared only with those authorized to have health information about a patient).

Conversely, the concept of **privacy** refers to the patient's right for his or her health information to remain confidential and to be released only with his or her consent.

Any health care provider involved directly in a patient's case—the circle of care—legally has access to that patient's information. In the hospital setting, the circle of care may include the doctors, nurses, social workers, physiotherapists, and other members of the health care team who are instrumental in the patient's care and rehabilitation. Administrative personnel also have access to a person's health information and likewise must keep it confidential. Almost all places of employment—particularly in the health care sector—require employees to sign a confidentiality waiver (see Web Resources on Evolve for a link to a sample waiver) and to adhere to the principles and policies within the document. Every facility will have protocols for protecting the patient's right to confidentiality, from the fact that he or she is seeking care to any and all health information, in all forms, including oral exchanges between or among health care providers. As a rule, health care providers should never discuss health information with anyone other than members of the health care team responsible for the patient's care. It is unacceptable to mention to a friend that Sally just had a baby boy or that Pang broke his leg and has a cast (Box 4.5).

Privacy
The patient's right to control access to his or her body and personal information.

Box 4.5 Confidentiality: An Age-Old Concept

The concept of confidentiality was outlined in the Hippocratic Oath 2500 years ago as follows:

> Whatever, in connection with my professional practice, or not in connection with it, I see or hear, in the life of men, which ought not to be spoken of abroad, I will not divulge, as reckoning that all such should be kept secret. While I continue to keep this Oath unviolated, may it be granted to me to enjoy life and the practice of the art, respected by all men, in all times. But should I trespass and violate this Oath, may the reverse be my lot.

Source: The Internet Classics Archive. (n.d.) *The oath, by Hippocrates*. Retrieved from http://classics.mit.edu/Hippocrates/hippooath.html.

Health care providers, both morally and legally, must keep a patient's health information secure and restricted to only those who have the need to know and the right to access that information; however, under some circumstances, health care providers may have a moral and legal responsibility to *release* confidential health information (e.g., when an individual has harmed or is in danger of harming him- or herself or others). Also, some health conditions, such as communicable diseases, must be reported to the local public health authority.

A patient who discovers a breach of confidentiality can bring a lawsuit against the individual responsible for the breach, whether the breach was intentional or not (Case Example 4.7).

Case Example 4.7

While at a party, Alicia, a student nurse, was conversing with Ruby, who commented on how fast their mutual friend Heather delivered her baby boy last week. "Imagine," said Ruby. "Heather's delivery lasted only three hours. That's really fast for her first baby." Alicia responded, "But that wasn't her first delivery, and second babies usually come much faster." The damage was done. Heather had had a baby 10 years prior, as a teenager. She'd given the baby up for adoption and told no one. Now the secret was out, causing hurtful and damaging information to circulate among Heather's friends. Think of the possible implications if Heather's husband did not know her history!

SECURITY

Health records of any type must be kept in a manner that is both safe and secure, meaning they must be protected from fire and damage from environmental disasters such as flooding, among other possible scenarios. In the case of electronic records, the use of encrypted software and passwords is essential. All health information must be stored in such a manner that access is restricted to authorized persons. Hard copies of electronic information and copies of paper-based information must be carefully tracked. Anyone who has access to health information must be bound by confidentiality agreements (from physicians to administrators to nonregulated health care providers). Every functioning electronic system should have a functioning audit trail. Any health care worker who suspects an unauthorized person of trying to access health information, whether within a clinic or a hospital unit, should question the person's identity and intent. Most health care providers and health facilities have protocols for both storing and allowing access to health information they are responsible for.

ELECTRONIC HEALTH INFORMATION REQUIREMENTS

Both electronic and hard-copy records are subject to the principles of confidentiality and the protection of health information. However, the electronic environment poses unique challenges to maintaining confidentiality and privacy standards.

Electronic health records and electronic medical records are separate collections of the same material. Whereas **electronic medical records (EMRs)** are housed in one facility and pertain only to care received at that facility, **electronic health records (EHRs)** provide the "bigger picture." Compiled in a central database accessible to authorized persons for the purpose of providing care, electronic health records contain information from several different sources.

Since an electronic health record contains information from various sources, several people will have accessed the information. The more people involved, the more likely it is that a breach of confidentiality can result. As with all electronic information, the potential exists for information theft by hackers or by individuals who gain unauthorized access to information because of carelessness with passwords. The physical components of computers present the opportunity for files containing health information about thousands of people to be carried off by one person—quite within the realm of possibility compared with someone trying to walk off with thousands of files in hard-copy format.

Physical units storing health information may even go missing. Although electronic records are deemed more secure than paper records, neither is foolproof. In May 2008, four computer tapes containing confidential information about residents of New Brunswick and British Columbia who had received treatment outside of their own province disappeared while en route from New Brunswick to Health Insurance B.C. The devices were being transferred to British Columbia as part of the reciprocal agreement whereby provinces reimburse one another for health services administered in other provinces (with the exception of Quebec). The information, on magnetic tapes, was not encrypted. For three weeks, the fact that the tapes had not arrived in British Columbia went unnoticed. Not until two months after they had gone missing did the Ministry of Health notify the Office of the Information and Privacy Commissioner for British Columbia (Canadian Press, 2007). In 2011, Cancer Care Ontario reported that the health records of thousands of Ontarians were lost in the mail—an event that might have been avoided had the information been transferred electronically. The records contained names, provincial insurance plan numbers, and test results (Canadian Press, 2011).

The consent rules that apply to information stored in hard-copy format apply, too, to information managed electronically, according to *PIPEDA* and territorial and provincial health privacy legislation. The information custodian must disclose to the patient who will have access to the information and any auxiliary purposes for which the information may be used. The patient also has a right to know what safeguards the facility has in place to protect the information. Some information custodians believe that once people give consent to have their information stored on an electronic health record, implied consent allows for

Electronic medical record (EMR)
Health information obtained and stored at one facility, perhaps a dentist's, chiropractor's, or doctor's office.

Electronic health record (EHR)
Health information collected by more than one facility and shared electronically among health care service providers (e.g., a doctor's office, emergency department, and pharmacy).

other uses of that information. Not so. Any new, previously undisclosed initiative requires renewed consent from the patient.

Many health care facilities use patient information for research purposes. Strictly speaking, the health care facility should obtain the patient's consent, as well as provide clear and accurate information about the research.

With the support of the Canadian Health Information Management Association, several organizations, including the Canada Health Infoway, are working toward introducing electronic health information systems at a national level. (These organizations are discussed in more detail in Chapter 10.) Jurisdictions across Canada have reached various stages of implementing electronic health information systems. As these systems evolve, so, too, will concerns about and solutions for dealing with privacy, confidentiality, and security.

HEALTH CARE PROFESSIONS AND THE LAW

The regulation of health care providers is discussed in detail in Chapter 9. This section briefly looks at the significant legal applications of regulated health professions.

Regulated Health Care Providers

Most health care providers in Canada belong to a regulating body that assumes a high level of responsibility for the ethical, moral, and *legal* conduct of its members. All regulated professions have a system in place for dealing with complaints against their members and for dealing with members charged with an offence. Likewise, they have an obligation to protect their members when claims prove unfounded, and they do so in a collaborative manner when violations involve the courts.

Patients who have complaints against health care providers may launch a legal complaint as well as a complaint to the related regulatory organization. In the case of the latter, the organization's regulatory committee will assess the complaint and, if it finds the health care provider at fault, impose a penalty that may range from a reprimand or a suspension of the health care provider's licence to the permanent cancellation of his or her licence. The offending individual may also be subject to legal penalties.

Although litigation against health care providers happens far less often in Canada than in the United States, it is becoming increasingly common here; therefore, all health care providers should purchase some type of liability insurance. Many health care providers obtain malpractice or liability insurance through their professional college or the organization they work for.

Every profession has a **code of ethics** (see Chapter 5) that provides moral and ethical guidelines for health care providers to follow in their professional practice. However, codes are not legally binding documents. Rather, they advise the public what to expect from the health care provider. Adhering to the principles of one's professional code of ethics is a good way to avoid unethical or illegal practice.

"Sorry, I Made a Mistake"

Historically, an admission of error in medical care has led to litigation. Apology laws, which first appeared in the United States in the 1990s, offer another option. When an adverse event occurs because of human error, the physician has the legal and moral obligation to inform the patient of all relevant facts. Apologizing for the mistake has been seen as opening the door to impending litigation. One of the objectives of apology legislation is to reduce physician concerns regarding liability.

Currently, in Canada, eight provinces and one territory have apology legislation: British Columbia, Alberta, Saskatchewan, Manitoba, Ontario, Nova Scotia, Prince Edward Island, Newfoundland and Labrador, and Nunavut. The remaining jurisdictions have been urged by the Uniform Law Conference of Canada and the Canadian Patient Safety Institute to adopt some form of apology legislation but, to date, have not done so. The principles of the Canadian legislation are similar in all jurisdictions. According to the Canadian Medical Protective Association (2013), the legislation holds that an apology does not constitute an admission of fault or liability, must not be taken into consideration in determining fault or liability, and is not admissible as evidence of fault or liability. Protection offered by this legislation is effective in tribunals, college disciplinary committees, coroners' inquests, and before the courts.

The offer of an apology reduces the tendency of patients to resort instantly to litigation and allows health care providers to deal with their patients humanely—by recognizing the importance that an apology can play in settling disputes.

Ending a Physician–Patient Relationship

A physician becomes legally responsible for the care of a person when active treatment begins. If a physician or other health care provider refuses or ceases to care for a patient without due process (e.g., notifying the patient), he or she can be charged with abandonment. Unfortunately, a variety of situations will cause a patient and a physician to part ways, such as significant disagreement between the patient's expectations and the physician's ability to meet those expectations or aggressive or unacceptable behaviour on the part of the patient.

In most jurisdictions, the physician must address the termination of a patient–physician relationship in writing (often called a *Dear John letter*). The administrative assistant working for the doctor usually bears the responsibility of handling

Code of ethics
A set of values and responsibilities serving to guide the behaviour of the members of an organization or a profession.

this correspondence, which is most often sent by registered mail or courier to gain proof that the letter was received. Physicians must continue to provide care for any such patient until the patient has found another doctor—a challenge, given the current shortage of doctors in Canada.

Conversely, patients can simply walk away from their doctor—with no formal separation process—never to return.

Physician Authority: Involuntary Confinement

In all jurisdictions, under a provincial or territorial *Mental Health Act*, doctors have the power to temporarily commit a patient to a mental health facility under certain circumstances, whether acting either independently or in conjunction with the patient's family. Patients who pose a danger to themselves or others and who are noncompliant with requests to receive treatment may be subject to a physician's enacting this authority. Most regions require the physician and a judge to sign a form, which designates a time frame (e.g., 72 hours) within which the patient will receive an evaluation. Afterward, the patient can be discharged; discharged and, if need be, readmitted on a voluntary basis; or readmitted as an involuntary patient. In the case of the last situation, to protect the rights of the patient, a physician other than the one who signed the original form would have to provide an assessment. In most jurisdictions, the patient and his or her family must also have access to a trained rights advisor or advocate, who may provide an avenue for appeal of the decision for involuntary commitment.

NONREGULATED HEALTH CARE PROVIDERS

Nonregulated health care providers are discussed in detail in Chapter 9. The current landscape and structure of health care in Canada increasingly uses nonregulated health care providers, primarily in community-based care. For the most part, hiring agencies provide liability insurance for nonregulated health care providers. Personal attendant caregivers, usually hired by the family of an ill person, however, may or may not have liability insurance, sometimes creating a grey area in which the family and the caregiver have little legal protection.

OTHER LEGAL ISSUES IN HEALTH CARE

THE USE OF RESTRAINTS

Restraints are most frequently used for patients who have dementia or psychiatric conditions or who are temporally and disproportionately disoriented and agitated for other reasons. Restraints should be used only when all other interventions have failed and when the patient's behaviour poses a danger to self or others or disrupts treatment. Restraints can be mechanical, environmental, physical, or chemical (medications). The use of restraints of any kind must be ordered by a physician, and in the best-case scenario, with permission from the patient's family or the person who has the power of attorney for personal care. The actual application of restraints falls primarily to the nursing domain.

Most facilities have a "least restraint policy," which means that health care providers must reserve the use of restraints as a last resort, employing every possible intervention to calm the patient before restraints are used. Only in rare and exceptional circumstances should a health care provider apply restraints without an order.

Injury can result from using restraints, perhaps more easily than when they are not used in a situation. As well, litigation often results from the use of restraints, even when physical injury to the patient has not occurred. The legal issues relate to obtaining informed consent from the proper people, legal authorization, the rights of the patient, the safety of the patient and others, and the use of the least amount of restraint.

Patient Self-Discharge From a Hospital

Unless confined under legislation, any **inpatient** can leave a hospital at any time without a physician's permission. Typically, a doctor will decide to discharge a patient when he or she feels that hospital care is no longer required because the patient can manage at home or in an alternative facility. The doctor writes a discharge order on the patient's chart, and the patient leaves.

When a patient decides to leave a hospital without a doctor's permission, the facility should have the patient sign a form releasing the hospital, the physician, and other members within the patient's circle of care from responsibility for that patient's well-being. Once the patient leaves, he or she assumes all responsibility for any unforeseen effects of this action.

> **Inpatient**
> An individual remaining in a health care facility (e.g., an acute care hospital) overnight or longer.

Good Samaritan Laws

Good Samaritan laws legally protect anyone who offers to help someone in distress if something goes wrong—as it did in Case Example 4.8. Most jurisdictions in Canada have some form of Good Samaritan legislation. For example, Manitoba, British Columbia, and Ontario have Good Samaritan acts, and Alberta has its *Emergency Medical Aid Act*. Under Quebec's Civil Code, every citizen must act as a *bon père de famille*, meaning that every person must act wisely and in a

> **Good Samaritan law**
> A law protecting individuals who attempt to offer help to a person in distress.

reasonable manner to help someone in distress if it does not pose a serious threat to the person. In other words, any person responding to an urgent situation is expected to do so within his or her scope of practice, knowledge, and level of expertise. A person with no medical training would be held less accountable than would a nurse or a doctor.

Case Example 4.8

Greg was having a heart attack. Ishim found him on the ground with no vital signs. Trained in first aid, Ishim began CPR. Greg survived but suffered a punctured lung as a result of a rib that was broken when Ishim initiated cardiac compressions. In provinces with a Good Samaritan law, Ishim would likely be protected if Greg tried to sue him for causing the broken rib and collapsed lung.

WHISTLEBLOWING

Whistleblower
An individual who assumes responsibility for publicly divulging information about a wrongdoing or misconduct by another individual or an organization.

A **whistleblower** is a current or past employee or member of an organization who reports another's misconduct to people or entities with the power and presumed willingness to take corrective action. Unfortunately, whistleblowers often suffer a backlash, such as demotion, suspension, or termination for their efforts.

Provinces and territories remain at various stages of addressing the issue of whistleblowers; however, overall, whistleblowers currently receive little protection in Canada. The federal government provides legislation to protect public servants. Bill C-11, the *Public Servants Disclosure Protection Act* passed in 2005, covers the entire federal public sector and Crown corporations.

However, whistleblowers in both the public and private sectors must rely chiefly on the protection offered by common law. Under common law, an employee owes his or her employer the general duties of loyalty, good faith, and, in appropriate circumstances, confidentiality (*Public Service Whistleblowing Act*, 2002). When an employee breaches these duties by revealing a confidence or some information, believing it is in the public interest, the employer usually takes disciplinary action, which may include dismissal. In the face of such punishment, employees may seek protection from the courts or, if they are governed by a collective agreement, through a grievance procedure.

SUMMARY

4.1 In Canada, various levels of government are authorized to create laws, ranging from constitutional law to common and public laws. Most of these apply to health care but in varying degrees. Tort law, for example, is commonly applied when negligent acts on the part of health care workers occur or because of a compromised standard of care that may be the responsibility of a facility.

4.2 The federal government maintains legal authority over spending, issues related to criminal law, and issues related to laws that uphold "peace, order, and good government." For example, the control of narcotics and other drugs is regulated by the federal government. Under the Constitution, Health Canada can also exercise emergency powers through the *Quarantine Act* in the event of a national disaster or pandemic.

4.3 As the Canadian health care landscape changes, so do the expectations for our health care system. Many Canadians regard health care as a fundamental right, even though it is not specifically identified in the Canadian Charter of Rights and Freedoms. Challenges relating to the right to health care, however, often arise under sections 7 and 15 of the Charter.

4.4 Canada has always harboured some level of private health care, maintained restrictions on what types of health care can be delivered privately, and governed the services Canadians can purchase with private health insurance. The concept of "medically necessary" plays a huge role in what private clinics can legally offer. Private health care services have flourished more in some provinces than in others; whether it is complementary to or in opposition with the concept of universal health care remains a question.

4.5 Consent to treatment is a complicated and sometimes controversial subject. *Express consent* means that a person gives clear written or verbal consent for a procedure; *implied consent* is more ambiguous. Also contentious are the right for minors to make their own decisions and situations wherein parents make decisions for children that contravene what a health care provider deems best or essential.

4.6 Confidentiality, the protection of health information, and consent to treatment are issues covered, in some cases, by both federal and provincial and territorial legislation. The *Personal Information Protection and Electronic Documents Act (PIPEDA)* federally regulates how organizations may collect, store, and use personal information, including medical records, for commercial purposes. Hospitals and other health care facilities are largely exempt from this legislation but subject in most jurisdictions to similar legislation that specifically concerns health information.

4.7 Almost every major health profession has a self-governing body that controls such things as educational standards, provincial, territorial, or national registration protocol, and entry-to-practice requirements. Any member of the public wanting to launch a complaint against a health care provider would do so to the related regulatory body. Each profession also has a code of ethics, but such codes are not legally binding.

4.8 Some important legal issues in Canadian health care include the use of restraints, self-discharge from a health care facility, and whistleblowing. Legislation governing these areas is sometimes ambiguous. For example, the use of restraints is contentious, even in situations in which it is deemed in the best interests of the patient.

Review Questions

1. Explain the federal government's authority under the *Quarantine Act*.
2. What is the purpose of occupational health and safety legislation?
3. Identify some drug-seeking behaviours.
4. Why is the term *medically necessary* controversial?
5. What impact did the ruling in the *Chaoulli* case have on health care in Quebec?
6. Under what circumstances would a physician who owns a private health care facility be in conflict of interest?
7. List and describe three elements of informed consent.
8. Describe the purpose of a power of attorney for personal care.
9. How long must a health care provider or facility retain medical records?

References

Canadian Centre on Substance Abuse. (n.d.). *Prescription drugs*. Retrieved from http://www.ccsa.ca/Eng/topics/Prescription-Drugs/Pages/default.aspx.

Canadian Charter of Rights and Freedoms. (1982). Part I of the Constitution Act. *1982, being Schedule B to the Canada Act 1982 (UK)* c. 11.

Canadian Medical Protective Association. (2008). *Retaining medical records*. Retrieved from https://www.cmpa-acpm.ca/cmpapd04/docs/resource_files/infoletters/2005/com_il0520_2-e.cfm.

Canadian Medical Protective Association. (2013). *Apology legislation in Canada: What it means for physicians*. Retrieved from https://oplfrpd5.cmpa-acpm.ca/-/apology-legislation-in-canada-what-it-means-for-physicians.

Canadian Press. (2007, December 11). Confidential medical records go missing. *CTV News*. Retrieved from http://www.ctv.ca/servlet/ArticleNews/story/CTVNews/20071211/medical_records_071211/20071211?hub=Health.

Canadian Press. (2011, July 27). Lost medical records a big deal: McGuinty. *CTV News*. Retrieved from http://toronto.ctvnews.ca/lost-medical-records-a-big-deal-mcguinty-1.675786#ixzz2ZKhzdHir.

References

CBC News. (2012, June 15). The fight for the right to die. *CBC*. Retrieved from http://www.cbc.ca/news/canada/story/2012/06/15/f-assisted-suicide.html.

CBC News. (2013, June 12). Quebec tables bill on medically assisted death. *CBC*. Retrieved from http://www.cbc.ca/news/canada/montreal/story/2013/06/12/montreal-quebec-palliative-sedation-assisted-suicide-dying-with-dignity-legislation.html.

Ciarlariello v. Schacter. (1993). 2 SCR 119, La Forest CJC. Retrieved from http://scc-csc.lexum.com/scc-csc/scc-csc/en/item/996/index.do.

College of Physicians and Surgeons of Alberta. (2010). *Patient records*. Retrieved from *http://www.cpsa.ab.ca/Resources/StandardsPractice/PracticeManagement/patient-records*.

College of Physicians and Surgeons of British Columbia. (n.d.). *FAQs*. Retrieved from https://www.cpsbc.ca/for-public/faqs.

Constitution Act. (1982). *1982, being Schedule B to the Canada Act 1982 (UK)* c. 11, s. 92. Retrieved from http://laws-lois.justice.gc.ca/eng/CONST/INDEX.HTML.

False Creek Surgical Centre. (2014). *Vancouver surgical centre, plastic surgery & MRI/CT scan*. Retrieved from http://www.falsecreekhealthcare.com/.

Fenton, D. (2013, September 28). "Who owns my life?": Sue Rodriguez changed how we think. *The Windsor Star*. Retrieved from http://blogs.windsorstar.com/life/who-owns-my-life-sue-rodriguez-changed-how-we-think.

Flood, C. M., & Archibald, T. (2001). The illegality of private health care in Canada. *Canadian Medical Association Journal*, *164*(6). Retrieved from http://www.cmaj.ca/cgi/content/full/164/6/825#T135.

Fong, P. (2013, March 3). B.C. mother continues daughter Gloria Taylor's fight to legalize assisted suicide. *Toronto Star*. Retrieved from http://www.thestar.com/news/canada/2013/03/03/bc_mother_continues_daughter_gloria_taylors_fight_to_legalize_assisted_suicide.html.

Health Canada. (2005, August). *Drugs and health products: The distinction between advertising and other activities*. Retrieved from http://www.hc-sc.gc.ca/dhp-mps/advert-publicit/pol/actv_promo_vs_info-eng.php.

Medical Profession Act, CPSS Regulatory Bylaw and By-law #46.

Public Health Agency of Canada. (2004). *New Quarantine Act reintroduced in Parliament [News release]*. Retrieved from http://www.phac-aspc.gc.ca/media/nr-rp/2004/2004_54-eng.php.

Public Service Whistleblowing Act. (2002). *Bill S-6*. Retrieved from http://dsp-psd.tpsgc.gc.ca/Collection-R/LoPBdP/LS/362/s13-e.htm.

Chapter Five

Ethics and Health Care

Learning Outcomes

5.1 Define ethics, morals, values, and duties.
5.2 Discuss ethical theories that shape health care decisions.
5.3 Explain the ethical principles that are important to the health care provider.
5.4 Summarize the rights Canadians have with respect to health care.
5.5 Demonstrate an understanding of ethical behaviour in the workplace.
5.6 Discuss ethical considerations relating to end-of-life issues.
5.7 Discuss ethical considerations relating to the allocation of resources in health care.
5.8 Briefly discuss the moral and ethical issues related to abortion and genetic testing.

Key Terms

Active euthanasia, p. 174

Advance directive, p. 177

Autonomy, p. 159

Beneficence, p. 158

Compassionate interference, p. 169

Continuity of care, p. 163

Deontological theory, p. 156

Divine command ethics, p. 157

Double effect, p. 158

Duties, p. 155

Ethical principles, p. 158

Ethical theory, p. 155

Ethics, p. 151

Fidelity, p. 160

Fiduciary relationship, p. 159

Involuntary euthanasia, p. 174

Morality, p. 151

Morals, p. 151

Nonmaleficence, p. 158

Passive euthanasia, p. 174

Paternalism, p. 165

Physician-assisted suicide, p. 174

Rights in health care, p. 161

Role fidelity, p. 160

Self-determination, p. 152

Teleological theory, p. 156

Values, p. 153

Values history form, p. 177

Virtue ethics, p. 156

Voluntary euthanasia, p. 174

Health care providers are held to a high level of accountability because the personal and sensitive nature of health care demands it. Entering a health care profession means entering into a moral and ethical contract with patients, peers, and other members of the health care team. It requires a person to employ the highest standards of professionalism and ethical behaviour and to make a commitment to excellence in practising in one's chosen field. Anyone entering the health care field must respect the rights, thoughts, and actions of patients; advocate for them; put aside biases; and assist patients in their quest to achieve wellness. Finally, health care providers must work collaboratively with all health care team members, respecting their areas of expertise and scopes of practice.

People will often make ethical decisions that differ from ones another might make in the same situation, but different people can make different ethical decisions. This chapter briefly outlines four ethical theories that form the basis for most ethical decisions. Recognizing the perspective from which a person makes an ethical decision helps those who disagree with the decision to show tolerance. Understanding and supporting the patient does not require one to compromise his or her own beliefs and values.

Health care providers have a duty to adhere to six ethical principles that have particular relevance to the health care profession. This chapter addresses these principles from the perspective of clinical and administrative practice, emphasizing the importance of ethical behaviour, professionalism, and patient autonomy.

WHAT IS ETHICS?

Ethics is the study of standards of right and wrong in human behaviour—that is, how people ought to behave, considering rights and obligations, as well as virtues such as fairness, loyalty, and honesty. Various systems, approaches, and conceptual frameworks deal with how human actions are judged. Ethics examines the criteria we use to determine which actions are right or wrong (Alberta Health Services, n.d.; Online Ethics Center for Engineering, 2006; Washington Ethical Society, n.d.).

Ethics also involves values, duties, and moral issues. Ethics is neither religion nor determined by religion—if it were, nonreligious persons would be considered unethical. Ethics remains separate, too, from the law, although ethical and legal issues are at times closely connected. Ethical choices do not always fit with what is legal, and things that may be legal—or legal decisions—are not always ethical. Moreover, being ethical does not mean following social norms; behaviour considered ethical in one society may be deemed unethical in another (e.g., polygamy).

The term *ethics* also refers to a code of behaviour or conduct. Our behaviour reflects our belief system, which is shaped by many factors, including how we are parented, our home environment, and societal factors such as religion, friends, and school. Continually influenced by events and experiences, our ethical viewpoints change over time. Ethical standards are influenced by morals, values, and a sense of duty—all elements critical to ethical practice in health care.

MORALITY AND MORALS

Almost always linked to ethics, **morality** extends from a system of beliefs about what is right and wrong. It encompasses a person's values, beliefs, and sense of duty and responsibility. **Morals** are what a person believes to be right and wrong

> **Ethics**
> The knowledge of and rules about behaving according to set values, duties, and moral principles.

> **Morality**
> A code of conduct defined by a group of people, culture, society, or religion. Individuals may have a moral code that governs the way they live, behave, and interact with others.

> **Morals**
> A person's beliefs about right and wrong regarding how to treat others and how to behave in an organized society.

regarding how to treat others and how to behave in an organized society. For example, a person may have a moral belief that one must always tell the truth, regardless of the consequences.

Morals can be said to define a person's character. Ethics can be described as an individual's *collection* of morals. More broadly, ethics are a social system in which a collection of morals from a number of people are applied. As a professional code of conduct, ethics encompass the morality and moral beliefs of the profession. People bring their own moral code to their profession; it influences how they behave as professionals as well as the degree to which they honour their profession's code of ethics.

The differences between morals and ethics are subtle and may be best illustrated in an example. Suppose a client and physician have agreed to apply a do-not-resuscitate (DNR) status to the client's infant because of that infant's clinical condition. Amy, a registered nurse working in the pediatric unit, does not morally agree with the decision, believing that all attempts to save the infant's life should be applied, including cardiopulmonary resuscitation (CPR). However, ethically (i.e., out of respect for the client's choice, or his or her *autonomy*), Amy must abide by the decision of the client and the doctor and refrain from initiating CPR should she be present when the infant has an arrest.

Health care providers who understand their own values and moral standards come better prepared to deal with issues that may arise in their professional role. As well, they typically possess a better sense of their commitment to practise in an ethical manner.

Many grey areas exist in ethics and in beliefs regarding what is morally right. Often, no absolute right or wrong exists, and the health care provider's personal beliefs may affect how he or she deals with difficult situations or reacts to patients. Understanding and feeling comfortable with one's own beliefs in such areas can make accepting the decisions of others easier. Importantly, respecting the decisions of others does not mean compromising one's own values. Morally charged topics include the right to die, withholding treatment, DNR orders, withholding information from a patient, and interfering with the patient's right to **self-determination**—the freedom to make his or her own decisions.

Less dramatic moral issues are more common: Is it proper to accept a gift from a patient, or will the act bind a health care worker to providing the patient with preferential treatment? Is it morally acceptable to cover up a medication error that did not cause harm to a patient? Is it acceptable for a health care provider to chart on care not given because he or she was so busy that there

Self-determination
The freedom to make one's own decisions.

was time only to do the basics? Is it okay to take hospital supplies home for personal use as long as there are plenty left for the patients? How one decides what is acceptable and unacceptable behaviour will depend on his or her moral code and values.

VALUES

Values, beliefs important to an individual, guide a person's conduct and the decisions he or she makes. People can have personal values, social values, and work values. A person who greatly values friendship may consider his or her relationship with a particular person more important than, for example, a material object. And although a person may value friendship in general, one friend may be more valued than another. Context may also influence values and, therefore, behaviour (Case Example 5.1).

Values
Something a person holds dear, such as a quality or a standard by which to act or behave (e.g., loyalty, honesty).

Case Example 5.1

Tony, an occupational therapy student, clearly values professional conduct at work more than he does personal conduct at school. At work, he maintains an excellent attendance record, is never late, and does his job well. However, at school, he talks in class, hands in assignments late, does not study for tests, and has poor attendance—especially on Friday afternoons. As well, he often misses a day of classes prior to an exam or test. He may place more importance on work for several reasons, including earning money for rent and other amenities. He may not (at least not yet) value his education or see it as a means to an end—establishing a career and becoming financially secure.

In health care, particular value is placed on certain virtues—truthfulness (also referred to as *veracity*), respect for others, competency, and the right to proper medical care. For example, one cannot effectively establish therapeutic relationships with patients or trusting relationships with colleagues without truthfulness (the foundation for trust) and respect for others. All of these values were applied when a health care provider found a discrepancy in chemotherapeutic drug solutions being administered to patients in the hospital she worked in (In the News: Watered-Down Chemotherapy Drugs).

In the News   Watered-Down Chemotherapy Drugs

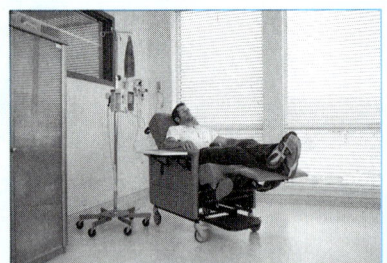

It was discovered in April 2013 that, over the course of a year, well over 1000 Canadians undergoing intravenous (IV) chemotherapy received drugs that were watered down. The premixed bags containing one or a mixture of drugs were diluted anywhere from 3% to 20% over the prescribed amount. These premixed IV bags were purchased by four Ontario hospitals and one in New Brunswick. What remains unknown is whether the reduction in the strength of the drugs the patients received will reduce the benefits of the treatment regime, ineffectively treating the cancer. Fortunately, experts believe that the chances of the solution proving ineffective are low.

According to the Ontario College of Pharmacists, the company that prepared these bags was not an accredited pharmacy and, therefore, does not hold any federal licences that would necessitate the company being subject to guidelines and inspections.

Source: Zlomislic, D., & Gillis, W. (2013, April 2). Wrong chemotherapy doses given to nearly 1000 cancer patients in Ontario. *Toronto Star*. Retrieved from http://www.thestar.com/news/gta/2013/04/02/wrong_chemotherapy_doses_given_to_nearly_1000_cancer_patients_in_ontario.html.

At times, another person will make a decision that violates one's moral beliefs and values. After all, health care providers face situations that challenge deep-rooted values and interfere with the preservation of life, as illustrated in Case Example 5.2.

Case Example 5.2

Jennifer seeks an abortion to terminate a pregnancy resulting from rape. Her primary nurse, Sanga (a new graduate), cannot understand how Jennifer could make that decision. Sanga values life more than anything. Had it been her, abortion would have been out of the question, regardless of the circumstances. However, Sanga also values trust, respect for others, and integrity. For that reason, she can give Jennifer the care and support she needs and respect Jennifer's right to make the decision best for her. She realizes that caring for Jennifer in a respectful manner does not compromise her own values and beliefs.

SENSE OF DUTY

Duties often arise from others' claims. If a patient depends on you (i.e., has a claim on you) for your professional services, you have a duty, or obligation, to deliver these services. As a member of the health care profession, you also have a duty to behave in an ethical, moral, and competent manner. Alternatively, duties may be self-imposed. For example, a person who values honesty will make it his or her duty to be truthful.

Health care providers, by the very nature of the field they work in, have a moral and ethical duty to care for their patients in a competent manner as well as a legal obligation, called the "duty of care." As discussed in Chapter 4, the legal component of this duty requires health care providers to provide patients with a reasonable standard of care in accordance with their professions' standards of practice. In terms of a moral obligation, health care providers are expected to provide care even in situations that may threaten their own lives or health; however, they may not be legally bound to do so.

> **Duties**
> Obligations a person has in response to another's claims on them. A duty may result from a professional or personal obligation or may relate to one's own morals or values.

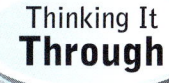

Thinking It Through

Suspected of having Middle East respiratory syndrome (MERS), a lung infection caused by a deadly and highly infective coronavirus similar to severe acute respiratory syndrome (SARS), Sasha has been placed in isolation. You have been asked to provide his treatment despite considerable risk of contracting the infection yourself.

1. Would you carry out your professional responsibilities because it is your duty to, or would you refuse to treat Sasha because of the risks involved?

2. Would your decision differ if Sasha was suspected of having the H1N1 virus?

ETHICAL THEORIES: THE BASICS

Health care providers face making ethical decisions that affect them individually, that affect other members of the health care team, and that affect their patients. These professionals also face exposure to ethical situations in which decisions made by others may affect them, perhaps not directly but emotionally.

An **ethical theory** guides people toward making an ethical decision. The discussion of ethical theories that follows, although not in-depth, will help you see how individuals make difficult decisions.

> **Ethical theory**
> A framework of ideas that provides a template for making decisions to justify a set of actions.

Teleological Theory

Teleological theory, also referred to as *consequence-based theory*, defines an action as right or wrong depending on the results it produces. Theoretically, the "right" action brings about the most benefit for the most people. Consider Case Example 5.3, a real-life situation.

> **Teleological theory**
> An ethical theory that defines an action as right or wrong depending on the results it produces; also called *consequence-based theory*.

Case Example 5.3

Postsurgery, it is discovered that a sponge was left inside a patient. The patient, a man with metastatic cancer, has a limited life expectancy. The staff members present, along with Nima, an operating room technician, decide it is in everyone's best interests to say nothing. The sponge will not hurt the man, but opening him up and removing it would hasten his death and cause him more pain. The family, already trying to cope with the man's impending death, would be distressed over the incident. It is a simple mistake—why get the surgeon and nurses into trouble?

In Case Example 5.3, to say nothing becomes the group's ethical decision. The individuals involved determine what they think would be the best result and make their decision accordingly. Of less importance to them is that, in taking this chosen action, they will conceal the truth (not to mention the legal implications of their decision—by law, in most jurisdictions a patient must be told when a medical error has occurred).

Deontological Theory

Deontological developed from the word *duty*. In the case of **deontological theory**, a moral and honest action is taken, regardless of the outcome. If, in Case Example 5.3, the team had used a deontological approach and did the "right" thing, they would have removed the sponge, or they would have told the family what had happened, explained the risks, and allowed them to make the decision.

> **Deontological theory**
> An ethical theory that calls for a moral and honest action to be taken, regardless of the outcome.

Virtue Ethics

Virtue ethics look at the ethical character of the person making the decision, rather than at his or her reasoning. This theory operates under the belief that a person of moral character will act wisely, fairly, and honestly and will uphold the

> **Virtue ethics**
> An ethical theory that operates under the belief that a person of moral character will act wisely, fairly, and honestly and will uphold ethical principles.

principles of justice. Therefore, virtue ethics, unlike teleological and deontological theories, do not provide guidelines for decision making.

In Case Example 5.3, several people were present for the postsurgery discovery. Person A may have decided that it would be best not to divulge the incident about the sponge, while Person B may have decided the incident must be exposed. Each person would make an individual decision based on his or her own set of values and morals. A common decision often, however, must be reached. When people disagree about the course of action to take, sometimes the majority will rule; other times, one person may have the authority to make a call. However, each person should still feel comfortable with his or her own actions because each person might have to take responsibility for such actions. In the case example, individuals following the principles of virtue ethics may believe that the surgeon has high moral principles and will, therefore, refrain from questioning the surgeon's decision. In addition, they may believe that loyalty to the surgeon is a virtue. Then again, the act is both illegal and contrary to hospital policy, so these individuals may take a personal risk by complying with the decision not to report the incident. Ultimately, each person must weigh the situation, determine to whom he or she owes the greater loyalty, and decide according to his or her own conscience.

Divine Command

The most rigid ethical theory, **divine command ethics**, follows philosophies and rules set out by a higher power. For example, Christians must live by the Bible's Ten Commandments, a list of religion-based moral laws. Muslims follow the rules outlined in the Koran, such as maintaining a just society and engaging in "appropriate" human relationships. In Case Example 5.3, followers of divine command ethics would without question decide that the incident should be reported because honesty makes up a significant part of the divine command theory.

Divine command ethics
An ethical theory believing that ethical philosophies and rules are set out by a higher power.

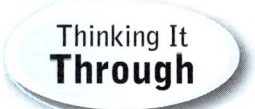

Dr. Kowalski decides to lie to Jake (an older patient with no relatives or emotional support system) about the nature of his illness—amyotrophic lateral sclerosis (ALS), which causes progressive paralysis eventually leading to the inability to swallow or breathe. The physician believes that she is sparing Jake unnecessary grief, at least for the short term.

1. Is Dr. Kowalski justified in her decision to lie to Jake?

2. Would it make any difference if Jake had family or friends to support him?

ETHICAL PRINCIPLES AND THE HEALTH CARE PROFESSION

> **Ethical principle**
> An acceptable, usually highly valued and moral, standard of human behaviour—for example, honesty, truthfulness, and fairness.

Common to all ethical theories, **ethical principles**—acceptable standards of human behaviour—provide guidance for decision making and, therefore, form the basis of ethical study. Ethical principles can be personal or professional in nature. In the best-case scenario, individuals practise similar principles in both their personal and professional lives. Personal principles predominantly guide a person's actions and form the foundation from which professional principles evolve. People who believe in showing kindness and helping those in need in their personal life will likely do the same in their professional life. Those with an uncaring, indifferent attitude toward others in their personal life are unlikely to show support, respect, or adequate care to a patient.

Outlined below are a number of ethical principles that lend themselves particularly well to health care. These important elements of ethical decision making almost always appear in the codes of ethics adopted by health care professions.

BENEFICENCE AND NONMALEFICENCE

> **Beneficence**
> The act of doing good or being kind.
>
> **Nonmaleficence**
> Doing no harm.

The foundation of health care ethics, **beneficence** refers to showing kindness to or doing good for others. No matter what ethical theory is used, beneficence guides the process toward a morally right outcome. Often treated as a separate principle from beneficence, **nonmaleficence** refers specifically to causing no harm, whereas beneficence encompasses the duties to prevent harm and to remove harm when possible. All health care providers have a duty to do good, to prevent harm, and to not cause harm.

> **Double effect**
> Acting in a manner that brings about the most good or the least harm.

Similar to beneficence, the principle of **double effect** requires a person to choose the option that achieves the most favourable outcome or that causes the least harm. When secondary, potentially negative outcomes or side effects can be predicted, these must not be the intended outcome of the action. For example, Augusta, who has terminal cancer, takes high doses of morphine sulphate controlled-release (MS Contin), which has proven to be the only means of controlling her pain. However, she now experiences respiratory distress—a known side effect of MS Contin—which could well lead to her death. Despite this, making Augusta comfortable is considered, ethically and morally, the action of choice.

RESPECT

Another key ethical principle is respect. All patients have the right to be treated with respect by those who care for them. Health care providers and their colleagues also have this right. Respecting others involves honouring their right to autonomy (see below), being truthful, not withholding information, and honouring their decisions, whether stemming from personal, religious, cultural, or societal influences.

Autonomy

Autonomy comes from the Greek *autos*, meaning self, and *nomos*, meaning governance. The ethical principle of **autonomy** underscores a person's right to self-determination. Autonomy recognizes the right of a mentally competent individual, given all of the relevant facts, to make independent decisions without coercion (i.e., pressure or force). Health care providers may try to influence a patient's decisions, often unintentionally, thinking they know what is best. However, patients have the right to choose their own course of treatment or to refuse treatment altogether.

Autonomy
The right to self-determination.

Truthfulness

Truthfulness (also referred to as *veracity*), a valued principle that patients should expect of a health care provider, contributes to building a bond of trust vital to any patient–health care provider relationship. Without this bond, an effective relationship is impossible. Rarely justifiable, withholding the truth shows disrespect and works against a person's autonomy and rights.

A special relationship, called a **fiduciary relationship**, exists between health care providers and their patients. To some degree, the health care provider retains a position of power over the patient, considering the patient's dependence on the health care provider for his or her care. In such a relationship, patients should expect the health care provider to care about them as well as for them to be honest and trustworthy.

Fiduciary relationship
A relationship based on trust.

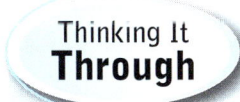
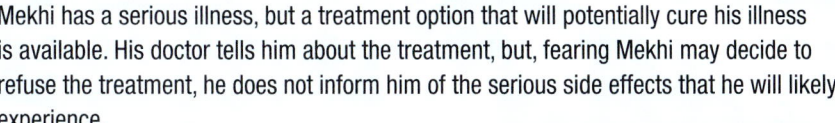

Mekhi has a serious illness, but a treatment option that will potentially cure his illness is available. His doctor tells him about the treatment, but, fearing Mekhi may decide to refuse the treatment, he does not inform him of the serious side effects that he will likely experience.

1. Do you think the physician is showing respect for Mekhi?

2. What ethical principles has the physician breached?

Fidelity

Fidelity
The quality of being faithful.

Role fidelity
In health care, meeting the reasonable expectations of members of the health care team, patients, their families, and employers by being loyal, truthful, and faithful; by showing respect; and by earning and maintaining trust.

The principle of **fidelity**—faithfulness or loyalty—requires health care providers to adhere to their professional codes of ethics and the principles that define their roles and scopes of practice, as well as to fulfill their responsibilities to patients by practising their skills competently. The term *fidelity* comes from a Latin root word meaning to be faithful. Fidelity, therefore, requires faithfulness and loyalty to patients, colleagues, and employers (Case Example 5.4). Health care providers are also expected to uphold the rules and policies of the organization (or person) for which they work. In the workplace, **role fidelity** becomes an important ethical principle for health care providers as they work to honour patients' wishes and to earn the trust essential to the professional–patient relationship.

Case Example 5.4

Cecelia, who owns a number of urgent care clinics, is on a bus and overhears a conversation between two young women in the seat in front of her. "That clinic is the worst," says one. "They expect me to do everything they ask, and they want it done, like, yesterday."

"Yeah," responds the other, "I know what you mean. I bet you hate working there. It sounds like that manager is a real dragon. I'd never go to that clinic—unless I was dying and there was nowhere else to go!"

Cecelia recognizes one of the women as an employee. Needless to say, the clinic staff will be subject to a discussion about loyalty the next day.

Justice

The principle of justice applies, in one way or another, to most ethical situations. In health care, for example, it raises questions such as the following: Do all patients get the appropriate (i.e., just) treatment? Are health care resources fairly distributed? Are the patient's rights honoured? The three main types of justice are distributive, compensatory, and procedural. *Distributive justice* deals with the proper and equitable distribution of health care resources. Distribution may not be equal because it is prioritized and based on need. *Compensatory justice* relates to the paying of compensation for wrongs done (e.g., if a person can prove that he or she developed cancer from working with asbestos, the company may have to compensate that person financially for pain and suffering and cover pertinent medical expenses). *Procedural justice* points to acting in a fair and impartial manner (e.g., seeing patients on a first come, first served basis; not giving preferential treatment to a friend).

The *Canada Health Act* entitles all Canadians to equal access to prepaid health care and physician and hospital services. However, with resources stretched to their limits and long waiting lists for many services, equal access, as well as other principles of the Act, is compromised. Health care providers, therefore, must do what they can to provide the best services to their patients.

Health care providers must practise within the boundaries of the law and report any actions that break the law or compromise the health or safety of a patient. Most organizations set up a process for reporting unethical or illegal behaviour. It is important to learn this process and to follow it, no matter who— an employer, a peer, or a superior—one finds acting unethically. By simply having knowledge of an illegal or immoral act and not reporting it, a person may be considered guilty in the matter. Consequences can range from a tarnished professional and personal reputation to legal action and patient harm. In Case Example 5.3, therefore, Nima may disagree with the decision not to report the missing sponge, but, by not reporting it, she could share the guilt in any ensuing legal action.

Justice in health care also considers the allocation of health care resources, which raises questions about whether health care services are spread evenly across Canada. The allocation of resources is discussed in more detail later in this chapter.

PATIENTS' RIGHTS IN HEALTH CARE

Numerous moral controversies surround **rights in health care**, such as the right to die, the right to self-determination, the rights of a fetus, the rights of women to abortion, smokers' rights, and the rights of an individual to health care. These are addressed in one way or another under the *Canada Health Act* and the Canadian Charter of Rights and Freedoms (see Chapters 1, 4, and 7). Technological advances has raised questions about an individual's right to certain health care services and procedures, including, for example, in vitro fertilization (IVF). Depending on the jurisdiction, the cut-off age in Canada for IVF ranges from 45 to 50 years old. But is it fair to place such limits on who may receive the procedure? Should older women be given a right to it? Should the number of embryos implanted be limited? If such limits are put in place, and a woman travels out of the country to have multiple embryos implanted, should her provincial or territorial plan be responsible for her medical costs? In vitro fertilization in older women and the implantation of multiple embryos into a woman's uterus, regardless of her age, both present significant risks to mother and baby

Rights in health care
Entitlements, or things that can and should be expected of health care providers and the health care system. Rights may be tangible (e.g., the right to receive a vaccination covered under the provincial or territorial plan) or intangible (e.g., the right to be treated with respect).

(or babies). When complications arise, they cost the health care system millions of dollars. Ethical storms brewed in 2009 when a 60-year-old gave birth to twins, prompting discussion about implementing clear guidelines for in vitro fertilization (In The News: Should Age Be a Factor?).

In the News: Should Age Be a Factor?

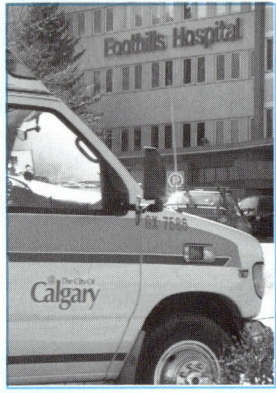

In February 2009, a 60-year-old Alberta woman, Ranjit Hayer, delivered twins by Caesarean section at Foothills Hospital in Calgary. She conceived through in vitro fertilization, which she had done in India because clinics in her home province refused her the procedure. She is the oldest woman known to have borne children in Canada.

This case gives way to ethical questions regarding how old is too old for in vitro fertilization. Will this mother be around to care for her children? Will she be capable of caring for them as they grow? According to Hayer and her husband, who had been trying for decades to have children, in India, children are considered a blessing, and few married couples do not have them. The couple views the birth of their twin boys as having completed their family. Fertility centres across Canada set their own flexible guidelines considering such things as the age and health of the woman and the age of the eggs (frozen when the woman was younger or donated by another woman). Most clinics, however, will not sanction IVF for a woman over age 50.

Sources: Reuters. (2009, February 5). Canadian woman, 60, gives birth to twins: Report. *Reuters.com*. Retrieved from http://www.reuters.com/article/2009/02/05/us-twins-idUSTRE5145BP20090205; 60-year-old woman gives birth to twins in Calgary. (2009, February 9). *Calgary Herald*. Retrieved from http://www.calgaryherald.com/health/year+woman+gives+birth+twins+Calgary/1256889/story.html.

Photo credit: The Canadian Press/Jeff McIntosh.

Patients' rights fall into three categories: the rights Canadians have *within* health care, the right *to* health care, and the right to *timely* health care (Flood & Epps, 2002):

1. Rights *within* health care, established in law in most provinces and territories, include patients' right to their own medical records, the right to confidentiality concerning their health affairs, and the right to informed consent. Other rights are vaguer, such as the right to be treated with respect, compassion, and dignity, the right to privacy, and the right to a reasonable quality of care, including

continuity of care. Usually contained in the codes of ethics of health care professions, these latter rights tend to be described more as elements health care providers must deliver, rather than as rights the patient is entitled to.

2. Although difficult to enforce and, at times, subjective, the principles of the *Canada Health Act* address Canadians' right *to* health care (with limitations). Services offered within each province and territory vary, with some jurisdictions offering services that surpass the requirements of the *Canada Health Act*. Some newer procedures, however, remain uncovered by provincial or territorial plans, resulting in those who cannot afford them doing without, thus creating the basis for the argument that a person's right to adequate health care is violated.

3. A growing movement claims that Canadians should also have the right to *timely* health care—that is, reasonable wait times for both urgent and nonurgent medical services (In the News: Wait Lists: Do They Work?). Improving wait times for services would require further government financing, increased human health resources, and a redistribution of health care services; thus, it is an issue not easily addressed. Currently, no legislation guarantees a person's right to prompt medical care, and only limited legal avenues exist for a patient to pursue a related complaint. Despite commitments from the federal, provincial, and territorial governments to shorten wait times, waiting lists are, in most regions, actually getting longer (see Chapter 10).

Many countries have developed a patients' bill of rights—a statement of the rights patients are entitled to when they receive medical care—that usually include rights to information, fair treatment, and autonomy over medical decisions. Legislation in countries such as Norway, New Zealand, the United States, England, Spain, Sweden, and Italy supports these bills of rights. In some other countries, patients' bills of rights exist only as guidelines, not laws. In Canada, provincial and territorial governments have adopted a range of approaches:

- Quebec implemented legislation defining patients' rights in 1991.
- In Ontario, a private member's bill (Bill 27), called the *Tommy Douglas Act*, was introduced in 2002 to provide a patients' bill of rights that would standardize levels of care and ensure whistleblower protection for health care providers who report inadequacies within the system. This bill, however, was defeated by the Conservative government later that year.
- In New Brunswick, the *Health Charter of Rights and Responsibilities Act*, the first such act in Canada, was introduced to the legislature in April 2003.
- Other provinces have set health care goals, objectives, and expectations in planning and policy documents for patients' bills of rights, but these have not been formally legislated.

> **Continuity of care**
> Health care based on the treating practitioners' having all required information to optimize the care the patient receives. Having access to the individual's health records and maintaining excellent communication among all parties involved in the patient's care are ways to ensure continuity of care.

Most hospitals create their own patients' bills of rights. Many include a section outlining the responsibilities of the patient, which include sharing accurate health information with health care providers; taking an active role in their health care; being courteous to health care providers, other patients, and staff members; and respecting hospital property.

In the News — Wait Lists: Do They Work?

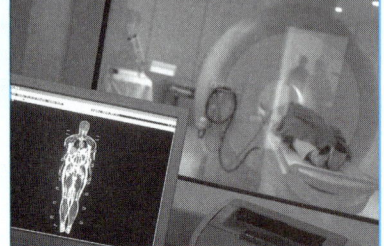

To deal with a patient's right to timely care involving hospitalization, most provinces and territories now post wait times online (accessed through the Ministry of Health Web page). Individuals can log on to find out the length of wait for admission for certain procedures and can possibly seek the necessary service in an area with a shorter list. The Canadian Institute for Health Information (2014) reported that the 2014 wait times for priority procedures such as joint replacement and radiation therapy had improved substantially over the past decade. Other procedures with benchmark time frames have remained virtually unchanged since 2010. Half of the provinces reported longer wait times for two or more procedures. Increases in volume—the number of people seeking procedures—are cited as part of the problem.

Photo credit: © Haak78/Dreamstime.com.

DUTIES AND RIGHTS

If a patient has a right *within* health care or *to* health care, for the most part, the health care provider has the responsibility, or duty, to grant that right. At the heart of patients' rights in health care is the principle of autonomy, which has prominence over most other things. Thus, duties, rights, and autonomy are necessarily joined.

To fulfill one's duty to honour patients' rights, the health care provider must either act to carry out a responsibility or refrain from acting or interfering in a situation. In other words, a patient's right to something may require one to take steps to provide a service (e.g., educate the patient to aid his or her decision making); alternatively, it may require one to do nothing (e.g., refrain from pointing a patient toward a particular treatment option). Patients' rights include noninterference regarding some aspects of their health care.

Autonomy and the Patient

The principle of autonomy serves as the basis for the principles involved in informed consent and self-determination regarding treatment choices. As discussed in Chapter 4, patients must be mentally capable and fully informed about their situation to be able to make autonomous and knowledgeable decisions about their health care. It falls upon the health care provider to ensure that patients have the appropriate information, to help patients understand the information, and to answer patients' questions regarding their situation. Patients also have the right to seek a second opinion.

Attitudes toward patient autonomy have changed over the years—health care has shifted from being physician-directed (paternalistic) to patient-centred. A society that embraces **paternalism** allows the doctor to assume the responsibility of decision making on behalf of patients or to sway patient decisions in choosing treatments. Because the concept of paternalism may restrict a person's rights, it clashes with modern theories and philosophies. This attitude change has resulted in a contemporary version of the Hippocratic Oath that is more aligned with modern concepts, philosophies, and practices (Box 5.1).

> **Paternalism**
> The attempt to control or influence another's decision regarding medical care. Paternalism does not honour the patient's right to autonomy.

Box 5.1   A Modern Version of the Hippocratic Oath

I swear to fulfill, to the best of my ability and judgment, this covenant:

I will respect the hard-won scientific gains of those physicians in whose steps I walk, and gladly share such knowledge as is mine with those who are to follow.

I will apply, for the benefit of the sick, all measures [that] are required, avoiding those twin traps of over-treatment and therapeutic nihilism.

I will remember that there is art to medicine as well as science, and that warmth, sympathy, and understanding may outweigh the surgeon's knife or the chemist's drug.

I will not be ashamed to say "I know not," nor will I fail to call in my colleagues when the skills of another are needed for a patient's recovery.

I will respect the privacy of my patients, for their problems are not disclosed to me that the world may know. Most especially must I tread with care in matters of life and death. If it is given me to save a life, all thanks. But it may also be within my power to take a life; this awesome responsibility must be faced with great humbleness and awareness of my own frailty. Above all, I must not play at God.

I will remember that I do not treat a fever chart, a cancerous growth, but a sick human being, whose illness may affect the person's family and economic stability. My responsibility includes these related problems, if I am to care adequately for the sick.

I will prevent disease whenever I can, for prevention is preferable to cure.

Continued on next page

> I will remember that I remain a member of society, with special obligations to all my fellow human beings, those sound of mind and body as well as the infirm.
>
> If I do not violate this oath, may I enjoy life and art, and be respected while I live and remembered with affection thereafter. May I always act so as to preserve the finest traditions of my calling and may I long experience the joy of healing those who seek my help.
>
> Written in 1964 by Louis Lasagna, Academic Dean of the School of Medicine at Tufts University.
>
> Source: Nova Online. (n.d.). *The Hippocratic oath: Modern version*. Retrieved from http://www.pbs.org/wgbh/nova/doctors/oath_modern.html.

As a result of this shift toward patients' independently determining what is best for themselves, physicians committed to beneficence may face moral dilemmas when, for instance, a patient refuses life-saving treatment. In most cases, however, health care providers both respect and uphold patients' decisions. When, on occasion, they do not, significant stress and often litigation result.

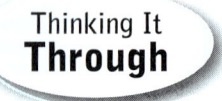

Patients frequently ask health care providers for advice based on their specific professional knowledge and expertise. For example, Jennifer, an asthmatic, may ask a respiratory therapist whether she should use her inhalers as often as prescribed.

1. Is it acceptable for a health care provider to give treatment advice to a patient based on his or her own judgement and experience—for example, "If I were you, I would do this"?

2. Where do you draw the line between strongly suggesting the patient follow your advice and allowing the patient to make an independent choice?

TRUTHFULNESS

All patients have a right to the truth, and health care providers, as discussed above, have a duty to provide it. Expecting that others will be truthful and honest is central to trust, even in our daily lives.

In the past, physicians would often choose to withhold "upsetting information" from a patient, or family members would ask a physician to withhold such information (Case Example 5.5). The modern, patient-focused (not physician-focused) approach to treatment requires physicians to keep the patient fully and truthfully informed. Denying patients information or lying to them causes more harm than good in most situations.

Case Example 5.5

Ira, 86, has terminal lung cancer. He has other chronic health problems that have reduced both his quality and his enjoyment of life. Unsure how capable Ira is, mentally and physically, to deal with the news of his cancer, the physician tells Ira's family first. His wife and grown children do not want Ira to know, believing that it would be best that he enjoy some degree of quality in the last months of his life without having to face the stress related to the diagnosis. Ira worries excessively about his health. The doctor, against his better judgement, agrees to remain silent. Only days before he dies, Ira learns of the diagnosis of several months before. Bitter, he feels that had he known, he could have put his affairs in order, come to terms with dying, and better prepared his children for his death.

PARENTAL RIGHTS, ETHICS, AND THE LAW

When a patient is considered an adult, self-determination takes precedence over paternalistic intervention, even when the patient's life is at stake. However, paternalism and the legal system sometimes join forces when life-saving treatment is thought to be necessary for a minor yet is refused—for example, when parents make decisions for their minor children that the health care provider believes will compromise the health or life of the child, as in the case of Jehovah's Witness parents refusing a blood transfusion that would save their child's life. In these cases, the parents' or guardians' rights are not absolute, and the provincial or territorial courts will almost always obtain legal custody for the child and allow the recommended treatment. Numerous cases have surfaced over the past few years involving children from newborns to teenagers (In the News: Rights of the Individual Versus Medical Advice).

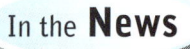

Rights of the Individual Versus Medical Advice

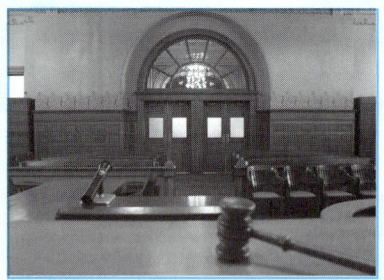

In 2014, an 11-year-old First Nations girl in Ontario refused recommended chemotherapy for acute lymphoblastic leukemia at McMaster Hospital in Hamilton, Ontario. This type of leukemia is a common type to affect children and has approximately an 80% cure rate when treated with chemotherapy. The girl made the decision to stop chemotherapy after experiencing the unpleasant side effects of chemotherapy; as well, she said that she had a spiritual encounter supporting her decision. She opted for treatment with traditional Aboriginal medicine, with the full support of her family and community. As required by Ontario law, the authorities at the hospital notified the affiliated Children's Aid Society (CAS). The girl's lawyer argued that having the capacity to understand the risks and benefits of her treatment options gave the girl the legal right to self-determination. After investigating, the CAS decided not to bring the girl into care or pursue the case. "The more we looked at it, we realized that this is a warm, loving family," said Andy Koster, executive director of the Children's Aid Society of Brant. "We don't believe that bringing her into care, taking her away from that family—which is her support—and forcing chemotherapy is going to be in any way emotionally sound for her, or psychologically or even spiritually."

Source: Hopper, T. (2014, May 15). Eleven-year-old's choice to treat her cancer with indigenous medicine instead of chemo may be legal, experts say. *National Post*. Retrieved from http://news.nationalpost.com/2014/05/15/eleven-year-olds-choice-to-treat-her-cancer-with-indigenous-medicine-instead-of-chemo-may-be-legal-experts-say/; Clarke, K. (2014, May 20). Girl, 11, with cancer is free to refuse chemotherapy, Children's Aid officials rule. *National Post*. Retrieved from http://news.nationalpost.com/2014/05/20/girl-11-with-cancer-is-free-to-refuse-chemotherapy-childrens-aid-officials-rule/.

Photo credit: © iStock.com/ftwitty.

All involved parties want what is best for the patient, but what one considers best may differ from what another considers best. Values, cultural and religious beliefs, and ethical codes can conflict. Who is to say which path should be followed? Do parents not have the right to make decisions for their underage children? Do doctors not have a legal obligation to preserve life? For physicians, cases such as the one cited in the In the News box on page 168 differ significantly from withdrawing life support for a terminally ill patient. Jehovah's Witnesses do not want their children to die, nor do they refuse all medical treatments—only those involving blood products.

Patients who refuse a blood transfusion, even in the face of death, are following the divine command theory. Their religious beliefs dictate their course of action. Physicians, on the other hand, observe duty ethics; their duty is to treat the patient. Some might argue for a teleological approach—treating the patient saves the patient's life and, in the end, benefits everyone involved. Could that outcome be argued, however, if the patient is ostracized by his or her community for having had a blood transfusion and if the patient feels wronged for having been forced to do something contrary to his or her religious beliefs? What do you think?

Rights and Mental Competence

Conflict with a patient's autonomy frequently arises when a question of mental competence exists. Consider a person with anorexia nervosa, a devastating eating disorder that primarily affects young women, although both men and women of all ages are vulnerable. It is often caused by another physiological disorder, or vice versa. Conditions associated with anorexia include obsessive compulsive disorder, borderline personality disorder, bipolar disorder, post-traumatic stress disorder, and depression. The nature of these diseases often hinders the patient's ability to make rational decisions.

Does a person whose illness skews his or her ability to make rational decisions have the right to self-determination? Concerns over such situations led psychiatrist Marian Verkerk (1999) to propose the concept of **compassionate interference**, which allows physicians to treat individuals against their will. Dr. Verkerk argues that treatment restores patients to a sound physical and mental state, allowing them then to make informed decisions.

As discussed, parental authority has been removed when parents or guardians refuse medical treatment deemed necessary to save a child's life. These cases can become even more complex—for example, when the child in question also refuses treatment but is considered mentally unfit to make such a decision, as illustrated in the case below (In the News: When Does a Child Have a Right to Autonomy?).

Compassionate interference
The act of imposing treatment against a patient's will when deemed in the best interests of the patient.

ETHICS AT WORK

All regulated health care professions have codes of ethics, as do many places of employment. Review the one belonging to your profession or organization. If none exists, you should consider recommending that one be implemented. Many ethical situations arise in the health care industry, and codes of ethics significantly help professionals make appropriate decisions.

> In the **News**

When Does a Child Have a Right to Autonomy?

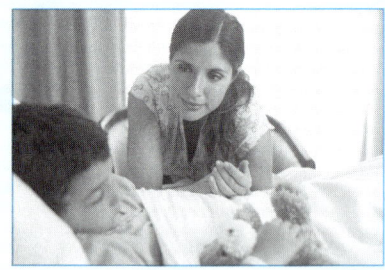

In 2004, an 8-year-old boy living in Hamilton, Ontario, was successfully treated for leukemia. The father described the treatments as "hell." The boy lost his hair, had sores all over his body, had to wear diapers, and could not keep food down. In 2008, the leukemia returned. This time, his father and stepmother refused further treatment, claiming they would rely on spiritual healing and the outcome determined by their Creator. The boy, then 11, claimed he did not want the treatment because he was not prepared to experience the overwhelming side effects again. The boy, who suffers from fetal alcohol syndrome and attends special education classes, was assessed as incompetent to make such a decision.

The court obtained statements from two of the country's top specialists in the field of leukemia, both of whom felt that treatment was Dillon's only hope and that a reasonable chance of a positive outcome existed. The boy was made a ward of the Children's Aid Society, and treatment was imposed.

Sources: Canadian Press. (2008, May 10). Boy undergoing chemotherapy against his wishes. *CTV News*. Retrieved from http://toronto.ctv.ca/servlet/an/plocal/CTVNews/20080510/unwanted_chemotherapy_080510/20080510/?hub =OttawaHome; Canadian Press. (2008, May 13). Forced chemo treatment of child "heavy-handed" decision: Bioethicists. *CBC News*. Retrieved from http://www.cbc.ca/news/canada/toronto/forced-chemo-treatment-of-child-heavy-handed-decision-bioethicists-1.717082.

Photo credit: © OJO Images/Fotosearch.

THE CODE OF ETHICS

A formal statement of an organization's or profession's values regarding professional behaviour, a code of ethics provides guidance for ethical decision making, self-evaluation, and best practices policies. Most codes cover expectations related to professional conduct that, if violated, can result in loss of the person's professional licence, dismissal from employment, or legal action.

Special Boundaries and Relationships

With Patients

Personal relationships between patients and health care providers in any discipline are, for the most part, prohibited while the formal relationship remains and, sometimes, even for a period of time after the professional relationship ends. Codes of ethics for physicians clearly outline these boundaries. Doctors may not establish personal relationships with patients under their care. In most circumstances, a physician may not date a former patient for one year after the termination of the patient–physician relationship. Most other health care professions take a similar, though often not as strict, stand on developing personal relationships with patients. For example, no formal objection exists to a physiotherapist starting a relationship with a former patient several weeks after their professional relationship has ended.

Often, especially in small towns, a patient admitted to hospital knows many of the staff members. Depending on the nature of the relationship, this may or may not cause concern. If the health care provider feels uncomfortable caring for a particular patient, or the other way around, however, it would be in the best interests of both to have someone else assume that patient's care.

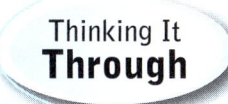

Thinking It Through

In the workplace setting, you will meet a wide range of people, some of whom you are drawn to and feel a natural desire to want to develop a friendship with.

1. Is it ethical for a health care provider to exchange phone numbers with a patient with the intent of dating after the patient is discharged?

2. Does it make a difference if the exchange of phone numbers is for the purpose of developing a platonic friendship?

With Colleagues

Inevitably, you will develop friendships in the workplace. Unless these friendships interfere with how you do your job, doing so is not considered unethical. However, you must remain impartial and not choose favourites among the staff. Developing alliances by forming cliques at the expense of others is both unprofessional and destructive. Tight-knit groups in the workplace make it difficult for new staff members to integrate and feel welcome. Starting a new job is difficult enough. A warm and inviting environment goes a long way toward helping new employees fit in and begin to function competently as a member of the health care team.

Personal business has no role in the workplace, either. Discussing last night's party, tomorrow's trip, or someone's recent breakup remains inappropriate in any work environment.

In the Hospital Setting

Health care providers employed in a hospital setting are expected to carry out their duties in a professional, legal, and ethical manner. All health care facilities have procedures, policies, and guidelines governing ethical conduct. As well, employers expect health care providers to uphold the ethical codes of their individual professions. Although members of the health care team should support each other, overstepping certain boundaries can breach ethical conduct (e.g., moving a colleague's family member up a wait list).

Health care providers also have an obligation to report fellow health care providers' misconduct or incompetence, whether regarding their job performance or a violation of the principles of confidentiality. Most health care environments develop procedures outlining what to report and whom to report it to. Ethical issues unresolved at a lower level, in most facilities, will be reported to an ethics committee.

Rationale for Boundaries

Trust

A health care worker providing medical services for a patient does so within a therapeutic relationship. Patients trust the health care provider to perform his or her professional services impartially and competently. Not only is changing the nature of that relationship ethically and morally wrong; it can also interfere with the care and compromise the ability of the health care provider to fulfill his or her professional duties. The higher the professional's level of responsibility (e.g., a physician versus a physiotherapist, respiratory therapist, or medical secretary), the more damaging such a change can be.

Vulnerability

The patient occupies the vulnerable position within the patient–health care provider relationship. As a result of this vulnerability, the patient may exhibit sick role behaviour (see Chapter 2) and feel dependent.

Balance of Power and Transference

In a physician–patient relationship, decisions made by the physician can have a significant impact on the patient's health and recovery. Along with feeling vulnerable, the patient may be in awe of the physician and misread feelings for him or her. Patients somewhat commonly feel a sense of "falling in love" with physicians or other health care providers. The health care provider has a responsibility to recognize the relevant signs and to ensure the relationship remains formal. In some cases, physicians have to stop providing care for the patient.

All health care providers dealing with patients should be aware of the possibility of such situations. Patients have a right to equitable and fair care—and to trust that they receive it. Any personal ties with a patient, therefore, have the potential to interfere with the care of that patient or others, to interfere with a trusting relationship, and to put the patient in a vulnerable position.

Accepting Gifts

Patients often give gifts to health care providers who have cared for them, usually as an expression of gratitude. Little literature is available about the ethics of accepting gifts. A box of chocolates for the nursing station when a patient leaves the hospital, some flowers sent to the office, or a card with a small ornament are examples of acceptable gifts. Accepting anything more is inappropriate and may place the health care provider in a difficult position because the patient may expect favouritism, such as access to special treatment or an appointment whenever he or she wants it. Some health care providers make it a policy not to accept anything—ever. If an employer or regulatory college has guidelines about accepting gifts, these must be followed.

Seasonal gifts may be an exception. During the holidays, patients often give health care providers and their office staff gifts, such as home baking, wine, or other tokens of appreciation—usually with no strings attached. Some people get a true sense of satisfaction from the opportunity to express gratitude. Common sense and familiarity with the patient are the best guidelines when accepting seasonal gifts if the workplace or regulatory college does not address the issue.

The Ethics Committee

An ethics committee consists of a group of people—often volunteers—who listen to, evaluate, and make recommendations about acts perceived as unethical. Members of such committees usually come from a variety of backgrounds and may include doctors, nurses, social workers, physiotherapists, lawyers, ethicists, and members of the public. Public members do not require special qualifications other than the ability to listen and assist with making fair and unbiased decisions. Members remain on the committee for designated time frames.

Aside from evaluating unethical acts, ethics committees may provide health care providers with guidance in making controversial medical decisions and compile research for policy development within the facility. In the health care

END-OF-LIFE ISSUES

End-of-life issues that raise ethical concerns include patients' wishing to withdraw life-saving measures, issuing DNR orders, and requesting supportive or palliative care in the face of a terminal illness. The phrase *allow natural death* (AND) is sometimes used as an alternative to DNR and is deemed less harsh and perhaps more appropriate. In Canada, end-of-life issues have were brought into the news in June 2014 when Quebec's controversial Bill 52 was passed in a free vote at the National Assembly. This legislation allows medical aid in dying (euthanasia) (Gollom, 2014).

EUTHANASIA

The purpose of euthanasia (also called *aid in dying, assisted suicide,* or *physician-assisted suicide*) is to deliberately end a life in order to relieve pain and suffering due to an incurable disease. Various categories of euthanasia exist. **Voluntary euthanasia** occurs when a person causes the death of another with the dying person's consent—often in the form of a living will or advance directive (see page 177); **involuntary euthanasia** occurs when a person causes the death of a dying person without the latter's consent. **Active euthanasia** refers to the taking of deliberate steps to end another's life (e.g., with a lethal injection); **passive euthanasia** refers to the process of allowing a person to die by removing life support or other life-sustaining treatment. In the case of **physician-assisted suicide**, the doctor provides the patient with the means to end his or her own life; the patient, however, carries out the act.

With the exception of passive euthanasia, the act of ending or assisting to end a person's life is illegal in most countries. Euthanasia, a highly controversial concept, has both legal and ethical implications. The act conflicts with the moral values of most societies, which respect the sanctity of life and the duty of the health care provider to save or preserve life. On the other hand, allowing euthanasia respects the autonomy of the person who wishes to die.

The possibility of legalizing euthanasia raises fears of misuse of the process—for example, ending Aunt Sally's life to inherit her money or putting Dad to sleep because he is too difficult to care for. Euthanasia has also been proposed to end lifelong suffering, even when death is not imminent (In the News: The Latimer Tragedy).

Voluntary euthanasia
A person's bringing about the death of a dying person with the dying person's consent.

Involuntary euthanasia
A person's bringing about the death of a dying person without the dying person's consent.

Active euthanasia
The taking of deliberate steps to end a dying person's life.

Passive euthanasia
The process of allowing a person to die by removing life support or other life-sustaining treatment.

Physician-assisted suicide
The taking of one's own life with means provided by a doctor.

In the News The Latimer Tragedy

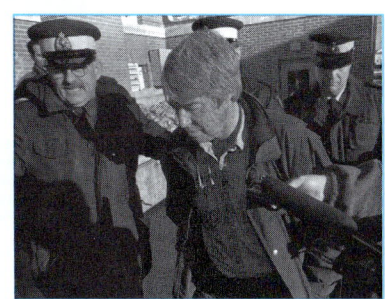

A noteworthy and historic case of involuntary active euthanasia, with ramifications that persist today, is that of Robert Latimer, a Saskatchewan farmer who killed his daughter, Tracy, in 1993 by placing her in a car and rerouting exhaust fumes to euthanize her. Tracy, a 40-pound, 12-year-old quadriplegic with cerebral palsy, functioned at the level of a 3-month-old. According to most reports, she suffered constant and severe pain. Her father could not bear to see her life continue indefinitely in this manner. Convicted of second-degree murder, Mr. Latimer was sentenced to life in prison (which was a mandatory minimum sentence of ten years), with a chance of parole after ten years. Parole was granted in 2010 with some conditions. In July 2013, the Parole Board of Canada lifted the requirement that Mr. Latimer continue with one-to-one psychological counselling, stating that he was now able to manage his emotions. He is still prohibited from caring for a disabled person and must apply to the parole board if he wants to travel outside of the country.

Source: Canadian Broadcasting Corporation. (2008, March 17). "Compassionate homicide": The law and Robert Latimer. *CBC Archives.* Retrieved from http://www.cbc.ca/news/canada/compassionate-homicide-the-law-and-robert-latimer-1.972561; QMI Agency. (2012, September 17). Robert Latimer granted parole exception for trip to England. *Toronto Sun.* Retrieved from http://www.torontosun.com/2012/09/17/robert-latimer-granted-parole-exception-for-trip-to-england; CBC News. (2013, July 8). *Parole condition lifted for Robert Latimer.* Retrieved from http://www.cbc.ca/news/canada/saskatchewan/story/2013/07/08/sk-robert-latimer-parole-condition-lifted.html.

Photo credit: The Canadian Press/1997 (str-Kevin Frayer).

Debate over the ethics in the Latimer case and the severity of the sentence Mr. Latimer received continues to this day. At Mr. Latimer's second trial, ordered because of jury interference in the first trial, the jury upheld the charge of second-degree murder but recommended Mr. Latimer be eligible for parole after one year. In this trial, Justice Ted Noble tried to distinguish between murder and mercy killing. He called Tracy Latimer's murder a "rare act of homicide that was committed for caring and altruistic reasons. That is why for want of a better term, this is called compassionate homicide" (CBC News, 2010). Does Robert Latimer present a danger to society? Most would say no. However, in 1998, the Saskatchewan Court of Appeal overturned Judge Noble's ruling, imposing the mandatory minimum sentence: 25 years, with no parole for ten years. Latimer's first bid for parole in 2007 was denied because he maintained his belief that he killed Tracy for her benefit and would not express remorse. Groups championing the rights of disabled persons argued that showing leniency would endanger disabled persons and rate them as second-class citizens. Canadians with disabilities continue to campaign for protection of what they deem a fundamental human right—the right to life (CBC News, 2010).

Another widely known case is that of British Columbia resident Susan Rodriguez, who suffered from ALS (also called Lou Gehrig's disease). For months, Ms. Rodriguez petitioned the courts for permission to die legally with medical assistance. The courts refused (*Rodriguez v. British Columbia*, 1993). In the end, she terminated her own life in 1994 with physician assistance. The physician was never named or charged. See the Web Resources on Evolve for a link to videos of Susan Rodriguez petitioning the courts.

In another case, Nancy B. developed Guillain-Barré syndrome, which left her incapable of movement, including breathing, although her mental capacities remained. She petitioned the Superior Court of Quebec to have her respirator turned off. The court upheld Nancy B.'s right to consent or to withhold consent to any medical intervention (*N.B. v. Hôtel-Dieu de Québec*, 1992).

Some of the most complicated cases involve individuals in a vegetative state who are kept alive by respirators, feeding tubes, or both. Often the family cannot agree on a course of action—some family members want life-sustaining measures withdrawn, and others want them continued. Depending on the situation, after the withdrawal of life-sustaining measures, death can take days to occur or can occur almost immediately.

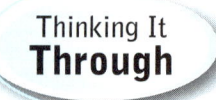

The cases of Susan Rodriguez and Nancy B. illustrate two individuals wanting the right to die—one being refused this right, and the other being granted it.

1. Why do you think the courts ruled differently?

2. Should the person or persons who assisted Ms. Rodriguez to die face legal action?

THE RIGHT TO DIE

People suffering from a poor quality of life as a result of illness, usually a terminal illness, may request the right to die (i.e., passive euthanasia). As discussed earlier, mentally competent adult patients have the right to refuse medical treatment, to request a DNR order, or to ask for only comfort measures in the face of a serious, possibly terminal, illness.

Older people and those with debilitating diseases commonly request that they not be resuscitated (through a DNR order) if they suffer a cardiac arrest (i.e., heart attack). These people are not pursuing euthanasia; they simply do not want any intervention if a major health event occurs. Health care providers are legally bound to honour such requests, which can be difficult for those who believe that active measures should be taken at all costs. Importantly, a person can reverse his or her DNR request at any time.

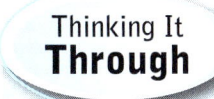

Currently hospitalized, Pierre suffers a cardiac arrest. His nurse, Nayla, is in his room at the time and knows that he has a DNR order because he was constantly reminding the staff of it. However, because of Nayla's religious beliefs, she feels that saving a person's life takes precedence over everything else. Not resuscitating Pierre is a difficult choice for her to make, but resuscitating him would violate the patient's personal request and, thus, his right to autonomy. What should Nayla do?

An **advance directive**, also called a *living will* or *treatment directive*, specifies the nature and level of treatment a person would want to receive in the event that he or she becomes unable to make those decisions at a later time. People prepare advance directives so as to ensure their wishes are known and honoured by family and loved ones and carried out by medical caregivers. Advance directives that appoint a power of attorney for personal care are most likely to result in the person's instructions being followed.

A **values history form** is a comprehensive document that guides people in thinking about treatment options they would or would not want in the event that they were to become unable to make decisions about their own health care. People can detail their feelings, thoughts, and values as they relate to medical interventions. The form may also assist loved ones who might have to make decisions on the person's behalf, as well as clarify the person's choices if disagreements among loved ones occur (Case Example 5.6).

Advance directive
A legal document that specifies the nature and level of treatment a person would want to receive in the event of later being unable to make those decisions. Also called a *living will* or *treatment directive*.

Values history form
A document that helps people think about the health care choices they would want made for them.

> **Case Example 5.6**
>
> Sam, a 67-year-old who recently suffered a severe stroke, created an advance directive expressing his wish to receive no active intervention if he has another stroke. However, concerned that another stroke may leave him unable to communicate and on a respirator, he begins to have doubts about his decision, fearful that if he has a change of heart, he would be unable to communicate it. (Many people who have decided against intervention change their minds when actually facing death.) Some family members know of his recent second thoughts about his advance directive. Sam decides to complete a values history form to clarify his feelings and thoughts about medical intervention. This form *might* help Sam's family if they ever have to make treatment decisions for him.

A patient in hospital can request varying levels of care in the event of a life-threatening incident, ranging from comfort measures only to active treatment but no CPR to full and active treatment (e.g., every possible intervention to preserve the person's life). Rating systems vary among agencies, but "comfort" or "supportive" measures usually include pain control and any other intervention to prevent suffering, whereas "active" treatment may refer simply to, for example, the administration of an IV for hydration and pain medication but no antibiotics or the use of any and all medications that will sustain life and end the crisis. Some individuals refuse their daily medications (e.g., antihypertensive medication, diuretics) in an attempt to accelerate their demise. Such refusal is perfectly legal but may pose moral questions for those involved in the individual's care.

PALLIATIVE CARE

Palliative care, an increasingly important component of medical care in Canada, addresses the physical and emotional needs of those who are dying. Individuals opposed to any kind of interference with the natural course of death believe that palliative care can facilitate a peaceful and painless natural death. Whether delivered in a hospital, in a hospice, or at home, palliative care can aid any person at any age and at any stage of a life-threatening illness. Teams of experts work with patients and their families to manage physical discomfort and psychological distress and to meet spiritual needs. Palliative care offers terminally ill people an alternative to facing death alone and an end to the fear of a painful death that strips them of human dignity. Many consider palliative care an important alternative for those who might consider ending their lives by other means.

ALLOCATION OF RESOURCES

The term *allocation of resources* refers to who gets what, when, and for what reason. Rising health care costs, expensive technologies, and limited access to many services have made the allocation of resources an increasing concern in the health care industry. And limited resources mean that "Who gets what?" becomes a huge ethical problem. A brief discussion of select limited resources follows, with the intent of promoting thought and discussion.

ORGAN TRANSPLANTATION

The advancements that led to the ability to transplant organs, a scarce resource, have introduced several ethical issues. Consider Case Example 5.7.

Case Example 5.7

The transplant team at a large hospital has just received word that a liver has become available. The list of approved critical candidates includes both Joe and Olga. Joe, despite living a very healthy lifestyle, suffers from an autoimmune disease that has destroyed his liver. Olga, an alcoholic, has advanced liver disease and generally very poor health. Her history suggests that she remains at high risk for returning to drinking—a setback that would surely damage the new liver should she receive one. All other things being equal (age, family situation, finances), which candidate do you think should get the liver? Should Olga be considered a less desirable candidate than Joe because of her disease?

In Case Example 5.7, Olga has been unable to overcome the disease of alcoholism. Although she has managed to give up drinking for limited periods of time, her ability to maintain sobriety remains questionable. A return to drinking would sharply decrease her chances of maintaining even reasonable health with a transplanted liver. Should she therefore be denied a chance at a new life? Joe, on the other hand, lives a healthy lifestyle yet has contracted a disease typically considered less preventable than alcoholism. But what if, as is debated in modern medicine, alcoholism were more commonly considered a disease, rather than a moral failing? Would Olga then be in a more favourable position to compete for the liver? Would she be on equal footing with Joe?

Other considerations from a medical perspective encourage the following questions: Who would be more likely to see significant improvements in his or her health with the new liver? What damage has alcoholism done to Olga's overall health? Alcoholics tend to have lower success rates with transplantation since their general health is usually poorer. A return to drinking would interfere with compliance with the necessary post-transplant treatment regime, which requires taking immunosuppressant drugs. Nonetheless, do any of these factors provide a solid reason to deny Olga?

FINANCES AND RESOURCES

In Canada, the demand for health care resources—including finances, health care providers, and medical services such as diagnostic tests and hospital beds—sometimes exceeds supply. The allocation of resources in health care presents an ethical problem because it raises questions about fairness and justness. Priorities should be based on need, but how does a person, organization, or government assess need?

Health care funding in Canada, for the most part, is distributed in such a way that each region can set its own priorities and make decisions about how best to meet the health care needs of the populations it serves. If funds increase, however, how are they distributed? If funds decrease, which services are maintained, and which are sacrificed? How can someone make a decision, for example, to fund expensive treatment for a small number of autistic children if that same amount of money might be spent on cancer treatment that could save thousands of lives?

All levels of government and an army of health care providers collaborate to implement strategies they believe will be the most cost-effective. The recent thrust toward preventive care has directed funding toward raising awareness of the importance of, for example, periodic physical examinations, breast screening and Pap smears for women, immunizations for children, colon cancer home tests, and a healthy lifestyle (e.g., a proper diet, regular physical activity, and avoidance of self-imposed risk behaviours such as smoking). The healthier the

Canadian population is, the fewer health care dollars ultimately need to be spent. Although many consider immunizations among the most important advances in preventive care, others argue that vaccines pose more risks than do diseases such as polio, measles, mumps, typhoid, and rubella, suggesting that immunizations have caused autism in some Canadian children (no definitive proof of this claim exists).

Many groups compete for health care dollars—some for treatments for rare conditions that would empty the health care pot of millions of dollars. Teleological theorists, however, would suggest that funds should go to those services that meet the needs of the most people. Most Canadians take the stand that treatment should be available to all Canadians and that governments should ensure such universal availability without imposing financial hardship on an individual or family.

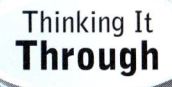

Thinking It Through

Thousands of Canadians suffer from relatively rare conditions that are incurable but that can be treated with some success. These treatments, however, are often extremely expensive—sometimes drugs are not covered by the public plan, and sometimes treatments do not fall within the definition of "medically necessary."

1. Is it ethical to spend a large amount of money on a few individuals when that money could be used to improve health care services for a much larger group?

2. Does each life not deserve the same consideration?

New technologies have introduced treatment modalities that preserve and prolong life, and Canadians feel a sense of entitlement to these technologies. However, funds are limited; if every life-saving or treatment measure were offered to every person in need, the health care system would collapse. For example, significant (and costly) advancements have been made in sustaining life for very premature babies; however, these infants often have little hope of recovery or a satisfactory quality of life if they do recover (Case Example 5.8). With health care costs rising, Canadians may ultimately be asked to consider the expense of their choices.

Case Example 5.8

Raja delivered a baby, Damian, at 23 weeks gestation. Damian was transported to the nearest neonatal intensive care unit. Three days later, the doctors told Raja that her baby had a 30% chance of survival and that if he did survive, he would likely be blind, require multiple heart surgeries, suffer from a seizure disorder, and have cerebral palsy. They asked whether she wanted them to continue treatment to attempt to save the baby's life. The cost to the health care system would be enormous, and the quality of life the baby would have, questionable. Left to make her very difficult decision, Raja had to consider the small margin of hope that her son would live and, if he did survive, the complications he would have to endure. The last thing on her mind was the expense of the treatments—they were covered by the health care system.

NORTHERN ACCESS TO HEALTH CARE

Providing health care resources for the population of Canada's northern communities is very costly. Remote Aboriginal reserves and villages with few resources result in a large percentage of available health care dollars being spent on transportation costs to larger centres. (Such services are covered under federal, provincial, and territorial health plans in accordance with the principles of the *Canada Health Act*.) Canada's Inuit population in the Arctic especially lacks adequate health care. See Chapter 10 for more discussion on access to health care in Canada's northern communities.

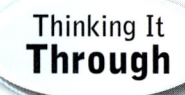

Is it moral or ethical that Canada's Inuit population endures health care conditions that Canadians in more southern, populated communities would consider unacceptable?

OTHER ETHICAL ISSUES IN HEALTH CARE

ABORTION

One of the most longstanding and controversial issues in health care, abortion has remained without restrictions in Canada since 1988, when the Supreme Court of

Canada declared that the law could not forbid abortion because doing so would violate Section 7 of the Charter. Moreover, this court decision held that the then current restrictions on access to abortion were unfair and unreasonable. Section 7 states that "everyone has the right to life, liberty and the security of the person and the right not to be deprived thereof except in accordance with the principles of fundamental justice" (Canadian Charter of Rights and Freedoms, 1982).

In Canada, abortions remain legal to the point of "viability" (defined as a fetus weighing more than 500 grams or having reached more than 20 weeks gestation) (Canadian Medical Association, 1988). Second-trimester abortions are allowed only under certain circumstances, usually when the mother's life is at risk. Third-trimester abortions may also be performed under such circumstances; however, new technologies have given most babies born at that stage a reasonable chance of survival. Babies born after 28 weeks gestation receive the best chance of achieving a healthy life.

Access to and coverage for abortion vary among the provinces and territories. In British Columbia, Alberta, Manitoba, Ontario, Quebec, and Newfoundland, the cost of an abortion is covered under the provincial plan regardless of where the procedure is performed (hospital or private clinic). New Brunswick provides no funding for abortions obtained in clinics but funds those done in hospitals. In Saskatchewan, the Northwest Territories, Nunavut, and Yukon, there are no private clinics, but in-hospital abortions are covered by the public plan. Prince Edward Island offers no abortion facilities at all. Women in P.E.I. wanting an abortion travel to out-of-province hospitals. To qualify for provincial health coverage, they must have a physician's referral; the request is then reviewed by the Medicare Medical Consultant before funding is granted. In early 2008, Quebec decided to fund abortions without limitations.

Since health care providers are not obligated to perform abortions, many will opt not to because of religious or moral beliefs, providing patients some limitations on access. Canadians in northern and other remote regions usually must travel long distances at their own expense to access abortion services.

The moral and ethical issues around abortion concern two main issues: the right of the fetus to life and the right of women to make decisions that involve their own bodies. These issues also include philosophical, religious, and political components.

Pro-life groups believe that personhood (i.e., the state of being considered a person) begins at conception—the moment the sperm meets the ovum. From a spiritual perspective, some believe that the soul enters the body at this point. Pro-lifers consider any deliberate interference that threatens the life of this "person" murder, believing that the fetus shares the same rights as all other humans, including the right to life.

Pro-choice groups argue that the mother has the choice to carry the baby to term or to end the pregnancy, maintaining that abortion is a constitutional right and that, therefore, safe and timely access in hospitals and clinics must be guaranteed. Views among pro-choice groups vary as to when the fetus becomes a person with rights. People who, for example, believe that personhood does not begin until the start of the second trimester or later assert that an abortion occurring prior to 13 weeks is both moral and ethical if it reflects the wishes of the pregnant woman.

The debate over whether abortion is right or wrong, ethical or unethical, will continue. The argument comes down to personal, moral, religious, and cultural values and beliefs.

Genetic Testing

Through genetic testing—the examination of one's deoxyribonucleic acid (DNA)—people can learn whether they carry any genes that put them at a higher risk for disease, such as certain types of cancer. Similarly, carrier testing determines whether the potential exists to pass on a genetic disease (e.g., sickle cell anemia) to offspring. A couple who undergo such tests and have positive results then must weigh the severity of the potential disease and the chances of its occurrence when deciding whether to bear children.

Prenatal diagnostic screening can determine a fetus's risk for certain genetic disorders, aid in earlier diagnosis of fetal abnormalities, and provide prospective parents with important information for making informed decisions about a pregnancy.

Genetic testing raises a number of moral and ethical questions, however. For instance, if an insurance company obtained records showing that a prospective patient carried a gene that put him or her at risk for developing cancer, would that person be considered uninsurable? Would an employer with access to similar information decide against hiring that person?

What the individual does with the information obtained raises further issues. For example, a woman who learns she has the breast cancer gene might elect to have her breasts and ovaries removed (see In the News: Angelina Jolie's Medical Choice in Chapter 3, page 79).

Canadians are encouraged to think carefully (i.e., to ask what the benefit is in knowing) before having genetic testing for presumed or established conditions. For example, would it help a person to know that he or she may develop Huntington's disease, an incurable neurological disorder? Such knowledge might provide relief from uncertainty and give a person an opportunity to get his or her affairs in order. On the other hand, the anxiety produced from living with the risk for an incurable disease can be overwhelming and debilitating in itself.

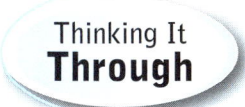

Thinking It Through

Assume that several members of your family have suffered from Alzheimer's disease. A genetic test will tell you whether you carry the inherited gene, which would increase the likelihood of your developing the disease.

1. Would you want to know if you carried the gene?

2. What advantages and disadvantages exist of either knowing or not knowing?

Although demand for genetic testing in Canada is growing, resources are limited, and individuals who turn to private laboratories usually surrender the advantage of receiving counsel from their own doctors. Results can be indefinite, stressful, damaging to family relationships, and harmful to careers. Genetic tests covered under public insurance in Canada include those for breast and ovarian cancer, colon cancer, high cholesterol, and Alzheimer's disease.

Provincial and territorial governments have questioned the cost-effectiveness of genetic testing (i.e., allocation of resources) and have agreed that the cost-effectiveness depends on the test. For example, genetic testing for colon cancer is probably cost-effective since individuals who test positive for a colon cancer gene can undergo regular screening (usually via colonoscopy) that can diagnose cancer in its early stages. Testing for lesser-known conditions is sometimes considered expensive and unlikely to save the health care system money in the long run.

Expert genetic counselling accompanies genetic testing in some Canadian jurisdictions, but not all. Genetic counselling aims to provide individuals with an understanding of the implications of a positive test, both for themselves and for their relatives, and to ensure individuals make an informed choice about taking the test.

PATENTING GENES

A very controversial issue in ethics is whether or not genes can be patented—for example, whether a company that discovered a gene would "own" it and all related rights to testing on it. Patents for discovered genes have been granted in the United States for nearly 30 years. In that time frame, American companies have been awarded patents for approximately 20% of the human genome (Lovgren, 2005). Companies who put millions of dollars into research argue that patents allow them to recoup the money spent discovering the genes. The question of allowing patents for human genes, though, raises moral, legal, and ethical questions. For example: Is it either legal or ethical for a company to "own" something that is naturally occurring in the human body? Is it fair for one company to have exclusive rights to diagnostic tests related to a human gene? Will restricting patents for discoveries that cost millions of dollars make researchers think twice about investing in research? Should publicly funded teaching hospitals be allowed to hold patents that ultimately restrict availability of a test? The U.S. Supreme Court weighed in on this issue in 2013 (In the News: Patents on "Products of Nature" Invalid).

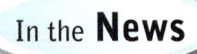

Patents on "Products of Nature" Invalid

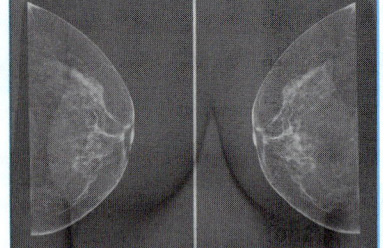

American firm Myriad Genetics was recently granted a patent for genes that the company discovered are markers for breast and ovarian cancer. Myriad subsequently marketed a test that identifies individuals at risk for developing these types of cancer. The test is very expensive, and because Myriad Genetics has a patent, the company sells the only breast cancer (BRCA) gene test. Without competition, the company sets the price—and individuals wanting the test have no choice but to pay that price.

This patent was challenged by two New York City advocacy groups, and in 2013, the U.S. Supreme Court ruled that no one could patent parts of naturally occurring human DNA (genes). This ruling rendered the patent on the BRCA1 and 2 genes illegal, opening the door to other companies to offer this test—and at a cheaper price. Two other companies, including Ambry Genetics, immediately marketed a similar test at a lower cost. Myriad Genetics and its associate companies have launched an appeal to protect their rights to the patent against Ambry Genetics. The Hospital for Sick Children in Toronto and a Quebec research firm have been named in the lawsuit as co-owners of the patent with Myriad Genetics.

Source: Crowe, K. (2013, July 18). SickKids Hospital dragged into U.S. breast cancer gene suit. *CBC*. Retrieved from http://www.cbc.ca/news/health/sickkids-hospital-dragged-into-u-s-breast-cancer-gene-suit-1.1338880

Photo source: © Can Stock Photo Inc./Flik47.

SUMMARY

5.1 Ethics is the study of what is right and wrong in how we behave. It encompasses a number of principles including fairness, loyalty, and honesty. The study of ethics examines people's morals, values, and sense of duty. *Ethics* also refers to a code of conduct expected of a person in his or her professional role. In health care, it is important to respect the decisions of others even when those choices may not be congruent with your personal ethical code.

5.2 Understanding your own moral and ethical beliefs, your values, and your method of making ethical decisions will help you to understand your responses to ethical problems encountered in your professional role. Four ethical theories (teleological theory, deontological theory, virtue ethics, divine command) define how most people make ethical decisions, providing some explanation for decisions that individuals make about their own health or the health of those they love.

5.3 Six principles (beneficence and nonmaleficence, respect, autonomy, truthfulness, fidelity, and justice) provide the foundation for ethics in health care. Beneficence—doing what is right and good for the patient—dates back as far as the practice of medicine itself and figures in the Hippocratic Oath. Establishing a trusting relationship with patients and being respectful, honest, and truthful allow the patient to make his or her own decisions. This approach also supports the principle of autonomy, or the patient's right to self-determination. In most circumstances, paternalism is no longer acceptable in health care. Patients retain the right to have active treatment withdrawn, to refuse treatment, and to die with dignity.

5.4 A person's right to health care is sometimes ambiguous. Rights generally considered viable include the following: access to one's own health information; the right to confidentiality; the right to informed consent; the right to timely health care deemed medically necessary; and the right to have health care needs addressed in a timely manner.

5.5 Health care providers must establish and maintain therapeutic and respectful relationships with their patients. The balance of power that exists between a health care provider and a patient puts the patient in a vulnerable position in which feelings can be misinterpreted. Health care providers faced with a relationship issue must respect the codes of ethics of their profession, their employer, or both.

5.6 The decisions a person makes with respect to end-of-life issues can be both complex and controversial. A person's decisions are usually based on their personal code of ethics and may be influenced by the nature of their illness. A person may decide to refuse treatment or seek active methods to end his or her life (which is illegal in Canada). It is important for health care providers to respect the decisions a person makes, even if the decision is incongruent with one they would make for themselves in similar circumstances.

5.7 With health care costs continuing to rise, provinces and territories have become more conscious about where, when, and how to distribute resources, particularly when related to cost. Should the allocation of resources be based on need, cost-effectiveness, or the principle of equal distribution?

5.8 Many areas of health care (e.g., abortion, genetic testing, and the right to patent genes) cause controversy in the application of morals, values, and ethics. For the most part, no right or wrong answers exist—only what beliefs and values dictate. It is essential for health care providers to maintain an open mind, respect the rights of others to make their own decisions, and recognize that such respect can be achieved without compromising one's own beliefs and values.

Review Questions

1. Differentiate among ethics, morals, and values.
2. What is the purpose of an ethical theory?
3. How do deontological and teleological ethical theories differ?
4. How are paternalism and the principle of autonomy in opposition to each other?
5. Is role fidelity the same thing as functioning within one's scope of practice? Explain.
6. What is meant by the "balance of power" between a health care provider and a patient?
7. Explain the difference between a values history form and an advance directive.
8. How can palliative care provide an alternative for someone who is terminally ill and contemplating euthanasia or is seeking physician-assisted suicide?
9. What is meant by the "allocation of health resources," and why does it present an ethical problem?
10. How would you define "personhood"?
11. What rationale did the U.S. Supreme Court give for striking down patents on human genes?

References

Alberta Health Services. (n.d.). *Ethics framework*. Retrieved from http://www.albertahealthservices.ca/9879.asp.

Canadian Charter of Rights and Freedoms. (1982). s. 2, Part I of the Constitution Act, 1982, being Schedule B to the Canada Act 1982 (UK) c. 11.

Canadian Institute of Health Information. (2014, March). *Wait times for priority procedures in Canada, 2014*. Retrieved from https://secure.cihi.ca/free_products/2014_WaitTimesAiB_EN.pdf.

Canadian Medical Association. (1988). *Induced abortion. CMA Policy*. Retrieved from http://policybase.cma.ca/dbtw-wpd/PolicyPDF/PD88-06.pdf.

CBC News. (2010, December 6). "Compassionate homicide": The law and Robert Latimer. *CBC*. Retrieved from http://www.cbc.ca/news/canada/compassionate-homicide-the-law-and-robert-latimer-1.972561.

References

Flood, C., & Epps, T. (2002, November 20). *A patients' bill of rights: A cure for Canadians' concerns about health care*. Retrieved from http://irpp.org/research-studies/a-patients-bill-of-rights/.

Gollom, M. (2014, June 9). Will the end-of-life-care bill turn Quebec into a euthanasia tourist destination? *CBC*. Retrieved from http://www.cbc.ca/news/canada/will-the-end-of-life-care-bill-turn-quebec-into-a-euthanasia-tourist-destination-1.2667383.

Lovgren, S. (2005, October 13). One-fifth of human genes have been patented, study reveals. *National Geographic News*. Retrieved from http://news.nationalgeographic.com/news/2005/10/1013_051013_gene_patent.html.

N.B. v. Hôtel-Dieu de Québec. (1992). *Q.J. No. 1*.

Online Ethics Center for Engineering. (2006). What is ethics? *Ethics in the science classroom: An instructional guide for secondary school science teachers*. Retrieved from http://onlineethics.org/CMS/edu/precol/scienceclass/sectone/chapt2.aspx.

Rodriguez v. British Columbia (Attorney General). (1993). *Lamer CJC* 3 SCR 519.

Verkerk, M. (1999). A care perspective on coercion and autonomy. *Bioethics, 13*, 358–368.

Washington Ethical Society. (n.d.). *What does "ethics" mean?* Retrieved from http://www.ethicalsociety.org/article/19/about-wes/ethical-culture-our-religious-heritage/faqs-about-ethical-culture/what-does-ethics-mean.

CHAPTER SIX

The Role of Health Canada and Other Federal and International Health Agencies

 Learning Outcomes

6.1 Understand the basic objectives and responsibilities of Health Canada.

6.2 Describe the organization and responsibilities of Health Canada at the ministry level.

6.3 Summarize the organization and responsibilities of the key departments, branches, and bureaus of Health Canada.

6.4 Discuss the function of some of the independent agencies that report to the minister of health.

6.5 Summarize the function of major international organizations that collaborate with Health Canada.

Key Terms

Best practice, p. 205

Branch, p. 197

Bureau, p. 197

Central agency, p. 199

Consumer price index (CPI), p. 209

First Nations, p. 194

Hypoglycemic reaction, p. 203

Inuit, p. 194

Pandemic, p. 214

Patented drugs, p. 209

Risk assessment, p. 215

Severe acute respiratory syndrome (SARS), p. 193

How much influence does the federal government have over our health care? Who pays for health care for refugees who have not established residency in Canada? Are there any conditions on the extent of health care they receive? What department is responsible for licensing health products that come onto the market, and who is responsible for overseeing the safety of food, the use of insecticides on our crops, the type and the cost of medications on the market? What is in the flu vaccine, and why should we get it? Who makes recommendations to give the flu shot to babies? How does the World Health Organization (WHO) actually track health threats? What level of government is responsible for making recommendations regarding the numbers of nurses required across the country? To answer most of these questions, one must understand the role of the federal government in health care.

The federal, provincial, and territorial governments all play a part in health care. As noted in Chapter 1, the responsibilities of each were originally outlined in the *British North America Act* in 1867. Today, the federal government possesses little power over the health care of individual Canadians and absolutely no legal power over health care delivered in provincial and territorial jurisdictions. The provinces and territories continually guard their authority over health care in their individual relationships with the federal government. On the other hand, the provinces and territories want and need federal financial support, which comes with stipulations. In fact, it is through its control over medical and hospital care funding that the federal government exerts most of its influence.

The federal government also provides leadership, advice, and direction on health care issues on a national and international front. International issues require Health Canada to interact regularly with global organizations, particularly the WHO. For this reason, this chapter includes an overview of WHO, which has become more visible over the past several years, especially with respect to issuing warnings and bulletins about regional and global health threats. The **severe acute respiratory syndrome (SARS)** crisis in April 2003 and the H1N1 outbreak in 2009 are examples of such global health threats. The WHO continues to track the H1N1 virus, which caused some concern again in Canada during the 2013–2014 flu season.

This chapter examines the role of the federal government in health care, the hierarchical structure of Health Canada, and the functions of the various government departments and agencies. The chapter begins by looking at Health Canada's mission statement, philosophy, and commitment to health care in Canada. These pledges provide the foundation upon which the ministry was built and the values with which it strives to function. Despite the best of intentions, however, many issues are not addressed effectively and consistently, so problems with the Canadian health care system persist today.

> **Severe acute respiratory syndrome (SARS)**
> A severe form of pneumonia that first swept across parts of Asia and the Far East before spreading worldwide in 2003.

HEALTH CANADA: OBJECTIVES AND RESPONSIBILITIES

Health Canada, formerly known as the Department of Health and Welfare, is the federal government department responsible for health matters. Headed by a minister of health, it consists of a number of sub-departments organized into functional and administrative branches, agencies, offices, and sub-organizations. Since Health Canada's organizational structure changes frequently, this chapter discusses only the ministry's major components, with a focus on the primary responsibilities of each. Refer to the Health Canada Web site for information about any recent changes to the organizational structure.

Health Canada's detailed mission statement includes information about its purpose, values, and activities. It states that Health Canada is "committed to improving the lives of all of Canada's people and to making this country's population among the healthiest in the world as measured by longevity, lifestyle and effective use of the public health care system" (Health Canada, 2011a).

With a mandate to provide national leadership for health care and to maximize health promotion and disease prevention strategies, Health Canada has committed to working collaboratively with the provinces and territories on joint ventures such as creating policies and financing projects. The ministry manages funding policies and oversees the transfer of money and tax points (explained in Chapter 1) to the provinces and territories for health, education, and social programs. Health Canada also plays an authoritarian role, ensuring the provinces and territories remain compliant with the *Canada Health Act* and enforcing penalties on those that function outside of the principles within the Act. Health Canada may restrict funding to noncompliant provinces and territories.

As a service provider, Health Canada is responsible for health care for **Inuit** and **First Nations** communities and offers a variety of health services to selected population groups including some immigrants and refugee claimants, armed forces veterans, and correctional services employees. *Refugee claimants* are citizens of other countries who arrive in Canada claiming refugee status because they need protection from a threat or danger in their country of origin. Until a refugee claim is settled, the federal government retains responsibility for the claimant's health care needs. As well, the federal government, until recently, has been responsible for the health care needs of members of the Royal Canadian Mounted Police (RCMP). In 2012, however, the federal government introduced legislation (Bill C-38) that would shift this health care responsibility to the provinces and territories. The legislation includes numerous changes to the current health care package afforded to the RCMP.

First Nations Canadians on reserves and Inuit receive supplemental benefits, including medications, dental care, vision care, medical transportation, medical supplies and equipment, crisis intervention, and health counselling. Health Canada also provides primary care services in remote and isolated areas when the provincial or territorial government cannot meet these needs. Recent changes have decreased the services offered through the Interim Federal Health Program (IFHP), which authorizes basic health care coverage for protected persons, refugee claimants, and others who do not qualify for provincial or territorial coverage (In the News: Failed Refugee Applicants and the Provision of Health Care).

A primary source of information for Canadians, Health Canada conducts research projects and provides feedback on policy development. The ministry interacts with other nations and with the WHO to keep Canadians up to date on health concerns around the world. In conjunction with the WHO, Health Canada issues travel alerts and warnings for areas where health issues present cause for concern. The ministry also participates in producing and implementing national campaigns for health promotion and disease prevention, such as active lifestyle and anti-smoking campaigns.

> **Inuit**
> Aboriginal people in northern Canada living generally above the tree line in the Northwest Territories, Northern Quebec, and Labrador.
>
> **First Nations**
> A Canadian term of ethnicity referring to indigenous Canadians. The First Nations comprise 633 First Nations bands (usually registered as "Indians" under the *Indian Act*), representing 52 cultural groups and more than 50 languages (Assembly of First Nations, 2002). Other terms used include *Aboriginal*, *Native*, or *indigenous people*.

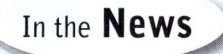 **Failed Refugee Applicants and the Provision of Health Care**

Canada's Interim Federal Health Program offers basic health care to some refugees, refugee claimants, and their dependents. In June 2012, the federal government changed the rules, reducing health care coverage for some refugee claimants and withdrawing even basic care for others. These changes affect individuals whose refugee claims have been rejected (including refugees from countries that are not recognized by the federal government as countries that produce refugees), leaving untold numbers of individuals in the country without access to basic health care. The coverage now includes only extreme emergency care and treatment for conditions that pose a threat to others. There are hundreds of stories of individuals badly needing care, going to a clinic or to the emergency department, and being told to either pay up front or leave. Most cannot afford to pay, so they leave without being seen.

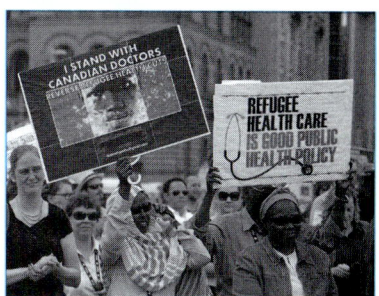

On January 1, 2014, Ontario and some other provinces implemented a temporary program allowing access to refugee claimants otherwise denied health care services, including most primary and urgent care services. The provinces will bill the federal government for services rendered. Then, in July 2014, the federal court ruled against the decision to cut back health care for refugee claimants, saying the decision was unconstitutional and amounted to cruel and unusual treatment.

Sources: Denying health care for refugees gives Canada a black eye [Editorial]. (2012, November 24). *Toronto Star*. Retrieved from http://www.thestar.com/opinion/editorials/2012/11/24/denying_health_care_for_refugees_gives_canada_a_black_eye.html; Canadian Council for Refugees. (n.d.). *Refugee healthcare: Interim Federal Health Program*. Retrieved from http://ccrweb.ca/en/ifh; Keung, N. (2013, December 9). Ontario reinstates basic health care for refugees. *Toronto Star*. Retrieved from http://www.thestar.com/news/canada/2013/12/09/ontario_reinstates_basic_health_care_for_refugees.html; Black, D. (2014, July 4). Court strikes down Conservatives' cuts to refugee health-care coverage. *Toronto Star*. Retrieved from http://www.thestar.com/news/canada/2014/07/04/court_rules_against_conservative_governments_refugee_health_cuts.html.

Photo Credit: The Canadian Press/Sean Kilpatrick.

HEALTH CANADA ORGANIZATION: MINISTRY LEVEL

The prime minister of Canada appoints an elected representative to head Health Canada as minister of health, a position that the prime minister can reassign at any time during the tenure of the party in power. The minister of health is responsible for "maintaining and improving the health of Canadians" (Health Canada, 2013). These responsibilities include overseeing more than 20 health-related laws and associated regulations. On occasion, the federal minister of health may also be responsible for other portfolios.

Responsibilities of the minister of health include:

- Overseeing Health Canada and other agencies, including the Public Health Agency of Canada, the Canadian Institutes of Health Research, the Hazardous Materials Information Review Commission, the Patented Medicine Prices Review Board, and Assisted Human Reproduction Canada
- Supervising the collection and analysis of information carried out under the *Statistics Act*
- Working collaboratively with the provincial and territorial governments

The federal minister does not routinely become involved in internal matters within the provinces or territories; however, establishing a positive working relationship with the first ministers (i.e., the provincial and territorial ministry heads) is essential for improving Canada's health care system across the country (Privy Council Office, 2011).

Rather than being an elected member of Parliament, the deputy minister of health is appointed from the civil service. The deputy minister works collaboratively with the minister of health, manages designated operations within the ministry, and may assume duties assigned to the minister of health if the minister is temporarily unavailable.

Several assistant deputy ministers of health and an associate deputy minister of health are also appointed from the civil service. Other agencies, such as the Departmental Secretariat and office of the chief public health officer, work collaboratively with the minister, deputy minister, and associate deputy minister. Their primary focus is to provide leadership to the Public Health Agency of Canada, whose principle mandate is to manage health promotion and health safety initiatives.

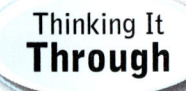

Officials of Health Canada are unelected employees that may work under the authority of many different governments. They are considered apolitical and remain in their positions even if a different party assumes power after an election.

1. Do you think having apolitical ministry employees is effective?
2. Would you rather see the deputy ministers of health be appointed from within the ranks of the party in power?

BRANCHES OF HEALTH CANADA

The organizational makeup of Health Canada is complex and sometimes confusing, in part because it features both an internal arm, which acts as a service provider for other groups under federal jurisdiction, and an external arm, which provides leadership for health care in the provinces and territories (see Figure 6.1).

More than 20 **branches**, offices, agencies, and **bureaus** operate within Health Canada. Some, such as the Departmental Secretariat, oversee the financing, function, and organization of Health Canada. Other divisions are more directly aligned with public initiatives and health care. The Audit and Accountability Bureau, the Chief Financial Officer Branch, and the Corporate Services Branch are responsible for, and work with, a number of sub-units. The following sections summarize only the most relevant functions of some of the branches.

Branch
A division of a main office offering extended or supportive functions.

Bureau
Government department responsible for a specific entity or duty.

INTERNAL SERVICES

Departmental Secretariat

An executive office to which other departments report, the Departmental Secretariat acts as the link between the executive (appointed) and the political (elected) levels of Health Canada. This department clarifies, redirects, or responds to communications received from other divisions of Health Canada (e.g., providing briefing notes for members of Parliament, providing answers to questions raised in the House of Commons, addressing requests that fall under the *Access to Information Act* and *Privacy Act*). Clients of the Departmental Secretariat include offices of the minister, deputy minister(s), and associate deputy minister.

Audit and Accountability Bureau

The Audit and Accountability Bureau (AAB) is Health Canada's internal monitoring system. The bureau conducts internal audits and reports to the Departmental Audit and Evaluation Committee. The AAB reviews different departments and bureaus to ensure that they are operating properly, in accordance with their mandate, and in a cost effective manner. Working with provinces and territories, the AAB ensures that money the government gives out as grants is used as intended.

Chief Financial Officer Branch

The Chief Financial Officer Branch (CFOB) is made up of several organizational units. The CFOB oversees the use of Health Canada's departmental resources and ensures finances are spent wisely and efficiently. It also ensures other departments and organizational units adhere to government policies and regulations; coordinates the management of risk; enhances performance measurement and

Figure 6.1 Health Canada Organizational Chart

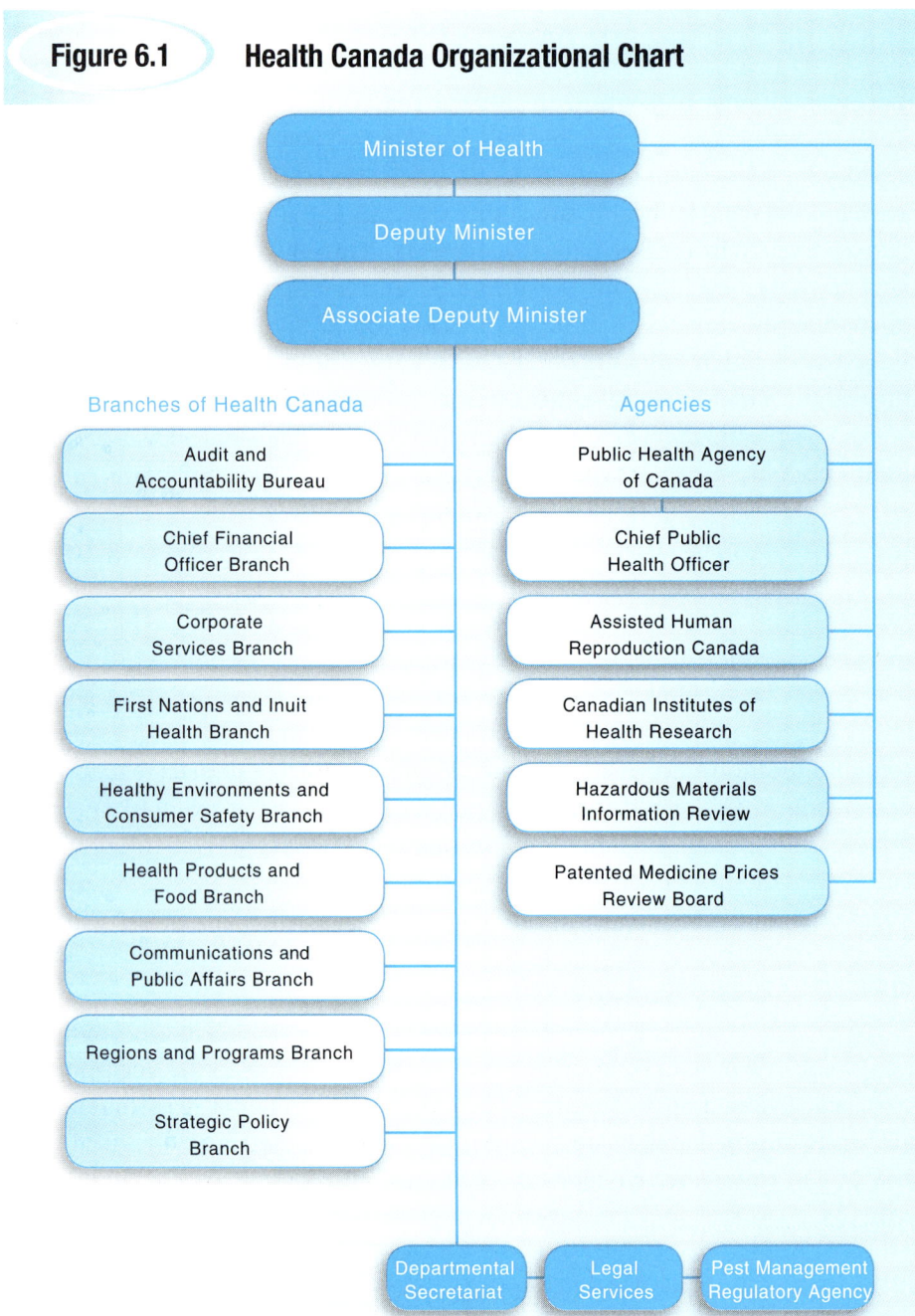

Source: Health Canada. (2014). *About Health Canada: Branches and agencies*. © All rights reserved. Health Canada. Reproduced with permission from the Minister of Health, 2014.

reporting; and monitors the execution of the accountability framework. As well, the CFOB oversees the financial management of **central agencies** including the Public Health Agency of Canada.

Corporate Services Branch

Composed of several directorates, the Corporate Services Branch (CSB) provides support and services to Health Canada in such areas as human resources management; occupational health safety, emergency, and security management; access to information and privacy matters; and information technology. This department also supports the *Official Languages Act*, providing language training and support and managing related complaints.

The CSB provides advice and guidance to the Human Resources Services Directorate on human resources management issues, and collaboratively manages occupational health and safety alongside occupational health and safety committees.

Working with the Information Management Services Directorate, the CSB helps to ensure effective use of the information technology used to deliver Health Canada's programs and services. The department also provides support for Health Canada infrastructure, including its computer systems, across the country.

Legal Services

Reporting to the Department of Justice, Legal Services employs lawyers to provide legal advice and other legal services to Health Canada. Through this unit, Health Canada can access specialized services provided by the Department of Justice, including advisory services relating to information privacy laws, administrative laws, and constitutional and criminal laws.

EXTERNAL SERVICES

Health Canada's external services consist of a variety of offices, directorates, branches, and other organizations. The structures, names, services, and related policies of these sub-departments change frequently. Several are discussed here. For current, more detailed information, visit Health Canada's Web site.

First Nations and Inuit Health Branch

The First Nations and Inuit Health Branch oversees the delivery of primary health care services to Aboriginal peoples, including public health and health promotion on First Nations reserves and within Inuit communities, as well as services provided to Aboriginal populations who do not live within Inuit communities or on reserves.

The branch also manages federal funding for health care services to these populations and works collaboratively with Aboriginal provincial and territorial councils to ensure high-quality health care. Providing adequate services remains

> **Central agency**
> An organization or department with the authority to direct or intervene in the activities of other departments. Central agencies aid with policy development and the coordination of activities.

a challenge, given Aboriginals' unique needs with respect to geography, demographics, population distribution, and other factors, such as lifestyle and mortality.

Strategic Policy Branch

The Strategic Policy Branch (SPB) develops and implements the federal government's and Health Canada's health care policies, including administering the *Canada Health Act*, creating health protection regulations and legislation, dealing with evolving problems on a priority basis, and authorizing new agencies to report information as required.

The SPB's programs are carried out by several offices and directorates, some of which are outlined below.

Health Care Policy Directorate

The Health Care Policy Directorate, an organization within the SPB, plays a key role in *reshaping primary health care delivery* with the objective of preserving the principles and conditions of the *Canada Health Act*. The directorate also assesses provinces' and territories' need for financial support for primary health care reform initiatives. The directorate monitors and analyzes the provision of community-based, continuing, and palliative care across Canada and gathers information that Health Canada uses to develop policies and initiatives that will assist the provinces and territories to improve health care in those areas.

Office of the Chief Scientist

The Office of the Chief Scientist helps to ensure that Health Canada has appropriate scientific information to make health-related decisions; provides leadership regarding decisions about potential health risks; and tracks the spread of diseases such as West Nile virus, SARS, mad cow disease (Creutzfeldt-Jakob disease), and the H1N1 virus.

Working with the Healthy Environments and Consumer Safety Branch and the Health Products and Food Branch, the Office of the Chief Scientist also helps to ensure that all products introduced to the Canadian market meet national standards of safety and abide by Canadian rules and regulations. The office assists 50 research and diagnostic laboratories across Canada, which conduct research in a wide variety of areas, including fields as diverse as natural resources and medicine.

Office of Nursing Policy

Created in 1999, the Office of Nursing Policy reflects the importance of nursing policy issues within health care. This office provides advice to Health Canada on select policy issues and programs from the nursing perspective and makes recommendations regarding the nursing workforce to help meet health care service needs. For example, it recommended hiring specially trained nurse practitioners to provide lower-cost comprehensive care in underserved areas. The Office of Nursing Policy also develops strategies to retain nurses by addressing issues such as burnout and frustration related to the occupational environment.

Health Products and Food Branch

The Health Products and Food Branch (HPFB) oversees several bureaus and directorates, including the Office of Nutrition Policy and Promotion, the Food Directorate, Health Products and Food Branch Inspectorate, and the Marketed Health Products Directorate. The branch reviews the health-related risks and benefits of drugs, vaccines, medical devices, natural health products, food, and veterinary drugs. The HPFB also grants licences for the sale, distribution, and use of products and for the application of therapies deemed safe and ensures Canadians have the information necessary to make independent, informed choices. Organizations and individuals must apply to have a product or device approved and licensed for use or sale in Canada. Such approval is necessary for both invasive (e.g., the collection of blood products through apheresis) and noninvasive products (e.g., recently introduced eSight glasses, one of the most significant technological advances for those with poor vision). Without the approval of Health Canada, such services and devices would not be marketable in the country. The many responsibilities and activities of the HPFB are carried out by several directorates and offices across the country, some of which are discussed below.

Office of Nutrition Policy and Promotion

The HPFB's Office of Nutrition Policy and Promotion develops the policies and standards for nutrition recommended in *Eating Well With Canada's Food Guide*. The food guide has evolved through years of research and collaboration with specialists from a variety of fields. A new guide adapted to the needs and lifestyles of First Nations, Inuit, and Métis populations has also been released (Box 6.1).

Food Directorate

The Food Directorate regulates the safety and nutritional quality of food in Canada. The directorate monitors additives used in food products (e.g., aspartame, vitamins, and other nutrients); genetically modified products; and methods of processing and packaging foods.

Therapeutic Products Directorate

Any company, group, or person wanting to introduce a new drug or medical device for use by Canadians must first receive permission from the Therapeutic

> **Box 6.1** **The First Ever Food Guide for First Nations, Inuit, and Métis**
>
> In April 2007, the first ever national food guide for First Nations, Inuit, and Métis populations, *Eating Well With Canada's Food Guide—First Nations, Inuit and Métis*, was launched in Yellowknife. "This is the first time that Canada's Food Guide has been tailored nationally to reflect the unique values, traditions, and food choices of Aboriginal populations," said then minister of health Tony Clement. "As a complement to the new 2007 version of Canada's Food Guide, this tailored food guide includes traditional food from the land and sea, and provides the best, most current information for eating well and living healthy."
>
> © All rights reserved. Health Canada, 2007. Reproduced with permission from the Minister of Health, 2014.

Products Directorate (TPD). The applicant must present an array of information about the product, including evidence regarding the related risks and benefits. The TPD oversees several branches and services, including the Medical Devices Bureau.

Marketed Health Products Directorate

Through the Marketed Health Products Directorate (MHPD), Health Canada collects information about adverse reactions to foods and food products and ensures that the public is aware of any identified risks. Through MedEffect, a program developed by the MHPD, Canadians can report adverse effects of and obtain safety information on health products and drugs (for online reporting, see Web Resources on Evolve). The Canada Vigilance Program—which functions under MedEffect and is the point of contact for health care providers and consumers—collects and assesses all reports of suspected adverse reactions to health products marketed in Canada (Health Canada, 2011b). Information can be submitted via an online form. This information allows Health Canada to continually gauge the safety of health products once they are available to consumers. And if, for example, a product's adverse effects outweigh its benefits, Health Canada will act to remove the product from the market, either to reassess and modify it or to ban it completely. Any medically related products and treatment options—therapies and products alike—rendered, used, sold, or otherwise distributed in Canada must be licensed by Health Canada (In the News: Revolutionary Eyewear Gives Visually Impaired People a New "Look" at Life).

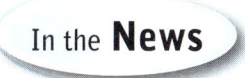

Revolutionary Eyewear Gives Visually Impaired People a New "Look" at Life

New high-tech glasses to aid the visually impaired were recently licensed for use and distribution by Health Canada. The glasses use a video camera, a computer, and LED screens to capture and process images in a manner that significantly increases the sight of individuals with central vision loss, including those with conditions such as macular degeneration, Stargardt disease, and diabetic retinopathy.

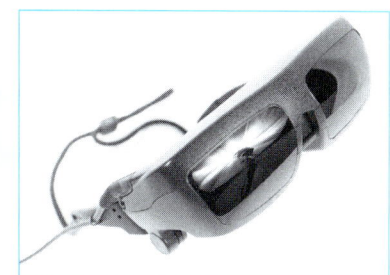

Sources: Ontario.ca. (n.d.). *Success stories—eSight: Groundbreaking digital eyewear helps the blind to see.* Retrieved from http://www.investinontario.com/en/Pages/OS_lifesciences_success_stories_esight.aspx.

Photo Credit: Courtesy of eSight Corp.

Natural Health Products Directorate

The Natural Health Products Directorate regulates all health products containing natural ingredients, including homeopathic medicines, vitamins and minerals, and traditional medicines. The regulations summarize and enforce licensing requirements for natural health products as well as stipulate packaging and labelling requirements—for example, product packaging must state health claims, ingredients, instructions for use, and potential adverse effects. Natural health product manufacturers must document and report any adverse reactions identified by consumers. Health Canada has the authority to request label changes and to remove any natural health product from the market at any time.

Despite these regulatory efforts, the use of natural products remains a concern to many health care providers across Canada. Not all consumers realize that a *natural* product may contain harmful ingredients or interfere with prescription medications. For example, combining a prescription antidepressant with St. John's wort (an herbal mood elevator) can cause nausea, vomiting, restlessness, dizziness, and headaches. St. John's wort can also reduce the effectiveness of oral contraceptives. Ginseng, another popular herbal medication, can increase blood pressure so should not be taken by someone with hypertension or someone on antihypertensive medication. Even garlic, when taken with hypoglycemic medications (used by people with diabetes), can cause a drop in blood sugar and, possibly, a **hypoglycemic reaction**.

Hypoglycemic reaction
A response to a drop in blood sugar levels. The symptoms may include mild weakness or dizziness; headache; cold, clammy, or sweaty skin; problems concentrating; shakiness; uncoordinated movements or staggering; blurred vision; irritability; hunger; fainting; and loss of consciousness.

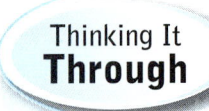
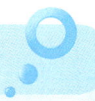

Thinking It Through

A patient tells you that she is taking a number of herbal medications, including synthetic estrogen preparations and metabolism boosters. She found on the Internet that these medications were recommended to combat fatigue and sluggishness. She believes it is unnecessary to tell her physician. As an allied health care provider, how would you respond?

Healthy Environments and Consumer Safety Branch

The Healthy Environments and Consumer Safety Branch (HECSB) develops and supports programs that promote a safe, healthy lifestyle and environment for Canadians. The HECSB provides information about the risks and benefits of various products and lifestyle habits with the goal of helping Canadians make constructive choices (e.g., an active lifestyle, healthy nutritional habits, and avoidance of self-imposed risks behaviours such as tobacco, drug, and alcohol use). The HECSB is also concerned with other matters, including drinking-water quality, air quality, and the use of smoke detectors. A number of programs operate within the HECSB. Some are discussed below.

Safe Environments Program

The Safe Environments Program (SEP) identifies and assesses health risks to Canadians posed by environmental factors in an effort to promote healthy living, working, and recreational environments.

Drug Strategy and Controlled Substances Program

The Drug Strategy and Controlled Substances Program regulates the use and distribution of narcotics and other controlled drugs in Canada, primarily through the *Controlled Drugs and Substances Act* and narcotic control regulations. The program's responsibilities include licensing pharmaceutical companies that manufacture and distribute drugs and controlled substances and tracking the movement of drugs and controlled substances inside and outside the country. When individuals seek special permission to use specific controlled drugs for a health condition—for example, marijuana to control pain—the Drug Strategy and Controlled Substances Program manages these requests. The process for obtaining such permission is discussed in more depth in Chapter 4.

Tobacco Control Program

The Tobacco Control Program aims to reduce tobacco use in Canada by regulating the manufacture and sale of tobacco products, which has included implementing rules about the labelling of packages (e.g., the graphic anti-smoking warnings on cigarette packages). The program also works with provincial and territorial governments on anti-smoking media campaigns.

Product Safety Program

Before they reach the Canadian market, most products—products as diverse as children's toys and cosmetics—are researched and assessed by the Product Safety Program. Responsibilities of this unit also include researching and evaluating ultraviolet radiation, radiation-emitting devices (e.g., those used in some diagnostic tests), and workplace chemicals.

Regions and Programs Branch

The Regions and Programs Branch of Health Canada comprises the regions, the Workplace Health and Public Safety Program, and the Programs Directorate.

Regions

Health Canada has divided Canada into eight regions: British Columbia, Alberta, Saskatchewan, Manitoba, Quebec, Ontario, the Atlantic Region, and the Northern Region. Each Health Canada region is headed by a regional director general, who reports to the assistant deputy minister of health. The regional director general ensures that services meet the needs of the region and are not duplicated. An important aspect of the regional director general's job is to maintain a positive working relationship with provincial or territorial groups.

Although the activities and programs (e.g., promotion of healthy environments and consumer safety, regulation of health products and food) launched by Health Canada in the various regions bear similarities, each region faces diverse challenges related to demographics and geography. For example, some regions have a greater need for alcohol- and drug-abuse prevention programs, drug and dental coverage, vision plans, and transportation services to treatment centres. In many northern regions, water quality and other environmental issues present particular concern, so Health Canada employs environmental health officers to deal with these problems.

Workplace Health and Public Safety Program

The Workplace Health and Public Safety Program promotes a **best practices** philosophy in the workplace with the goal of encouraging physically safe and emotionally positive workplace environments. The program recommends that managers and administrators ensure employees are healthy and fit enough to handle jobs assigned to them and encourages the implementation of office ergonomics: a well-designed desk and chair, appropriate lighting, and a safe computer workstation.

> **Best practices**
> Guidelines outlining treatments, procedures, or policies deemed to be most effective.

The Workplace Health and Public Safety Program also assumes responsibility for the health and safety of federal employees and for visiting dignitaries and politicians. To achieve this goal, the program collaborates with a number of departments, including the Emergency Preparedness and Response Unit, a group formed to respond to terrorist acts anywhere in Canada, be they biological, radiological, chemical, or nuclear.

Programs Directorate

Also under the umbrella of the Regions and Programs Branch, the Programs Directorate is responsible for a number of organizations, including the Canada Health Act Division, which provides policy advice related to the Act, monitors activities in the provinces and territories to assess their compliance with the principles and conditions of the Act, and reports any incidents of noncompliance to the minister of health. Any province or territory may engage in activities that are not compliant with the *Canada Health Act* as long as these activities are authorized by the provincial or territorial government. However, the consequence of noncompliance may be restriction of federal funding. The Canada Health Act Division produces a year-end report that details each province's or territory's obedience to the principles and conditions of the Act (Health Canada, 2011c).

Public Affairs, Consultation and Communications Branch

The Public Affairs, Consultation and Communications Branch (PACCB) performs a number of duties involving communication activities and responsibilities. Offices within this branch include Ethics and Internal Ombudsman Services and the Planning and Operations Division. Ethics and Internal Ombudsman Services acts as a confidential and unbiased resource for any employee within Health Canada, offering guidance and information about work-related concerns, regardless of occupation, title, or employment status. The Planning and Operations Division provides leadership to the PACCB with respect to human resources, contracts, finances, and strategic planning. Other offices of the branch are discussed below.

Public Affairs and Strategic Communications Directorate

The Public Affairs and Strategic Communications Directorate plays an important role in maintaining communication both within Health Canada and outside of it—that is, with the public, the provinces and territories, nongovernment groups, and international associations and governments.

Within this directorate, the Public Affairs Division, the ministry's first point of contact for the media, coaches and prepares Health Canada spokespersons to speak to the media. The Health Canada Web site provides a detailed list of telephone numbers and e-mail addresses to facilitate media contact with the organization.

Also within this directorate, the Horizontal Coordination Division manages communication across Health Canada; oversees external communication; and deals with issues related to access to information.

Marketing and Communications Services Directorate

The Marketing and Communications Services Directorate comprises the Web, Internal, and Corporate Communications Division; the Social Marketing Unit; and the Public Opinion Research and Evaluation Unit.

The Web, Internal, and Corporate Communications Division maintains the Health Canada Web site, which consists of more than 60,000 pages—an enormous task indeed. In 2005, the Web site was reorganized, with more than 100 sites being merged into one. This division also processes all public inquiries addressed to Health Canada.

The Social Marketing Unit manages all of Health Canada's advertising agencies. The unit is responsible for campaigns seeking to raise the public's awareness of certain disease risks and to encourage Canadians to develop healthy lifestyles.

Together with the Public Health Agency of Canada and Health Canada scientists, the PACCB publishes a bulletin called *It's Your Health*, which delivers information and articles to the general public on a variety of health-related topics.

The Public Opinion Research and Evaluation Unit conducts public opinion research, gathering information that is critical for helping Health Canada to understand Canadians' health-related needs, perceptions of health, and expectations about health.

Pest Management Regulatory Agency

Pesticides are used in various forms all across Canada—for example, to control species of mosquitoes that carry the West Nile virus, to protect agricultural crops from disease and infestation, and to keep lawns free from weeds, destructive insects, and other pests. Many pesticides, however, are harmful to the environment, wildlife, and humans.

The Pest Management Regulatory Agency (PMRA) evaluates all pesticides in Canada before allowing them on the market. They must meet Health Canada's safety standards and be used in accordance to instructions dictated by the PMRA. Products on the market are routinely re-evaluated to ensure they continue to meet safety standards.

AGENCIES OF HEALTH CANADA

Several independent agencies of Health Canada report directly to the minister of health. The functions of some are described below.

Canadian Institutes of Health Research

The Canadian Institutes of Health Research (CIHR) directs and funds research across Canada. CIHR distributes research funding based on priority and need, expanding research as required (e.g., in population health and health services research) and recruiting and training research scientists. CIHR is also responsible for ensuring that the research information gathered and analyzed is used properly—for example, to craft policies or to generate products and services for which a need has been determined.

CIHR operates 13 research institutes nationwide (Box 6.2 contains a list of these facilities) with a multimillion-dollar funding budget. More than 10,000 scientists and researchers in various hospitals, universities, and research institutes are involved with the agency. Targeted, ongoing, health-based research projects include those related to biomedical research, clinical science, and health care systems and services (Canadian Institutes of Health Research, 2014).

Box 6.2   CIHR Institutes Across Canada

Aboriginal Peoples' Health
Aging
Cancer Research
Circulatory and Respiratory Health
Gender and Health
Genetics
Health Services and Policy Research
Human Development, Child and Youth Health
Infection and Immunity
Musculoskeletal Health and Arthritis
Neurosciences, Mental Health, and Addiction
Nutrition, Metabolism, and Diabetes
Population and Public Health

Source: Canadian Institutes of Health Research. (2013). *CIHR institutes*. Retrieved from http://www.cihr-irsc.gc.ca/e/9466.html#a.

Hazardous Materials Information Review Commission

The Hazardous Materials Information Review Commission (HMIRC) aims to protect workers in the province while also protecting the participating industry's trade secrets. HMIRC is responsible for setting standards, policies, and rules for workplace safety.

The Workplace Hazardous Materials Information System (WHMIS), a combination of laws, regulations, and procedures, helps to reduce workplace injury and illness resulting from the use of hazardous chemicals. WHMIS represents a coordinated effort among the federal, provincial, and territorial governments to standardize workplace safety across the country. Through WHMIS, employers are obligated to supply employees with the training and knowledge to allow them to work safely with hazardous materials. Most individuals entering an occupational setting are required to take a WHMIS course and write a test before beginning employment.

Patented Medicine Prices Review Board

The Patented Medicine Prices Review Board (PMPRB), created in 1987, is a "watch" agency that monitors the prices of **patented drugs** to ensure fairness to both manufacturer and consumer. This board operates independently of other organizations within Health Canada that deal with product safety and inspection. The board reviews the prices at which the manufacturer sells patented drugs to wholesalers, hospitals, and pharmacies. Pricing is determined in several ways:

- Pricing is subject to guidelines in the *Patent Act*.
- Drugs used to treat the same disease are generally priced similarly. Revolutionary drugs, which have no measures of comparison, are priced in line with similar products used in other countries.
- Using the **consumer price index (CPI)**, the PMPRB considers previous prices of similar drugs against the current price of those same drugs.

If a manufacturer is thought to be overcharging for a drug, the board will first offer the manufacturer an opportunity to voluntarily adjust its pricing. If the company refuses, a judicial hearing may take place, with a binding federal court decision resulting.

The PMPRB is not involved with the pricing of generic drugs, which are traditionally significantly less expensive than "brand-name" drugs. However, what provinces and territories spend on generic drugs fluctuates dramatically. A recent agreement among jurisdictions to buy some generic drugs in bulk has reduced prices for selected drugs (In the News: Agreement Reduces the Cost of Generic Drugs).

Patented drugs
Drugs that are legally protected from generic production for a period of 20 years from the date of filing.

Consumer price index (CPI)
A method of determining changes in the cost of goods and services through the monitoring of selected items (e.g., food, rent, mortgages, gasoline) across Canada. Used to measure inflation, the CPI may affect such payments as social security, spousal support, and rent, which are periodically adjusted to reflect the CPI.

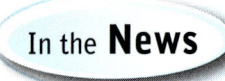

Agreement Reduces the Cost of Generic Drugs

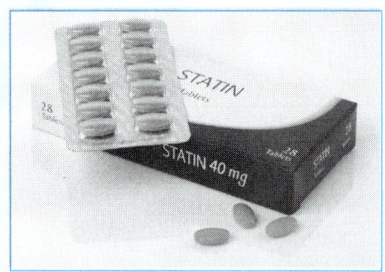

Under an agreement reached by the Council of the Federation's Health Care Innovation Working Group in 2013, provinces and territories (except Quebec) will pay less for six commonly used generic drugs by purchasing them in bulk. Currently, jurisdictions pay anywhere from 25% to 40% of the brand-name prices for these selected drugs. Under the new agreement, the price will drop to 18%, a savings across the board of $100 million annually. The six drugs involved are primarily for gastrointestinal ailments, depression, and heart disease.

Sources: Lunn, S. (2013, January 18). Provinces reach deal to save on 6 generic drugs. *CBC*. Retrieved from http://www.cbc.ca/news/politics/provinces-reach-deal-to-save-on-6-generic-drugs-1.1331370; Miller, S. (2013, January 18). Provinces reach a deal to buy six generic drugs at a lower cost. *Humber News*. Retrieved from http://humberjournalism.com/humbernews/provinces-reach-a-deal-to-buy-six-generic-drugs-at-a-lower-cost/7340.

Photo Credit: © Can Stock Photo Inc./rogera.

Public Health Agency of Canada

Created in 2004 and headed by Canada's chief public health officer, the Public Health Agency of Canada (PHAC) has a mandate to promote health and prevent diseases, including chronic infirmities such as cardiorespiratory conditions and cancer. The PHAC also aims to reduce accidents, prevent injuries, and respond to other public health issues, such as health emergencies and infectious disease outbreaks.

The PHAC promotes strategies for healthy pregnancies, campaigns for active lifestyles, and initiatives to combat childhood obesity and diabetes. In Canada, most Web-based data regarding health issues are organized and posted by the PHAC (a function formerly carried out by the Canadian Health Network, a national Internet-based health information service funded by the PHAC).

In terms of "health watch" activities, the PHAC tracks outbreaks of seasonal flu, tuberculosis, measles, and other illnesses and recommends corrective and preventive measures. Worth special mention is a branch called the Centre for Infectious Disease Prevention and Control (CIDPC), which has several departments, including the Blood Safety Surveillance and Health Care Acquired Infections Division and the Community Acquired Infections Division. CIDPC works closely with other agencies, such as the Centers for Disease Control and Prevention (CDC) in the United States.

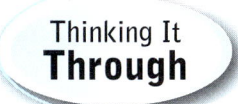

Billions of dollars are spent annually on research, development, and clinical trials to test the safety and effectiveness of new drugs. Patent protection allows pharmaceutical firms 20 years to make a profit on drugs they have brought to market. Companies that produce generic drugs, however, are pushing for a reduction in patent protection time so they can bring cheaper, generic brands of patented drugs to market earlier.

1. Do you think that the patent protection time frame should be reduced?

2. Bearing in mind the tremendous cost of bringing the original drug to market, should pharmaceutical firms receive compensation for the money lost to them if generic drugs are brought to market earlier?

Assisted Human Reproduction Canada

As of October 1, 2012, Assisted Human Reproduction Canada (AHRC) no longer functions as an agency reporting to the minister of health. The dissolution of this agency was in response to the 2010 ruling of the Supreme Court of Canada significantly reducing the federal role in developing policy and regulations related to assisted human reproduction.

INTERNATIONAL HEALTH AGENCIES WORKING WITH HEALTH CANADA

Health Canada collaborates with international health agencies and governments by sharing current information about new technologies and medications, identifying and tracking health risks, and helping to contain outbreaks of potentially damaging diseases.

World Health Organization

The United Nations' authority on health issues, the WHO provides leadership in health matters on a global level. The organization spearheads global research, provides technical support to members, monitors and assesses health trends, and sets standards within the fields of health and medicine. The WHO recommends policies and actions regarding population health initiatives to countries around the world. It is also instrumental in gathering information and producing statistics on health matters at an international level. In 2014, the Ebola outbreak in Africa prompted the WHO to issue a global alert. The WHO was then asked to make a decision on the ethics of using unproven vaccines to treat individuals with and in danger of contracting the disease. It ruled that using the vaccine was ethical, prompting Canada and other nations to ship vaccines to affected areas.

A total of 194 countries compose the membership of the WHO. Each member country of the United Nations may become a member of the WHO by accepting its constitution. Countries outside the United Nations may be admitted as members if their applications are approved by a majority vote of the World Health Assembly. Jurisdictions without responsibility for their international affairs (regions within a country, for example) may become associate members if approved.

To respond to an increasingly complex world, the WHO has developed a six-point agenda (Box 6.3).

Box 6.3   The World Health Organization: The Six-Point Agenda

1. *Promoting health development.* Giving priority to those countries and regions affected by poverty and socioeconomic inequities and other disadvantaged and vulnerable groups.
2. *Fostering health security.* Tracking and responding to outbreaks of epidemic-prone diseases and implementing measures to control and perhaps eliminate these threats.
3. *Strengthening health systems.* Working to extend health services to all those in need; implementing strategies to reduce poverty and to diminish those elements identified by population health initiatives that contribute to poor health.
4. *Harnessing research, information, and evidence.* Gathering and distributing relevant health information and using this information to set priorities, shape approaches and plans, and target outcomes.
5. *Enhancing partnerships.* Working collaboratively with organizations, including UN agencies, international organizations, and the private sector, to launch health initiatives and programs within countries; making the best use of available resources and facilities.
6. *Improving performance.* Working to continually improve each organization's effectiveness in meeting its goals and its many responsibilities.

Reproduced, with the permission of the publisher, from *The WHO agenda 2008*. World Health Organization. (2008). Retrieved from http://www.who.int/about/agenda/en/.

International Coding Systems

The purpose of an international coding system is to enable the **global** community to collect, classify, and compare health information (e.g., mortality statistics) in a consistent and standardized format.

ICD-10 is the Tenth Revision of the International Classification of Diseases (ICD). The classification system started in September 1983 and is the official international classification system. It is used primarily by WHO member states. ICD-10 addresses a broader scope of health information than previous versions. For example, it includes the classification of conditions and risk factors. Data is organized classified using a series of alphanumeric codes (e.g., Z56.3. is the code for a stressful work schedule). The latest version, ICD-11 should be complete by 2015. This version will be Web based and will better support the exchange of electronic information.

National Databases

Most countries also have coding systems that meet internal (national) needs, but with components that interconnect with the ICD system. For example, ICD-10-CA is an enhanced version of ICD-10 developed with the permission of the WHO and used exclusively in Canada to classify morbidity rates.

The companion classification to ICD-10-CA for coding procedures and interventions in Canada is the Canadian Classification of Health Interventions (CCI). Developed and maintained by the Canadian Institute for Health Information (CIHI), the CCI is used by most provinces and territories to categorize a broad range of health information (e.g., interventions for ambulatory care services, a variety of diagnostic procedures, counselling, and environmental assessments).

The Discharge Abstract Database (DAD) is a national database that contains information on all separations from acute care institutions in Canada, including discharges, deaths, sign-outs, and transfers. Over time, the DAD has also been used to capture data about day surgery procedures, long-term care, rehabilitation, and other services.

Another national database, the National Ambulatory Care Reporting System (NACRS), contains information on visits to emergency and ambulatory care clinics (e.g., outpatient clinics) in Canada. Ambulatory care services generate one of the largest volume-based activities in health care. The NACRS database includes demographic, administrative, and service-specific data elements. Although some jurisdictions across Canada use the DAD for collecting day surgery activity, the NACRS was developed to accommodate day surgery activity as well. Each province and territory determines the database to which it reports day surgery procedures.

These databases are just two of the databases that rely on ICD-10-CA and CCI classifications; they are exclusive to CIHI for national reporting.

ICD-10-CA and CCI codes are applied and organized by highly trained health information specialists throughout the country. Note that detailed information on all of these systems can be found on the CIHI Web site.

Pandemic Alerts

Outbreaks of influenza are recurrent but unpredictable events that can have serious effects on global and national economies as well as on the health of populations. It is the responsibility of the WHO to monitor the threat of potential global disease (a **pandemic**) and issue appropriate alerts based on specific criteria as outlined in its guidelines (often just referred to as Guidance). The Guidance for pandemic alerts, put together by health and policy experts, incorporates principles from other strategic initiatives, including principles from the WHO's all-hazards emergency risk management for health (ERMH) and from its International Health Regulations (IHR). The new Guidance reinforces the ERMH assertion that member states must have the ability to respond to all health hazards. The IHR is a legally binding agreement for member states that details procedures and policies for managing public health threats. The WHO has revised its pandemic guidelines three times since 1999 and most recently in 2013, incorporating lessons learned from the 2009 AH1N1 pandemic. Changes include the following:

- Four phases of alert (instead of six), which have been simplified and streamlined (Box 6.4).

> **Pandemic**
> A sustained, worldwide human-to-human transmission of disease.

Box 6.4 WHO 2013 Four-Phase Alert System

Interpandemic phase: This is the period between influenza pandemics.

Alert phase: This is the phase when influenza caused by a new subtype has been identified in humans. Increased vigilance and careful risk assessment, at local, national, and global levels, are characteristic of this phase. If the risk assessments indicate that the new virus is not developing into a pandemic strain, a de-escalation of activities towards those in the interpandemic phase may occur.

Pandemic phase: This is the period of global spread of human influenza caused by a new subtype. Movement between the interpandemic, alert, and pandemic phases may occur quickly or gradually as indicated by the global risk assessment, principally based on virological, epidemiological, and clinical data.

Transition phase: As the assessed global risk reduces, de-escalation of global actions may occur, and reduction in response activities or movement towards recovery actions by countries may be appropriate, according to their own risk assessments.

Reproduced, with the permission of the publisher, from *Pandemic influenza risk management: WHO Interim guidance*, p. 7. Geneva, Switzerland. World Health Organization. (2013). Retrieved from http://www.who.int/influenza/preparedness/pandemic/GIP_PandemicInfluenzaRiskManagementInterimGuidance_Jun2013.pdf?ua=1.

- A greater emphasis on the **risk assessment** rather than on geographic location, allowing affected regions to respond accordingly, instead of at the highest level to a threat resulting in unnecessarily stockpiling antiviral medications and vaccines. The severity of an outbreak in one area is likely to be different from that in another, and responses should be levelled to suit the national, regional, or local conditions.
- Improved communication among countries and decision-making bodies, particularly between those making risk assessments, and improved communication with the general public about regional outbreaks (e.g., containment issues, severity, progress, treatment protocols).
- Emphasis on the importance of having national and regional strategies in place to deal effectively with outbreaks, rather than relying exclusively on global strategies. During the 2009 pandemic, some member states responded immediately to the WHO's pandemic phase alerts, triggering such reactions as high-volume purchases of vaccines only to find that the numbers purchased were far in excess of what was needed.

> **Risk assessment**
> The assessment or examination of a condition or a situation to determine the potential harm or hazards (risk) related to it (e.g., the risk for having an accident if you drive a car in a snowstorm).

SARS, the WHO, and Canada

The WHO warnings first affected Canada in a significant and direct way during the SARS crisis of 2003. Although this event occurred more than a decade ago, it has had a prolonged and profound effect on emergency preparedness in Canada, as well as in other countries. SARS did not become a pandemic.

Estimates state that SARS affected 8000 people worldwide, killing 800, 44 of those in Canada out of the 375 recorded cases, all in Ontario (Ontario Ministry of Health and Long-Term Care, 2004). SARS brought Ontario and much of Canada economically to its knees when the WHO issued an alert warning people against travel to Canada. Canada clearly was not ready to effectively handle this calamity. With many questions unanswered regarding Canada's response to, containment of, and management of the crisis, Mr. Justice Archie Campbell was charged with investigating the country's response to the SARS crisis. His final report was released on January 9, 2007. He concluded that the handling (or mishandling) of the situation fell on the shoulders of many individuals, as well as on departments and agencies across the health care system. He concluded that the SARS crisis was further worsened by inadequate, ineffective policies and procedures—in effect, the health care system itself—which led to errors in judgement, treatment, and containment (through isolation), as well as to inadequate protection for health care workers, especially nurses (SARS Commission, 2006).

It has been over ten years since the SARS outbreak. Canada, along with countries around the world, claims to have learned valuable lessons from this event. Foremost is a continued commitment to adhere to the principles of the

International Health Regulations established in 2005. The IHR's plan of action to enhance global health safety includes the ability of a country to respond to all emerging health threats and to exhibit transparency in doing so.

Lessons Learned

Health Emergency Preparedness

Individual Canadians faced with any health-related emergency are initially responsible for their own protection. Depending on the complexity and seriousness of the threat, however, various levels of government become involved as resources, and more expertise becomes necessary to deal with the event. Under 1985's *Emergency Preparedness Act (EPA)*, each federal department must have an emergency response plan relating to its areas of responsibility. Such plans include the National Counter-Terrorism Plan and the Canadian Pandemic Influenza Plan. Each province and territory has its own legislation to deal with emergencies within its boundaries. However, in the event of a national emergency, federal plans under the *EPA* would take priority and be implemented collaboratively with each jurisdiction. The SARS crisis emphasized the importance of all levels of government working together to effectively deal with such an event.

To address national emergencies such as SARS, the Canadian government has taken steps to ensure rapid, effective responses and, in 2004, created two organizations for this purpose—Public Safety Canada and the Public Health Agency of Canada. As well, the federal government developed the National Security Policy and National Emergency Response System (NERS). The establishment of these organizations and policies addresses a wide variety of emergencies and concerns that Canadians may encounter. The PHAC, in particular, is charged with both recognizing and responding to public health threats.

The PHAC's key goals are public awareness, ongoing surveillance, early detection, prompt action to contain viruses, effective communication across the health care system, and collaboration among health care providers, organizations, and agencies at all levels of government. The government has created a Web site for the Centre of Emergency Preparedness and Response to provide access to resources in every province and territory.

With the outbreak of the H1N1 virus, Canada and most other developed nations appeared more prepared to respond, in terms of surveillance, testing, containment, and treatment.

The H1N1 Virus

In April 2009, an outbreak of a flu-type virus appeared to originate in Mexico. Clinical specimens of the virus were sent to Canada's National Microbiology Laboratory in Winnipeg, Manitoba, for analysis. The lab confirmed the virus as a human swine influenza—new but related to others, such as the AH1N1 human swine virus. The virus causes a respiratory illness with symptoms similar to those of seasonal flu. The virus was deadly, killing an estimated 80 Mexicans within the first few days of its appearance and affecting young, healthy individuals. Reporting of this outbreak was prompt, and the response was swift. Within days, Mexican officials closed schools, museums, and libraries in Mexico City and cancelled any activities involving crowds. Canada and other countries immediately implemented measures to monitor individuals returning from Mexico.

Initially, the WHO called the swine flu outbreak in Mexico and the United States a "public health emergency of international concern" and asked countries around the world to step up their reporting and surveillance of influenza. Using its then six phases (replaced with four phases in 2013—see Box 6.4) of categorizing the risk for such an outbreak, within a week, the WHO placed the alert level at phase three since human-to-human transmission was very limited. By June 11, 2009, however, with nearly 30,000 confirmed cases reported in 74 countries, the WHO raised the pandemic alert level to phase six (the highest level in the previous system), placing the world at the start of an influenza pandemic.

Influenza Vaccines

Using epidemiological information, the WHO meets twice a year to make recommendations for the formulation of the seasonal flu vaccine used around the world. Although the "swine flu" pandemic is over, the H1N1 strain that caused it is still around. The flu vaccine that has been formulated over the past few years has contained the H1N1 strain. In Canada, the National Advisory Committee on Immunization recommends that all Canadians over age 6 months get a flu shot and advises the shot is especially important for individuals in high-risk categories, including those with chronic diseases and diseases affecting the immune system, pregnant women, health care providers, older Canadians (over 65), and small children over 6 months of age. The Canadian Paediatric Society recommends two injections for children under the age of 9 who have never had a seasonal flu vaccine. The flu vaccine is deemed 70% to 90% effective, and if a vaccinated person does succumb to the flu, symptoms are usually milder. The need for the flu shot remains somewhat controversial, with many, including some health care providers, claiming that it is ineffective.

World Health Assembly

The World Health Assembly is the policymaking body for the WHO. The assembly's executive board comprises 34 members, all with qualifications in the health care field, who are elected for a three-year term. Each year, in Geneva, the assembly meets with representatives from member nations to discuss policies of the

WHO and to approve a budget for proposed programs for the upcoming year. The executive board tables reports that require further action, study, or investigation, as well as ensures that planned activities for the upcoming year are implemented.

Pan-American Health Organization

The Pan-American Health Organization (PAHO) aims to improve health and living standards in the Americas. Among other activities, this international public health agency serves as the Regional Office for the Americas of the WHO and functions as part of the United Nations. Member countries include the 35 nations that compose the Americas. Because many member states lack basic health care, clean drinking water, and adequate sanitation, one of the PAHO's main priorities is to promote current, effective, and community-based primary health care strategies.

Organisation for Economic Co-operation and Development

The Organisation for Economic Co-operation and Development (OECD) consists of 30 member countries (including Canada) that adhere to the principles of democracy and a free market economy. Through the organization, governments compare policy experiences and seek answers to common problems. The organization, among other things, measures the quality of medical care in member countries and rates health outcomes. For example, a report called *Health at a Glance 2013:* OECD Indicators provided valuable information on different aspects of health care performance in member countries. It also identified variations in indicators of health status and health risks and compared these to standards of practice in related health care systems (Organisation for Economic Co-operation and Development, 2013).

Summary

6.1 Through its complex and frequently changing hierarchical structure, Health Canada works to fulfill its mission to make Canadians among the healthiest populations in the world. Contrary to the belief of many Canadians, the federal government has little legal power over health care in the provinces and territories. Health Canada plays an authoritarian role in enforcing compliance with the *Canada Health Act* in that it can withhold federal-to-provincial transfers of funds when a province or territory breaches the principles and conditions of the Act.

6.2 Health Canada is led by the minister of health, who is supported by a deputy minister, assistant deputy ministers, an associate deputy minister, a chief public health officer, and the Departmental Secretariat. The minister of health is appointed by Parliament; deputies and assistant deputies are not. The primary responsibilities of the minister of health include overseeing other agencies, supervising the collection and analysis of information carried out under the *Statistics Act*, and working collaboratively with the provincial and territorial governments.

6.3 The many branches, offices, bureaus, and agencies that make up Health Canada work both independently and collaboratively within and outside of the organization. The Audit and Accountability Bureau, the Chief Financial Officer Branch, the Corporate Services Branch, and Legal Services have primary responsibilities supporting the internal workings of Health Canada. External branches of Health Canada include the First Nations and Inuit Health Branch; the Health Products and Food Branch; the Healthy Environments and Consumer Safety Branch; and the Public Affairs, Consultation, and Communications Branch. These branches are responsible for activities more directly aligned with the public's health and safety.

6.4 Several autonomous agencies work collaboratively with Health Canada, reporting directly to the minister of health. These agencies include the Public Health Agency of Canada, the Canadian Institutes of Health Research, the Hazardous Materials Information Review Commission, and the Patented Medicine Prices Review Board. The PHAC plays a significant role in health promotion and disease prevention initiatives; tracks outbreaks of seasonal flu, tuberculosis, measles, and other illnesses; and recommends corrective and preventive measures. The CIHR is instrumental in directing research projects in over 13 sites across the country.

6.5 Health Canada is active on an international level, working with a number of organizations to improve health at both a national and an international level. The World Health Organization, a key player in such initiatives, provides leadership on health matters globally. The WHO recognizes health threats such as the H1N1 virus and initializes pandemic alerts in response to information gathered. The Pan-American Health Organization aims to improve health and living standards in the Americas. The Organisation for Economic Co-operation and Development measures the quality of medical care in member countries and rates health outcomes.

Review Questions

1. What are the primary objectives of Health Canada?
2. In terms of health care, which population groups is Health Canada responsible for?
3. Explain the primary responsibilities of the minister of health and the deputy minister of health.
4. List and describe some of Health Canada's most important internal services.
5. Discuss the major branches of Health Canada's external services.
6. List the main agencies that report to the minister of health and describe their primary responsibilities.
7. Explain the functions of the World Health Organization, the Pan-American Health Organization, and the Organisation for Economic Co-operation and Development.

References

Assembly of First Nations. (2002). *Top misconceptions about Aboriginal peoples. Fact sheet*. Retrieved from http://tricitiesecd.ca/files/4013/3599/2965/FACTSandMisconceptions.pdf.

Canadian Institutes of Health Research. (2014). *Home page*. Retrieved from http://www.cihr-irsc.gc.ca/e/193.html.

Health Canada. (2011a). *About Health Canada: About mission, values, activities*. Retrieved from http://www.hc-sc.gc.ca/ahc-asc/activit/about-apropos/index-eng.php.

Health Canada. (2011b). *Drugs and health products: Canada vigilance program—collecting and assessing adverse reaction reports*. Retrieved from http://www.hc-sc.gc.ca/dhp-mps/pubs/medeff/_fs-if/2011-cvp-pcv/index-eng.php.

Health Canada. (2011c). *About Health Canada: Canada Health Act division*. Retrieved from http://www.hc-sc.gc.ca/ahc-asc/branch-dirgen/spb-dgps/chad-dlcs/index-eng.php.

Health Canada. (2013). *About Health Canada: Health portfolio*. Retrieved from http://www.hc-sc.gc.ca/ahc-asc/minist/portfolio/index-eng.php.

Ontario Ministry of Health and Long-Term Care. (2004, April). *Diseases: Severe acute respiratory syndrome (SARS). Health update*. Retrieved from http://www.health.gov.on.ca/en/public/publications/disease/sars.aspx.

Organisation for Economic Co-operation and Development. (2013). *Health at a glance 2013: OECD indicators*. Retrieved from http://www.oecd.org/health/health-systems/health-at-a-glance.htm.

Privy Council Office. (2011). *Accountable government: A guide for ministers and ministers of state*. Ottawa: Privy Council Office.

SARS Commission. (2006). *Spring of fear: The SARS Commission final report*. Toronto: Author.

CHAPTER SEVEN

The Role of Provincial and Territorial Governments in Health Care

Learning Outcomes

7.1 Discuss the common structural elements among the provincial and territorial governments.

7.2 Describe the purpose and general structure of regionalization initiatives.

7.3 Explain how provincial and territorial health care is financed.

7.4 Discuss provincial and territorial health insurance coverage for those who meet eligibility criteria.

7.5 Explain how drug plans help cover the cost of medications.

Key Terms

Copayment, p. 246

Deductible, p. 250

Dispensing fee, p. 250

Drug identification number (DIN), p. 251

Enhanced services, p. 243

Formulary list, p. 250

Methicillin-resistant *Staphylococcus aureus* (MRSA), p. 251

Vancomycin-resistant *Enterococcus* (VRE), p. 251

Vancomycin-resistant *Staphylococcus aureus* (VRSA), p. 251

This chapter provides an overview of the structure of the provincial and territorial health care systems, emphasizing the common elements among them and outlining their differences. While not every detail can be covered, the chapter will give a general understanding of the 13 health care systems across the country and how they operate. To better understand specific details about a certain province or territory, answer the Review Questions at the end of the chapter and visit the Web site of the provincial or territorial department or ministry of health.

This chapter follows two families who are new to Canada as they navigate their way through their respective provincial health care systems: the Jaeger family in British Columbia (Case Example 7.1) and the Wongs in Nova Scotia (Case Example 7.2).

Case Example 7.1

On January 1, 40-year-old Joseph Jaeger and his family arrive in Toronto from Germany and are en route to British Columbia. Joseph and his wife, Helga, 36, have three children: Anna, 16; Luca, 10; and Alois, 3. Although delighted to be in Canada, the family has little general information about their new country and even fewer details about an area of real concern to them—their health care. Anna is 3 months pregnant, Luca has asthma, and Alois requires updated immunizations. Joseph, who is overweight and on medication for high blood pressure, is a bricklayer and was told that, due to a shortage of skilled tradespeople in Canada, finding a job would be easy.

> **Case Example 7.2**
>
> Quang Wong, 36, and his wife, Ling, 35, arrive in Sydney, Nova Scotia, on January 15 with their two children: a son, Huan, aged 10, and a daughter Niu, aged 6. Quang, a doctor, plans to certify in Sydney; Ling is an architect. The family has no outstanding health problems.

PROVINCIAL AND TERRITORIAL HEALTH CARE PLANS

DIVISION OF POWERS

Both Canadians and non-Canadians often ask, "Does Canada have a national health insurance plan?" The answer is *no*, Canada does not have a national health insurance plan. Rather, Canada has 13 separate insurance programs run by 10 provinces and three territories, loosely bound together by federal agreements and the *Canada Health Act*. As mentioned in Chapter 1, these programs are frequently referred to collectively as *medicare*.

Although the federal government works in partnership with the provinces and territories to deliver health care, the provinces and territories maintain the bulk of the responsibility for health care. Under the *Constitution Act* (Box 7.1), provincial and territorial governments oversee matters relating to the personal health of their populations—the promotion of good health, preventive care, and health maintenance and the diagnosis and treatment of health problems. To receive continued federal funding for health care, however, provinces and territories must abide by the principles and conditions of the *Canada Health Act*, which obliges them to operate a health insurance plan that covers hospital care and medically necessary treatment for eligible residents. The Act is not concerned with the specifics of public or private health care delivery and does not address coverage of diagnostic services such as positron emission tomography (PET scans), magnetic resonance imaging (MRIs), and computed tomography (CT scans). Each province and territory controls which services are covered and how they are delivered.

> **Box 7.1** **The *Constitution Act*: A Clarification**
>
> The original *British North America Act* of 1867 became the *Constitution Act* in 1982, when Britain surrendered the power to make Canada's laws, including its Constitution. Among other things, the *Constitution Act* outlines the division of health care responsibilities.

STRUCTURE OF THE HEALTH PLANS: AN OVERVIEW

Within each provincial and territorial government is a ministry or department of health (titles vary) assigned to managing health care. The health ministries or departments oversee a variety of sub-divisions, branches, agencies, and programs that assume responsibilities for various matters and types of health care. Ministries also work with other service partners in the community—some government-funded, others private or nonprofit, and others a combination of government and private initiatives.

Each ministry is headed by an elected member of Parliament appointed by the premier to the position of minister of health (MOH). Typically, a government also appoints a deputy minister of health (sometimes more than one), who is not an elected member of Parliament. One or more associate deputy ministers and a management committee may also be assigned. Ultimately responsible for the health care system in the province or territory, the MOH has numerous organizations within the ministry reporting to him or her. These organizations provide leadership, direction, and support to service delivery partners, which include regional health authorities, physicians, and other health care providers.

One of the ministries' greatest responsibilities is implementing and regulating the provincial or territorial health insurance plan—that is, overseeing hospital and medical care. In some jurisdictions, this responsibility belongs to a single authority. In others, two administrative bodies share the duty—one handles hospitals and other health care facilities; the other, medical care. For example, in British Columbia, the Medical Services Commission administers the medical care plan, and the government, through the Ministry of Health Services, administers hospital services under the *Hospital Insurance Act*, reimbursing facilities for the medically necessary services they provide. But in Prince Edward Island, Health PEI administers both the hospital and medical services plans The provincial and territorial ministries must also oversee the negotiation of salaries and other policies with physicians' professional associations. Committees are typically created to manage these negotiations.

All provinces and territories provide three general categories of health care—primary, secondary, and tertiary—which are discussed below. The interaction between these categories is illustrated in Figure 7.1.

1. *Primary care* refers to "first contact" services to which the public has direct access, including family doctors, nurse practitioners, counselling services, clinics, emergency care services, and telephone helplines for health care advice. Primary care professionals diagnose and treat health concerns, make referrals to secondary health care services when required, and

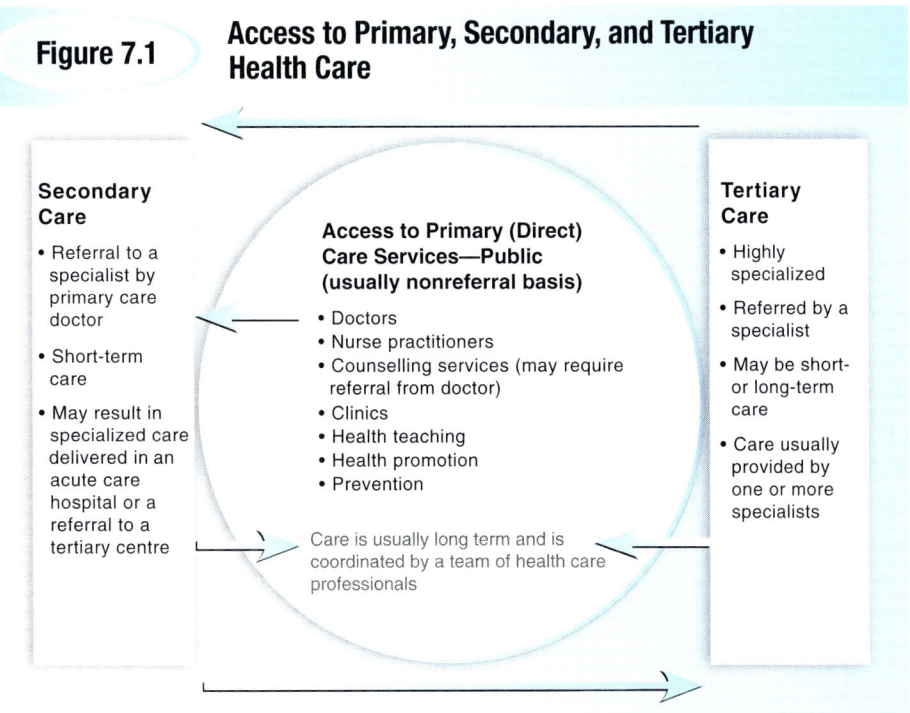

Figure 7.1 Access to Primary, Secondary, and Tertiary Health Care

provide preventive care, health promotion, and health education. Although typically long term and comprehensive in nature, primary care does not usually include hospitalization. Primary care should not be confused with the concept of *primary health care*, which encompasses essential medical and curative care received at the primary, secondary, or tertiary levels.

2. A patient must obtain a physician referral to access *secondary care*, including consultation with a specialist, such as a dermatologist, urologist, internist, or orthopedic surgeon. A specialist assists the primary care physician to diagnose a patient's problem and to provide specialized treatment, but the specialist's involvement is usually short term. Secondary care may involve admission to a general hospital or referral to a highly specialized facility, which provides tertiary care.

3. Highly specialized *tertiary care* also requires a referral. A cancer centre or cardiology centre, for example, would provide tertiary care. In a tertiary care setting, the patient may receive care from the referring specialist or from another specialist. Once care is considered complete, the patient may be sent back to the referring specialist, who will then discharge the patient back to his or her family doctor. Alternatively, the tertiary care centre itself may refer the patient back to the family doctor.

Although ultimately accountable for all aspects of health care, the provincial or territorial ministry or department of health assigns responsibilities to various departments. The most common method of delivering primary, secondary, and tertiary care is under a regional model using organizations commonly called *regional health authorities* (RHAs).

REGIONALIZATION INITIATIVES ACROSS CANADA

In the early 1990s, because of the rising cost of health care and the increasing demand for services in a variety of settings, many governments conducted public forums, reviews, and other studies to determine a way to improve health care delivery. The conclusion: to decentralize decisions about health care issues through regionalization (Box 7.2), a concept of assessing the need for specific types of care and delivering that care within a given jurisdiction. The regional approach was based on the belief that involving the community in decisions regarding health care needs would both increase public participation in health care initiatives and enable the ministry to address the unique needs of each community in a more effective, streamlined, cost-effective manner.

Box 7.2 Regional Health Authorities: A Definition

Regional health authorities (RHAs) are autonomous health care organizations responsible for health care administration in a defined geographic region within a province or territory. Through appointed or elected boards of governance, RHAs manage the funding and/or delivery of community and institutional health care services within their regions.

Source: Ferrell, B., & Coyle, N. (2006). *Textbook of palliative nursing*. New York: Oxford University Press.

Regionalization took different forms across the country, but every province and territory eventually became involved, with Ontario the last to regionalize care, in 2006. Each regional health authority is run by a board; in some regions, the provincial government appoints the board members; in others, board members comprise a mix of elected and appointed officials. The RHAs across Canada differ in terms of size, structure, responsibility, and name.

In most provinces and territories, RHAs are arm's-length agencies under the umbrella of the related ministry. Although, for the most part, they have the authority to disburse funds and direct services, they ultimately answer to the ministry and must provide financial statements and performance reports regarding services they have funded. In most jurisdictions, RHAs oversee long-term care, residential and acute care services, and, in some regions, public and mental health, addiction, and health promotion programs.

Over the past 15 years, most provinces and territories have altered the original structures of their health care delivery systems, merging or eliminating some RHAs and shifting some responsibilities among the ministry, other departments, and the RHAs.

BRITISH COLUMBIA

In British Columbia, the Ministry of Health assumes ultimate authority for the delivery of health care in the province. The MOH establishes performance guidelines for the RHAs (referred to as *provincial health authorities* in B.C.) and both evaluates and monitors operational outcomes. British Columbia has five regional authorities that oversee planning and delivery of care in their geographic areas. Another regional authority, the Provincial Health Services Authority, collaborates with the five RHAs to implement provincial programs. A seventh, formed in 2012, the First Nations Health Authority, has assumed responsibility for the care of First Nations people in the province (which was formerly overseen by Health Canada's First Nations Inuit Health Branch—Pacific Region).

Each RHA has an appointed board and is managed by an executive team, which participates in decision making at the operational level. The RHAs also manage community health councils (CHCs), which offer a variety of services throughout the province, including primary care clinics, health promotion, addictions services, home care, community mental health services, and specialized services, such as assistance for new immigrants, support for new mothers, and youth health drop-in centres. The range of services each CHC offers reflects the needs of the community it serves.

ALBERTA

In 2008, the government of Alberta reduced the nine regional health authorities to one, a new agency called the Alberta Health Services Board. The board also assumed responsibility of the Alberta Mental Health Board, the Alberta Cancer Board, and the Alberta Alcohol and Drug Abuse Commission. Since that time, there have been five regional health zones: South (zone 1), Calgary (zone 2), Central (zone 3), Edmonton (zone 4), and North (zone 5).

This new governance model aims to strengthen Alberta's approach to managing health care services, including surgical access, long-term care, chronic disease management, addiction and mental health services, and primary care access.

In 2012, in addition to the province's 42 primary care networks, AHS introduced the unique concept of family care clinics (FCCs). FCCs provide direct access to a variety of nonemergency services. FCCs do not have to be headed by a physician, and individuals can see any team member without a physician referral.

Saskatchewan

In 2002, Saskatchewan implemented the *Regional Health Services Act*, creating 12 RHAs (frequently called *health regions*), which provide the bulk of health care to the province's residents. The RHAs oversee hospitals, emergency response and ambulance services, long-term care and home care programs, community health services (including public health), and mental health and rehabilitation services.

Established in 2007, the Saskatchewan Cancer Agency plans and implements most of the cancer services in the province. The agency's duties include evaluating and developing guidelines for standards of care, treatment, and health promotion initiatives.

The Athabasca Health Authority (not an RHA) provides health care for five major communities in northern Saskatchewan, including two First Nations communities.

Manitoba

In 2012, Manitoba's 11 RHAs were reassigned into five regions: Northern Health, Prairie Mountain Health, Winnipeg–Churchill Health Region, Interlake Eastern RHA, and Southern Health. Each is overseen by a board of directors headed by a chairperson reporting ultimately to the Ministry of Health. The RHAs assess and prioritize community needs and deliver hospital care, long-term care, home care, public health services, rehabilitative services, ambulance services, and laboratory services. Manitoba also delivers health care services (e.g., medical care, counselling, health education) through community health centres, divisions of the RHAs run by local community boards.

Ontario

In Ontario, the Ministry of Health and Long-Term Care (MOHLTC) is responsible for health care in the province and is accountable for the provincial health plan, ambulance services, provincial drug programs, public health, and primary care. Reporting to the MOHLTC are 14 corporations called Local Health Integration Networks (LHINs). These nonprofit organizations are funded by the province through the MOHLTC and operate within the scope of agreements made with the ministry and reviewed annually. They determine, plan, and fund the health services deemed necessary within their designated regions. LHINs are responsible for hospitals, community care access centres (CCACs), community support service organizations, mental health and addiction agencies, community health centres (CHCs), Aboriginal health access centres (AHACs), and long-term care facilities. There over 100 CHCs and AHACs in the province. These community health centres are unique in that, using a team approach, they address the health and social needs of high-risk populations based on the determinants of health in each community. AHACs address the specific needs of Aboriginal people in the province in a variety of languages. Services include access to primary care, health promotion programs that interface with traditional healing, cultural programs, and social support services.

QUEBEC

In Quebec, the ministère de la Santé et des Services sociaux (MSSS) is responsible for both health and social services. The MSSS shares these responsibilities with Quebec's 18 RHAs—15 health and social services agencies and three regional associations in northern parts of the province (the Centre régional de santé et de services sociaux de la Baie-James in the Nord-du-Québec region, the Nunavik Regional Board of Health and Social Services in the Nunavik region, and the Cree Board of Health and Social Services of Baie-James). Responsibilities of the RHAs include hospitals, long-term care, home care, public health, mental health, rehabilitation, social services, and laboratory and ambulance services—a more comprehensive list of responsibilities than those of most other jurisdictions.

In 2004, 95 local service networks were established across the province to work under their respective regional health authorities. These networks provide comprehensive, accessible health care services to the populations in their region. At the heart of these local networks lie health and social services centres, created by merging local community health centres, residential and long-term care centres, and general and specialized hospital centres. By constructing service agreements with partners and stakeholders within the local services networks (e.g., rehabilitation centres, physician groups, medical clinics, youth protection centres, mental health organizations, university hospital centres), these centres ensure seamless access to primary, secondary, and tertiary care and adequate follow-up for the populations they serve.

NEW BRUNSWICK

The Department of Health (DOH) in New Brunswick is responsible for all health care in the province, including overseeing the funding, planning, and delivery of selected health care services through the province's two regional health authorities (Vitalité Health Network and Horizon Health Network). A board of directors oversees the operation of each RHA. Each board has 15 members—eight appointed and seven elected. These RHAs are responsible for hospital services, community health centre services, extramural services, most public health services; and mental health and addictions services. Included also are some tertiary services such as cardiac care and neurosurgery. The DOH retains responsibilities for other services such as long-term care and Ambulance New Brunswick.

Nova Scotia

Nine district health authorities (as RHAs are called in Nova Scotia) and the Izaak Walton Killam (IWK) Health Centre, an independent women's and children's tertiary care hospital, provide the bulk of Nova Scotia's health care services. Four medical officers of health oversee the regions within the district health authorities. District health authorities are responsible for hospitals (including staffing both acute and tertiary hospitals), public health, mental health, rehabilitation, and laboratory services. The district health authorities receive funding from the Department of Health and Wellness; in return, they prepare financial statements and service summaries for the ministry at designated intervals.

Nova Scotia's medical services insurance plan (MSI) is administered by Medavie Blue Cross (formerly Blue Cross), an agency that reports to the Department of Health. Medavie Blue Cross has the authority to determine the eligibility of health care providers who bill the provincial plan, to receive money from the province to pay physicians, and to provide educational seminars for physicians about their entitlements and responsibilities under the medical insurance plan. The Department of Health and Wellness is responsible for the Hospital Insurance Program, which covers the cost of hospital care.

Prince Edward Island

The Department of Health and Wellness in Prince Edward Island established Health PEI in 2010 to promote the concept of a "one island" health care system. The island formerly delivered health care under a regionalized delivery model. Health PEI is overseen by a board of directors who are appointed by the minister of health and wellness for a three-year term. Health PEI consists of two divisions: frontline services and systems supports. Frontline services include community hospitals and primary health care, including five primary health care networks; home and long-term care; management of chronic diseases, including prevention and early detection (e.g., care management of patients with stroke or diabetes; colorectal cancer and cervical cancer screening); and mental health and addictions services. Systems supports include responsibility for financial services, the management of health information (e.g., electronic health records), medical affairs (e.g., residency programs, tissue and organ donation, out-of-province referrals), and corporate development and innovation (e.g., interactions with the media, risk management, employee development). In 2010, Nova Scotia introduced Collaborative Emergency Centres to address the problem of emergency department closures and long waits for primary care appointments in rural and remote settings. Nurses and paramedics staff the centres at night, with a physician available remotely for consultation. The concept has been so successful that other jurisdictions, including Saskatchewan and P.E.I., are adopting this model for emergency department care.

Newfoundland and Labrador

The Department of Health and Community Services in Newfoundland and Labrador delivers provincial health care through four regional health authorities, which are responsible for health promotion and disease prevention initiatives, family and rehab services, addictions and mental health, public health, ambulance services, and both acute and long-term care. Also operating under this department are numerous divisions with unique roles and responsibilities (e.g., Memorial University Medical School, the Newfoundland and Labrador Centre for Health Information Services, the Department of Health and Wellness, and the Medical Services Division). The Department of Health and Wellness provides leadership, policies, planning, and direction for the delivery of health care in the province. As well, the department oversees health-related legislation and finances. The Medical Services Division is responsible for the delivery of medical, pharmaceutical, and dental services in the province. Physicians may work within an RHA or set up an independent practice. The RHAs have the authority to grant hospital privileges to qualified doctors.

Northern Regions

The spread-out populations and great distances between centres in the northern regions of Canada present unique and complex challenges in the delivery of health care. Technological advances (e.g., electronic health records, Telehealth, video links to large health centres) have contributed to significant improvements in the quality and accessibility of health care; however, care in the North remains woefully inadequate. Frequently, individuals must be air-lifted to a regional centre, such as Calgary, Edmonton, Winnipeg, or Sioux Lookout, to receive treatment that cannot be provided within the community—often despite the care of a visiting specialist or that provided by nurses and local physicians. Nurses play a significant role in delivering health care in Canada's North. There are over 600 First Nations communities alone, serviced by over 70 nursing stations and nearly 200 health centres. Nurses, more often than not, are the first point of contact for health care in the North. They are employed by the federal government or, in communities that, through a transfer agreement, assume responsibility for their own health care, by the band council.

This vast area comprises the Northwest Territories, Nunavut, Yukon, and the northern regions of other provinces, particularly British Columbia, Alberta, Saskatchewan, Manitoba, Ontario, and Quebec.

The federal government funds much of the health care for northern Inuit, Métis, and First Nations populations (In the News: Funding to Improve Care to Remote First Nations Communities). Health and health care services in Canada's North are discussed further in Chapter 10.

In the News: Funding to Improve Care to Remote First Nations Communities

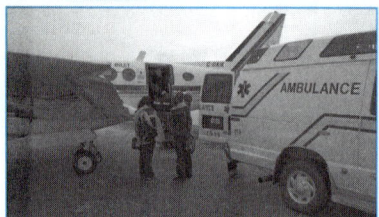

In 2013, the Department of Aboriginal Affairs and Northern Development announced the allotment of $48 million over a two-year period to expand the use of electronic health services in remote First Nations communities across Canada's northern regions. Another $4 million will be infused to improve mental health services and increase the presence of trained mental health professionals. A previously created Non-Insured Health Benefits Program will also continue to receive funding.

Source: Aboriginal Affairs and Northern Development Canada. (2013). *Budget 2013 highlights—Aboriginal and Northern investments*. Retrieved from http://www.aadnc-aandc.gc.ca/eng/1363964630328/1363964850834.

Photo source: © ColsTravel/Alamy.

Northwest Territories

The Northwest Territories health and social services system is managed by the Department of Health and Social Services, under which eight Health and Social Services Authorities (similar to RHAs) operate. Nongovernment organizations and private groups, agencies, and health care providers also provide services through agreements with the department and authorities. Physicians and specialists from larger centres in more southern regions routinely visit the communities of the Northwest Territories.

Community health programs in the territory include daily drop-in clinics, public health clinics, home care, school health programs, and educational programs. As well as offering these programs, the department oversees social service programs, including early intervention and support to families and children; child protection services; adoption services; family violence prevention; mental health and addiction services; and corrections services.

One way that the province serves its remote population is through its Health and Social Services Web site, which provides excellent information about health promotion and disease prevention, focusing on issues prevalent in northern areas, including healthy eating, risks of tobacco use, the importance of vaccinations, and diseases such as diabetes and tuberculosis (TB). For example, a link to an explanatory video about TB produced by the PHAC tells of the risks for transmission and treatment.

Yukon

The vast territory of Yukon consists of fewer people than most mid-size towns elsewhere in Canada, with between 25,000 and 32,000 residents who are eligible for government-funded health care. The territory does not have RHAs or similar organizations. The Department of Health and Social Services (DHSS) manages and delivers all components of health care through the following divisions: Health Services, Social Services, Continuing Care, and Corporate Services. The Health Services division is responsible for community nursing and community health programs, including the community health centres, which deliver front-line care and are managed primarily by nurses. The Continuing Care branch oversees residential and home care as well as day care and palliative care programs. The territory has three hospitals, managed by the Yukon Hospital Association.

Nunavut

Nunavut spans one-fifth of Canada's land mass and has communities spread across three regions—Baffin, Kivalliq, and Kitikmeot. Approximately 85% of the territory's population of roughly 32,000 people is Inuit.

Health care funding is centrally managed and distributed, with a significant portion of expenses going toward medical travel and out-of-territory treatments. Many of the health-related programs available in Nunavut are jointly funded by the territory and the federal government. Others, such as the Canada Prenatal Nutrition Program, are funded by Health Canada but delivered by the government of Nunavut.

Under the authority of a minister and deputy minister of health, three regional offices (one in each region) manage care in the jurisdiction. Primary care is delivered through 26 community health centres. One hospital, the Qikiqtani

General Hospital, serves Nunavut and is located in Iqaluit. Replacing the Baffin Regional Hospital, Qikiqtani is a modern, full-service 35-bed hospital that services approximately a dozen communities in its Qikiqtaaluk region. Services include a birthing centre, diagnostic imaging, and day surgery. Human resources are managed by the territorial government. As in other northern communities, retaining a full complement of nurses and other health care providers is sometimes difficult. The hospital's medical team consists primarily of resident physicians, visiting specialists, and general practitioner locums. Pharmacists and nurses, including nurse practitioners and public health nurses, play a vital role in health care delivery. When a patient must be air-lifted out, the destination is either Ottawa or Montreal.

HEALTH CARE: WHO PAYS FOR IT?

Each province and territory has a method (e.g., premiums, payroll tax, general revenues) of financing health care services not covered by federal funding. Private and volunteer organizations provide significant revenue for specific services or hospitals. For example, when a community hospital builds a new wing, a government grant usually covers part of the expense, and volunteer groups and the municipal government frequently make up the balance. A formal building campaign, often launched by the hospital undergoing the expansion, provides a conduit for donations.

HEALTH CARE PREMIUMS

Only two provinces—British Columbia and Ontario—currently charge premiums for health care services (Albertans stopped paying health care premiums as of January 1, 2009). British Columbia and Ontario residents cannot use premium payments as income tax deductions. Each province and territory determines how it will pay for health care. Premiums and other tax revenues do not contravene the *Canada Health Act* as long as residents are not denied medically necessary physician and hospital services because of an inability to pay.

British Columbia

British Columbia charges a health care premium (in 2013) of approximately $67 per month for a single person, $120 per month for a family of two, and $133 per month for a family of three or more, at which point the premium payment is capped.

Those who have been residents of Canada for the previous 12 consecutive months may qualify for financial assistance (British Columbia Ministry of Health, n.d.b). The province offers two premium-assistance packages to those in need. Regular premium assistance covers from 20% to 100% of the premium cost, depending on the individual's or family's income, less certain deductions. For example, a person, couple, or family earning less than $22,000 per year would receive 100% coverage of their premiums through this plan. The temporary premium-assistance program offers total premium coverage on a short-term basis for families or individuals undergoing unexpected financial difficulties.

Ontario

The Ontario government introduced health premiums to Ontario in 2004. Individuals who have an annual taxable income below $20,000 pay no premium; for others, the premium rate is based on taxable income. Consider a marriage in which the wife, Sally, earns $50,000 a year, and the husband, Mark, $60,000 per year. Sally's premiums would be based on her taxable income of $50,000, and Mark's would be based on his income of $60,000. Their income is not combined to determine the premiums. If the household included other family members making less than $20,000 (e.g., dependent children, a stay-at-home parent), these members would not pay any premiums (Ontario Ministry of Finance, 2014). As in B.C., no eligible resident can be denied health care based on income.

Payroll Tax

Some jurisdictions, including Manitoba, Ontario, Quebec, and Newfoundland and Labrador, levy a payroll tax (Normandin Beaudry, 2012), a tax collected from employers that specifically raises funds for health care, education, and social services. Employers with a payroll below a certain amount may be exempt; others may pay a reduced amount based on their salary or wage payout. Note that, in Ontario, this tax is in addition to health care premiums paid by residents (discussed above).

The payroll tax in Manitoba—known as the Health and Post Secondary Education Tax Levy (HE Levy)—is an obligatory tax on employee wages paid by all employers with permanent residency in the province. The tax amount the employer pays depends on the total payroll. In 2008, the government of Manitoba exempted employers with an annual payroll of less than $1.25 million. Those with payrolls between $1.5 and $2.5 million pay 4.3% on the amount in excess of $1 million (the first $1 million is a deduction), and those with payrolls over $2.5 million pay 2.15% of the total payroll (the first $1 million is not a deduction in that payroll category) (Manitoba Taxation Division, n.d.).

In Newfoundland and Labrador, employers pay a health and postsecondary education tax. Employers whose annual payroll exceeds a predetermined exemption threshold must pay a tax of 2%. In 2011, the exemption threshold was increased to $1.2 million (Newfoundland and Labrador Department of Finance, 2014).

In Ontario, employer health tax contributions are based on a percentage of the yearly payroll. The higher the payroll, the higher the tax. For employers with a payroll from $200,001 to $400,000, the tax ranges between 1.101% and 1.829% (Ontario Ministry of Finance, n.d.). Private-sector employers have a health tax exemption for a portion of their payroll calculated on the annual total amount paid out.

In Quebec, employer contributions to health care services are paid at a rate of 2.7% of the payroll for payrolls under $1 million. Those with payrolls between $1 million and $4.999 million pay a rate ranging from 2.7% to 4.26% of the total wages paid. For employers with payrolls of $5 million and greater, the tax rate is 4.26%. Starting in 2013, employers who employ individuals over the age of 65 may claim a reduction in Health Services Fund (HSF) contributions—up to $1000 per employee by 2016 (Raymond Chabot Grant Thornton, 2013).

Other Sources of Funds

In addition to federal funding (discussed in Chapter 8), provincial, territorial, and municipal governments provide some funds for services such as preventive health measures, medical- and hospital-based services (both inpatient and outpatient), the treatment of chronic diseases, community-based rehabilitation care, and care for nursing home residents.

Provincial and territorial health ministries fund and regulate hospitals. They may also contribute financially to community health organizations, services delivered by certain health care providers (other than physicians), and teaching and research institutions.

Distribution of Funds

Precisely how finances are organized and administered varies among the provinces and territories. In some provinces, for example, the ministry responsible for health care may directly manage hospital and medical insurance and cardiology and cancer care. Other provinces or territories may establish separate public organizations to oversee and finance these services. Currently, most provincial and territorial governments provide funding—at least in part—to RHAs, which, in turn, finance hospitals and health care services within their regions depending on each area's particular needs. For example, an RHA responsible for hiring community nurses would contract with private nursing agencies to provide care in a certain region. Managing its own funds, each nursing agency would then hire the nurses and deliver the care.

In some jurisdictions, other ministries provide funds for additional health care–related services. For example, the Ministry of Labour might oversee occupational health matters, and the Ministry of Community and Social Services might provide services (e.g., counselling, group homes, special education) for those with specific health issues, such as learning and physical disabilities.

The provinces and territories also allocate funds to supplementary benefits (e.g., medical supplies, prescription drugs, hearing aids). These funds, most commonly distributed through the RHAs, finance regional facilities and services.

Some provinces charge premiums for health care; others do not.

1. Do you think that charging premiums is a fair way to offset the cost of health care?
2. Would you be in favour of your province or territory charging a tax that goes directly toward covering the cost of health care?

HEALTH INSURANCE

Health insurance coverage is provided by provincial and territorial plans and by private insurance companies.

Third-party health insurance plays a significant role in offsetting the costs of services not covered by provincial and territorial health services. Approximately 60% of Canadians carry private health insurance, either provided through group employment benefits or purchased personally (Drug Coverage, 2007). Usually including coverage for employees' families and dependents, employee plans provide benefits for health care services not covered by provincial or territorial plans, such as vision and dental care, private nursing services, assistive devices, and enhanced medical services (e.g., semi-private hospital room).

PROVINCIAL INSURANCE PLANS

Eligibility

All of the following criteria must be met for a person to be eligible for provincial or territorial health insurance:

- Canadian citizenship or permanent resident status
- Resident of the province or territory in which he or she is seeking health coverage
- Physically in that jurisdiction for at least six months of the year (this criterion varies slightly among jurisdictions), although babies born in a given province or territory are insured from birth in most circumstances

People with study or work permits, issued under the federal *Immigration and Refugee Protection Act*, may be considered residents. Terms and conditions for insuring other population groups can be obtained from the provincial or territorial health Web sites. No Canadian can be denied medically necessary hospital or physician care under any circumstances.

Application for Coverage

In each province and territory, newcomers must apply to the ministry or department of health for health insurance coverage. The application process and documentation required can vary. Specific instructions for applying for health care coverage can be found on the Web sites of the provincial and territorial health departments. The application processes of Nova Scotia and British Columbia are illustrated as our two families, the Jaegers (Case Example 7.3) and the Wongs (Case Example 7.4), apply for provincial health coverage.

Case Example 7.3

In British Columbia, the Jaegers have several means of obtaining application forms:

- Forms can be downloaded from the Medical Services Plan, filled out, and mailed in or completed and sent electronically.

- Paper forms can be obtained from the Medical Services Plan or through the province's access centres. The Jaegers can call a toll-free number to be connected to the nearest Service B.C. Centre.

- A forms-by-fax service is available from the provincial government 24 hours a day, 7 days a week.

If Mr. Jaeger were employed, his employer would likely complete a group insurance form for him so that he could receive supplementary benefits.

Case Example 7.4

To apply for health insurance in Nova Scotia, the Wongs can call the Medical Service Insurance plan's registration department. The Wongs will receive application forms, which they must complete and submit with the required documentation—a copy of their landed immigrant papers and a copy of their permanent resident cards. Upon approval, each member of the Wong family will be issued a health card, which will expire every four years. When their health cards expire, the Wongs will call the same number to get a renewal form.

Documents required for provincial or territorial health insurance applications vary. Usually, a citizen of Canada must present proof of that citizenship, proof of residency in a particular province or territory, and further (or supporting) proof of personal identification (all original documents). To prove citizenship, a birth certificate, passport, citizenship card, or similar documentation is acceptable. To show residency, an income tax assessment, a child tax benefit statement, or a utility or property tax bill is acceptable. Proof of personal identification includes a credit card, an employee ID card, or a driver's licence.

Under the *Canada Health Act*, the waiting period is not to exceed three months, so in most provinces and territories, health coverage begins within three months of a person moving to a new jurisdiction. In New Brunswick, Ontario, Quebec, and British Columbia, however, newcomers are required to wait the full three months before they can enroll in the provincial program, thus many newcomers purchase interim health insurance. The Jaegers (Case Example 7.5) and the Wongs (Case Example 7.6) had different experiences in their respective provinces.

Under the reciprocal agreement (Box 7.3), health card holders qualify for health care services anywhere in Canada (other than Quebec), barring some exceptions; for example, people may not seek elective surgery in another province or seek a service that is uninsured in their province or territory of origin.

Case Example 7.5

In British Columbia, new residents are eligible for coverage after a waiting period that consists of the balance of the arrival month plus two months. If the Jaeger family arrives in British Columbia on January 5, they will be covered as of April 1. However, if Mr. Jaeger arrives January 5, and Mrs. Jaeger and the children follow on February 5, family coverage will not begin until May 1. Note that when Anna Jaeger delivers her baby, the baby will be insured from birth.

When one family member arrives at a later date, it is the latest arrival that determines when coverage for the whole family will start. The family will need supplementary health insurance until their three-month wait ends.

Case Example 7.6

The Nova Scotia health insurance plan covers the Wong family as soon as their applications are approved, presumably shortly after their arrival. (Individuals from within Canada moving to Nova Scotia must wait three months.) In Nova Scotia, the family will not have to pay premiums for their health care coverage.

Box 7.3 Reciprocal Agreement

The reciprocal agreement supports the principle of health insurance portability (see Chapter 3) among the provinces and territories. Through the agreement, a person's province of origin will pay for required health services in another province or territory at the rates imposed by the host province. This interprovincial agreement is not mandatory. For example, Quebec has not signed it.

As a result of this agreement, Canadians, for the most part, will not face point-of-service charges for medically required hospital and physician services when they travel within Canada. In most cases, a person can receive care in a host province by simply presenting his or her health card, and the patient's province of origin will pay the host province for services delivery.

Source: Health Canada. (2007). *Health care system—Canada Health Act.*

Thinking It Through

You are considering immigrating to Canada. You find out that some provinces and territories have no wait time before you would qualify for health care coverage, and others do, and that some provinces charge health care premiums, and others do not.

If you have a choice of where you will settle, would these factors sway your decision?

Health Cards

Once an application is approved, the ministry or department of health issues the applicant a health card, identified by a number, for the province or territory in which he or she resides. Some jurisdictions assign a number to a whole family and then, when the children reach a certain age, issue the children an individual health number. Other jurisdictions issue a personal health number to each person. In Ontario, for example, babies are issued an individual health number at birth.

Using a Health Card

Almost without exception, health care facilities require individuals to present their health cards at the point of service. If the health card does not contain a picture, the person may also be asked for photo ID (e.g., a driver's licence) with a current address. (Note that, in many jurisdictions, only providers of provincially or territorially funded health care can ask a person to produce a health card; the card itself should never be used for identification purposes.) The card may be validated at that time. If an "invalid" message appears (e.g., if the card has expired or was reported lost, or if an address change has since occurred), the cardholder may be asked to pay for the service he or she is seeking. After finding the health card or renewing an invalid one, the person can submit the receipt to the ministry for reimbursement. An invalid health card is much like an expired credit card.

In 2013, British Columbia started phasing in the BC Services Card to replace the BC CareCard. Those with driver's licences can get a dual-purpose Services Card that is recognized both as a driver's licence and health care card (British Columbia, n.d.).

Health Card Fraud

Health card fraud is a significant problem across Canada, resulting in an enormous cost—in the millions of dollars—to the provinces and territories. It is virtually impossible to detect fraudulent use of older health cards that have no special security features or photo identification (e.g., Ontario's old red and white cards). Most jurisdictions now have photo identification health cards for those over a certain age—usually 15 or 16—and increased security measures, such as a holographic topcoat and hidden ultraviolet ink printing that can be viewed only under UV light, to protect the information on the cards. These cards must be renewed at designated intervals, unlike the older-style cards, which never expired. Some cards also require signatures. A magnetic strip on the health card contains coded information, such as the holder's name and address. It is a serious offence in all provinces and territories to knowingly facilitate the illegal use of a health card. Health care providers are encouraged to watch for and to report anything suspicious—for example, a patient unable to provide his or her address or a person who looks decidedly different from the picture on the health card. Many jurisdictions have a hotline for health care providers or the public to call if they suspect fraudulent use.

Lost cards must be reported immediately, as must changes of address or name. All provinces and territories have a protocol to follow for lost or misplaced health cards. As soon as a card is reported lost or missing, it is invalidated, and the user is issued a new card with a new number or other variation, such as a version code.

INSURED AND UNINSURED SERVICES

Provincial and territorial governments are responsible for administering the health care insurance plan in their jurisdictions. They must decide on a multitude of things, including the need for different types of hospital beds (e.g., acute care, rehabilitation, long-term care), the mix of professional health care staff, and the structure of the system that will best serve various regions within the province or territory. In addition, the governments approve hospital budgets and negotiate physicians' fees with medical associations.

Under the *Canada Health Act*, medically necessary hospital and medical services are insured everywhere in Canada. The *Canada Health Act* also requires the provinces and territories to insure extended health care services, which include "intermediate care in nursing homes, adult residential care service, home care service and ambulatory health care services" (*Canada Health Act*, 1985).

Some provinces and territories may choose to provide supplementary benefits and services outside of the *Canada Health Act*. The governments then determine eligibility guidelines for specific services, funding formulas, and the length of time these services will be insured. Supplementary benefits include health care services, such as optometric, dental, and chiropractic services, that are insured by the province or territory but not mandated by the *Canada Health Act*.

All provinces and territories provide specific services (e.g., eye care, dental care, drug benefits) to certain population groups, such as those receiving income assistance or guaranteed income supplements, adults over age 65, and disabled persons. Many jurisdictions also provide some of these services to children of low-income families.

As noted in Chapter 6, the federal government, rather than the provincial and territorial governments, finance the majority of health care provided to First Nations and Inuit populations living on reserves. Other groups for whom the federal government bears responsibility (e.g., federal public service employees) receive coverage under plans separate from the provincial and territorial ones.

Contrary to what many Canadians believe, private health care has existed in some form or another since before the inception of the *Canada Health Act*. Despite some strictly private clinics in Canada being perceived as illegal under the principles of the *Canada Health Act*, numerous such clinics and services exist across the country. They circumvent the legal principles of the Act largely by offering services not technically considered medically necessary, since they cannot charge for medically necessary procedures that are covered by the public health plan. For example, private clinics may provide patients with a wide range of diagnostic tests (noted as preventive screening), such as colonoscopies, 3-D imaging of fetuses for pregnant women, or MRIs that are not medically necessary for individuals wanting them. Other services include counselling, physiotherapy, sports medicine, travel health assessments, and genetic testing and pharmacogenomics testing. The emergence of these private clinics raises many concerns (Box 7.4).

Box 7.4 Private Clinics: Concerns

Significant concerns exist across Canada about private clinics. At the forefront lies the worry that the availability of private clinics will lengthen wait times for those using the public system because private clinics use the services of physicians and other health care providers who also work in the public system. The prevailing thought is that doctors' time in the public system will be lessened. Those making cases against this belief argue that physicians working in the private sector do so on their own time, thus not interfering with services offered in the public system. For example, an orthopedic surgeon may have only two days of operating room time available to him or her, leaving three days a week during which he or she cannot perform surgical procedures. On such days, the surgeon can see patients in a private clinic, perhaps doing knee or hip replacements, and, conversely, shorten the line in the public system.

Another concern is that patients paying for **enhanced services** will unfairly move to the top of wait lists because of the additional revenue for the clinic. For example, in many jurisdictions, in the public system, a patient requiring a hip replacement will receive offers of "upgrades" (e.g., titanium), which generate revenue for the hospital. Some claim that cases exist in the public system in which people purchasing such upgrades move up the list.

Bundled services, some claim, provide another method by which individuals can jump the queue. For example, a clinic performing cataract surgery can "bundle" an uninsured laser surgery with the insured cataract surgery. The patient paying for the laser portion of the procedure could be bumped up the list, while someone wanting cataract surgery only continues to wait. More often than not, the enhanced or bundled service will occur at a private clinic, having no impact on the corresponding public service.

Private clinics charge substantial fees to individuals using their services for non–medically necessary procedures. A growing trend, particularly within the past five years, has seen physicians and specialists pooling their services to offer routine and specialized care via "health packages." Such groups (e.g., the Copeman Healthcare Centres in Vancouver, Calgary, and Edmonton) charge an enrollment fee and an annual membership fee. In return for fairly steep fees ($29,000 per year for the "elite" program at Copeman), patients receive the guarantee of prompt access to an impressive team of health care providers, including family doctors, dietitians, psychologists, and specialists, along with an array of other services. Fees are generally tax deductible, and many of the services are covered by third-party insurance. Critics of this type of private health care point out that the fees are well out of reach of the average Canadian family.

To what extent a two-tier system will develop in Canada is anyone's guess. The availability of private clinics and services suggests that, in one form or another, a two-tiered system will continue to exist.

Enhanced services
Optional health services, such as choice in hospital rooms, enhanced medical goods and services, and services not covered by the public health insurance system, offered to the patient at a cost.

Hospital Services

In the hospital setting, insured services for inpatients include standard hospital accommodation, meals, certain medications (in some regions, patients are asked to bring their own medications), operating room and delivery room services, anaesthetic facilities, diagnostic and laboratory services, routine medical and surgical supplies used for hospitalized patients, routine nursing care, and certain rehabilitative services (e.g., physiotherapy). Provincial and territorial plans do not cover private nursing care unless a doctor orders it, at which point it becomes medically necessary and is covered. Note that the cost of a private room may be covered by the provincial or territorial plan under some circumstances (e.g., for infection control, isolation purposes, or compassionate reasons).

Insured outpatient hospital services include emergency treatment, day surgery, and diagnostic and radiological procedures at a hospital or specialized clinic (e.g., outpatient cancer centre, orthopedic clinic). As well, most jurisdictions insure physiotherapy, occupational therapy, and respiratory therapy services for a limited period if deemed medically necessary.

Medical Services

Under the *Canada Health Act*, medically necessary care provided by a medical doctor (i.e., family doctor or specialist) is an insured service, with some conditions. In Ontario, for example, a person can claim coverage for only one visit to a medical doctor per day unless the physician submits the claim for special review. What is deemed medically necessary may vary a little across the country but is fairly standard.

Rules also govern insured services provided by a specialist. For instance, in most provinces and territories, a doctor must refer a patient to a specialist; the patient may see the specialist again for the same problem within a calendar year. After that, or for a new symptom or complaint, the family doctor must provide another referral. In most jurisdictions, when a patient requests the opinion of a second specialist, the provincial or territorial plan will pay for that visit if the family doctor provides another referral request. After receiving a second opinion, however, the patient would usually have to pay for further consultations even if referred by his or her family doctor.

Each province and territory generates its own list of insured services, which is reviewed periodically by the ministry or department of health and the province's or territory's medical association. At this time, some services may be delisted, and others added. Since "medically necessary" is subjective, these services vary from one jurisdiction to another. For example, having wax removed from one's ear is insured in British Columbia, but not in Nova Scotia (although it is covered for children). Ontario's provincial plan no longer covers what used to be called an annual checkup but now recommends a less extensive assessment, called a periodic health visit, limited to one visit per patient per 12 month period. British Columbia and several other jurisdictions do not cover an annual health exam; rather, the extent of an examination is complaint-driven. Patients who request a complete physical can have one but must pay for it themselves.

Doctors may choose to offer services that are deemed not medically necessary by their provincial or territorial health care plan. For these services, physicians may bill patients directly, or they may bill a third party—an insurance company, the Workplace Safety Insurance Board (WSIB), or an employer or other payer. The amount a doctor charges for uninsured services depends on guidelines set out by the governing medical association (Box 7.5). Physicians must post lists of uninsured services they offer and the cost. Some doctors may use *block payments* or an *uninsured services plan*. Essentially, they charge the patient or family an annual fee for any and all uninsured services that might be rendered during the year.

Box 7.5 Uninsured (Chargeable) Versus Insured Physician Services

Uninsured Services
- Telephone prescription renewal
- Travel advice
- Missed appointments
- Form completion (e.g., passport, driver or pilot fitness test)
- Back-to-work or back-to-school note
- Faxing or transfer of medical records
- Nonmedical TB skin testing
- TB testing due to possible exposure
- Cosmetic procedures (e.g., breast reduction)
- Uninsured vaccinations
- Telephone advice (dependent on practice guidelines)

Insured Services
- Visit to a doctor and prescription written in the office
- Advice or counselling regarding health issues
- No charge if notice given for missed appointments
- Visit to the doctor and a diagnosis of an illness keeping patient home
- Doctor sending pertinent records to a specialist
- Breast reduction because heavy breasts were causing back and shoulder problems
- Routine childhood vaccinations
- Advice given on a primary care group Telehealth line

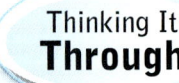

Thinking It Through

Physicians are required to inform patients of the price of any procedure, assessment, or treatment not covered by their provincial or territorial plan before carrying out any such procedure. Some doctors use what is called a *block payment plan*, whereby patients pay a lump sum annually that covers any uninsured procedure the physician performs during the course of the year, including third-party or camp medicals and return-to-school or -work notes.

1. If you had undergone an uninsured treatment provided by a doctor but did not learn until after the treatment was completed that you were required to pay for it, what would you do?

2. Would you be more likely to opt for a block payment plan or a pay-as-you-go plan for uninsured services?

Ambulance Services

In most jurisdictions, either land and air ambulance services are under regional management, and costs are shared with the provincial or territorial government, or these services are delivered privately through performance-based contracts. Because ambulance services are not addressed in the *Canada Health Act*, provinces and territories can establish their own guidelines, including fee schedules, for these services.

People using an ambulance even for medically necessary reasons may be responsible for a **copayment** (Case Example 7.7). However, fees are not usually charged for transportation between hospitals—whether the destination hospital is within a short distance, in another part of the province, in another province altogether, or outside of the country—as long as the transfer is for medically necessary reasons (Case Example 7.8). Interfacility transfers (e.g., from one nursing home to another) usually require a copayment. Most jurisdictions either reduce or eliminate the copayment for low-income individuals and families.

Copayments (also called *user fees* or *service fees*) vary, and all jurisdictions exempt some people from them, including individuals in long-term care homes or on provincial or territorial subsidized programs.

Copayment
A predetermined dollar amount or percentage of the cost of a health care service or medication that an individual must pay.

Case Example 7.7

While tobogganing with his children, Mr. Jaeger fell and broke his ankle. He was transported by ambulance to the local hospital for treatment. Mr. Jaeger was responsible for a copayment of $80 for the ambulance service.

Case Example 7.8

When Anna Jaeger went into labour eight weeks before her due date, her parents brought her to Vancouver General Hospital. Anna was carrying twins, who would require intensive care accommodation once they were born. No neonatal intensive care unit (ICU) beds were available in British Columbia, but Ontario had space. Anna was transported by air ambulance to Women's College Hospital in Toronto, where she delivered two healthy baby girls. Two weeks later, Anna and her babies were returned to Vancouver General Hospital. The British Columbia medical services plan covered the entire cost of the round trip air ambulance because the province was unable to meet Anna's medical needs at home.

Insured Health Care Providers Other Than Physicians

Some provinces and territories provide residents with limited insurance coverage for the services of health care providers other than doctors. A monetary limit may be imposed per calendar year, or coverage may be provided only for lower-income households. For example, Manitoba's residents receive partial coverage for up to 12 chiropractic adjustments per year. The covered portion increases for individuals living north of the fifty-third parallel (Manitoba Chiropractic Association, n.d.). Saskatchewan and Alberta also partially insure chiropractic care. The British Columbia Medical Services Plan will pay $23 per visit for a total of 10 visits per eligible person per year for chiropractic care, massage therapy, naturopathy, physiotherapy, and nonsurgical podiatry care for eligible residents (i.e., those on premium assistance) (British Columbia Ministry of Health, n.d.a). Coverage for other supplementary services such as optometric care and hearing tests varies by jurisdiction.

Extended Health Care Services

Long-term care homes offer 24-hour nursing care and support to individuals no longer able to live on their own. The terms *long-term care facility* and *old-age home* are often used interchangeably, but, in some provinces and territories, subtle differences may exist. For the most part, these facilities offer residents more intensive care than retirement homes provide. They may be owned and operated by private corporations (either profit or nonprofit), municipal councils, churches, or ethnic, cultural, or community groups. In most provinces and territories, these facilities are overseen by one or more pieces of legislation. In Nova Scotia, for example, nursing homes are under the governance of the *Homes for Special Care Act*. In Ontario, three acts—the *Aged and Rest Homes Act*, the *Nursing Home Act*, and the *Charitable Institutions Act*—were replaced by the *Long-Term Care Homes Act* in 2007.

The province or territory sets standards of care in long-term care facilities and performs regular inspections to ensure these standards are met. Long-term care facilities are encouraged to seek accreditation through Accreditation Canada (formerly known as the Canadian Council on Health Services Accreditation), an organization that conducts reviews on a three-year cycle. The Qmentum accreditation program introduced in 2008 has revised some assessment standards and added new ones, such as an improved survey process and more effective tools for measuring compliance. Assessments include reviews of patient care, staff management, information management, administrative management, and partnerships. Accreditation reflects a level of transparency and shows the public that the facility meets national standards of care and operation. More details about Accreditation Canada can be found in the Web Resources on Evolve.

Provincial and territorial governments design their own funding formulas for funding long-term care facilities. The funding of long-term care facilities is covered in more detail in Chapter 8.

Most provinces and territories offer a variety of other services:

- *Home care* helps individuals with basic personal care, meals, and household maintenance, allowing them to remain at home even once they find caring for themselves difficult.
- *Adult day programs* provide community day activities as well as respite care and in-home support to individuals with disabilities.
- *Respite care*, which allows nonprofessional caregivers some relief from caring for disabled family members, is often offered in long-term care facilities or the equivalent for a designated time frame.
- *Assisted living accommodation* helps to keep a person in his or her home by providing individualized support and care as required.
- *Group homes* allow persons with disabilities to live in an environment that provides supervision and assistance.
- *Hospice care* is provided in a homelike setting for those unable or unwilling to die at home. Individuals receive nursing and medical care, pain management, counselling, and other supportive care needed while dying.
- *Palliative care* provides care, medication, and some medical supplies for individuals dying at home.

Assistive Devices and Medical Products

Those in need of but unable to afford health care products and assistive devices—mobility devices (e.g., wheelchairs, walkers, motorized carts), prosthetic devices (e.g., post-mastectomy products, artificial limbs), bathing and toileting aids, and home care beds and accessories—can receive supplemental coverage; however, the coverage for such items varies across jurisdictions. In most jurisdictions, patients able to pay are responsible for a portion of the cost of selected assistive devices. For those that cannot pay, the cost is absorbed by the provincial plan.

Alberta offers two income-based programs: the Alberta Aids to Daily Living (AADL) and the Dental Assistance for Seniors programs. The AADL offers eligible Albertans with a long-term disability, chronic illness, or terminal illness financial support for the purchase of medical equipment and supplies. The dental assistance program provides required dental care to low- and moderate-income seniors to a maximum of $5000 for eligible services every five years. Other supplementary services, including audiology, physiotherapy, occupational therapy, and speech therapy, are delivered through Alberta Health Services, which assesses eligibility and prioritizes referrals based on service availability within each community.

In British Columbia, the Pharmacare Program, run by the province's RHAs, covers medical devices and equipment for designated population groups. A physician must make a referral, outlining the patient's medical eligibility criteria for the program.

Ontario's Assistive Devices Program covers more than most others in the country with respect to items insured and cost coverage (up to 75%). In addition, Ontario passed the *Accessibility for Ontarians with a Disability Act (AODA)* in 2005. The Act is one of Canada's most comprehensive; it phased in laws to which public and private businesses must comply over a number of years. The goal of the *AODA* is to make Ontario accessible to persons with disabilities by the year 2025. Implications range from having change rooms in a store modified for disabled people to training staff in a bank to communicate effectively with someone who is hearing impaired.

Manitoba offers similar assistance with medical supplies and assistive devices, delivered through the provinces five RHAs.

DRUG PLANS

Medications consume a huge portion of the health care dollars spent across Canada, second only to hospital spending. The immensity of this expenditure stems, in part, from the use of newer, more expensive drugs and an aging population with multiple health problems who are prescribed an astonishing array of medications.

As is the case with dental care, the majority of working Canadians have private or employer-sponsored insurance plans with drug benefits. Both types of plans may insure only certain medications. Publicly funded drug benefit packages (discussed below) and private insurance plans have copayments or **deductibles** (usually percentage-based) that beneficiaries pay, depending on their income and drug costs. Private insurance plans also require beneficiaries to pay **dispensing fees** themselves. For individuals on a public drug plan, the dispensing fee is either calculated as a percentage of the prescription cost or set at a flat rate, depending on the plan.

To qualify for provincial or territorial drug benefits, an individual must first apply for assistance. For example, residents in Nova Scotia, British Columbia, Manitoba, and Yukon apply to Pharmacare; in Ontario, to the Ontario Drug Benefit Program or the Trillium Drug Program; and in Saskatchewan, to the Drug Plan and Extended Benefits Branch of Saskatchewan Health. The organization would then assess the applicant's annual income, considering how many people that income supports, and calculate how much coverage the family should get for eligible prescription drugs.

Most jurisdictions require the family or individual to pay a predetermined deductible for prescription drugs. Once the deductible is reached, the public plan will pay a percentage of the beneficiary's eligible drug costs. Some jurisdictions also set a maximum amount, or a "cap," that the family or person must pay, after which point, the plan will cover 100% of the drug costs.

Some plans (both private and public) will cover only drugs prescribed from a **formulary list**. Formulary lists, although they include hundreds of drugs, are limited, containing, for the most part, cheaper, generic versions of common drugs. Some brand-name drugs may be covered, but only if there is not a less expensive alternative. Many combination drugs, time-release drugs, and so-called "lifestyle" drugs (e.g., sildenafil [Viagra], used for erectile dysfunction; orlistat [Xenical, Alli], used to treat obesity) are not available on most formularies. However, most plans will cover a nonformulary drug if the generic drug does not produce the desired therapeutic effect or causes adverse effects (Case Example 7.9). Doctors must seek approval to prescribe (and have covered) a nonformulary drug. These may include high-cost drugs or drugs with a high potential for misuse. Many private insurance plans offer an "open access" plan that will insure all prescription medications approved by Health Canada that are prescribed on an outpatient basis. Drugs are constantly being added to the formulary list, including, most recently, in many jurisdictions, rivaroxaban (Xarelto) and dabigatran (Pradaxa), which are new-generation drugs used to reduce clotting times. Unlike previously preferred anticoagulants, these drugs do not require routine laboratory monitoring.

> **Deductible**
> The amount of money that an individual or family is required to pay toward health care costs before an insurance plan will take over.

> **Dispensing fee**
> A service fee charged by a pharmacy for dispensing a prescription medication (i.e., reading the prescription and preparing the medication for the patient).

> **Formulary list**
> A list of prescription medications (often generic brands) selected for coverage by a public or private health insurance plan.

Case Example 7.9

Quang Wong is receiving assistance through Pharmacare because he does not yet have a job. He has developed an irregular heartbeat, and his doctor put him on Aspirin for its anticoagulant effects. Within days, Quang developed a pain in his stomach and other gastrointestinal (GI) symptoms. The doctor decides that the Aspirin is causing the GI upset and wants to switch Quang to clopidogrel bisulfate (Plavix)—another drug to prevent clots. This drug is on a limited use list (LU) on the Nova Scotia drug formulary list. The doctor fills out a special request form so that Pharmacare will cover the drug. He must note the **drug identification number (DIN)** and explain the situation.

Each formulary includes a limited use list (LU), which lists drugs deemed unsuitable or too expensive to be on the formulary list. These drugs may, however, have therapeutic benefits in special circumstances—for example, an antibiotic that can treat resistant bacteria such as **vancomycin-resistant *Staphylococcus aureus* (VRSA), vancomycin-resistant *Enterococcus* (VRE)**, and **methicillin-resistant *Staphylococcus aureus* (MRSA)**.

Some drugs are not on either the formulary or the LU list. The physician must seek special permission to have these drugs covered by a publicly funded drug benefit plan. Recently, Ontario implemented an Exceptional Access Program, which aims to provide easier and faster access to drugs that are not on the formulary.

SUMMARY

7.1 The *Canada Health Act* oversees 13 separate health insurance programs—one for each province and territory. Adherence to the principles and conditions of the CHA binds the provinces and territories to a set of predetermined obligations for health care delivery. Otherwise, each jurisdiction is free to deliver and pay for services deemed appropriate (e.g., assistive devices, long-term care).

7.2 Most provinces and territories deliver health care within a specific geographic area through regional organizations or authorities. These units assess the needs of the populations they serve and make decisions best suited for them.

7.3 Payment for health care services is provided in part by the federal government. A blend of taxes at the provincial and territorial level makes up the rest. Two provinces (British Columbia and Ontario) require their residents to pay health care premiums. Volunteer organizations across the country contribute significantly to the cost of some services and equipment.

Drug identification number (DIN)
A unique number assigned to each medication approved by Health Canada for use in Canada.

Vancomycin-resistant *Staphylococcus aureus* (VRSA)
A strain of *Staphylococcus aureus* that has become resistant to the antibiotic vancomycin.

Vancomycin-resistant *Enterococcus* (VRE)
A form of the bacteria *Enterococcus* that has become resistant to many antibiotics, including vancomycin—one of the most effective antibiotics to treat enterococcal infections.

Methicillin-resistant *Staphylococcus aureus* (MRSA)
A strain of *Staphylococcus aureus* that has become resistant to the antibiotic methicillin.

7.4 All those eligible for health care in each jurisdiction receive hospital and medical care deemed medically necessary. What is medically necessary is somewhat subjective, although most insured services are similar across Canada. For newcomers to Canada, as well as individuals moving from one jurisdiction to another, wait times (usually no more than three months) or other criteria apply.

7.5 Spending on medications is second only to hospital expenditures. All jurisdictions have a drug plan for individuals who meet specified criteria—for example, those receiving financial assistance, those with drug costs disproportionate to their income, disabled persons, and older adults. Almost everyone, including those with private drug insurance, must pay a deductible for prescribed medications.

Review Questions

1. What health care services are offered under the *Canada Health Act*?
2. What body or bodies administer the provincial or territorial health care plan in your province or territory?
3. What is meant by *regionalization of health care services*?
4. How can a drug formulary list reduce the cost of insured drugs for a province or territory?
5. Why does charging health care premiums not contravene the *CHA*?
6. Which provinces require a three-month wait before a newcomer to the province is covered by health insurance?
7. Explain the reciprocal agreement.

References

British Columbia. (n.d.). *The card for you.* Retrieved from http://www2.gov.bc.ca/gov/topic.page?id=1AFEC2D165B646AFBDD2D2420DF9A8D9&title=The%20Card%20for%20Youse used March 20 2014.

British Columbia Ministry of Health. (n.d.a). *Medical and health care benefits.* Retrieved from http://www.health.gov.bc.ca/msp/infoben/benefits.html.

British Columbia Ministry of Health. (n.d.b). *MSP premiums.* Retrieved from http://www.health.gov.bc.ca/msp/infoben/premium.html.

Canada Health Act. (1985). *RSC* c. C-6.

Drug Coverage. (2007). *Private insurance.* Retrieved from http://drugcoverage.ca/en-ca/private-insurance.

Newfoundland and Labrador Department of Finance. (2014). *Health and post secondary education tax (payroll tax).* Retrieved from http://www.fin.gov.nl.ca/fin/tax_programs_incentives/business/education.html.

Manitoba Chiropractors' Association. (n.d.) *Chiropractic health care coverage.* Retrieved from http://www.mbchiro.org/about_chiro/coverage.html.

REFERENCES

Manitoba Taxation Division. (n.d.). *The health and post secondary education tax levy*. Retrieved from http://www.gov.mb.ca/finance/taxation/taxes/payroll.html.

Normandin Beaudry. (2012). *Health insurance premiums and tax*. Retrieved from http://www.normandin-beaudry.ca/userfiles/file/Aide-memoire-2012_Quickfacts_2012_EN.pdf.

Ontario Ministry of Finance. (n.d.). *Employer health tax*. Retrieved from http://www.fin.gov.on.ca/en/tax/eht/.

Ontario Ministry of Finance. (2014). *Ontario health premium*. Retrieved from http://www.fin.gov.on.ca/en/tax/health-premium/.

Raymond Chabot Grant Thornton. (2013). Health services fund—Quebec. *Tax Planning Guide 2013–2014*. Retrieved from http://en.planiguide.ca/tax-planning-guide/section-13-social-programs-benefits/health-services-fund-quebec/.

CHAPTER EIGHT

The Dollars and "Sense" of Health Care Funding

Learning Outcomes

8.1 Explain the role of for-profit and not-for-profit organizations in the delivery of health care.
8.2 Outline the levels and mechanisms of health care funding in Canada.
8.3 Examine how hospitals are funded and what their major expenses are.
8.4 Explain how long-term health care accommodation is funded.
8.5 Describe the reasons for and the effect of rising drug costs in Canada.
8.6 Discuss health expenditures related to human health resources in health care.
8.7 Summarize the cost of advancing technology to the health care system.

KEY TERMS

Active ingredients, p. 278

Alternate levels of care (ALC), p. 274

Capitation-based funding, p. 281

Laparoscopic surgery, p. 270

Nonprofit organization (NPO), p. 272

Nursing home, p. 274

Organisation for Economic Co-operation and Development (OECD), p. 280

Positron emission tomography (PET) scanner, p. 284

Publicly funded health care, p. 257

Rationalization of services, p. 264

Renal dialysis, p. 268

Before you begin reading this chapter, write down—even if it is just a guess—what you think Canada spends on health care in one year and how much you think a visit to your family doctor for an intermediate assessment (for example, for an earache, a sore throat, or a cold) might cost. Next, write down how much you think a knee replacement, a hip replacement, and an appendectomy might cost. Keep these numbers handy to compare with figures you will see later in this chapter, and see the "Conclusion" section at the end of the chapter for the true costs of these services.

Can you imagine going to the doctor for an ear infection and having the administrative assistant ask for cash or a credit card to pay for the visit? Or a parent or aunt or uncle having cardiac bypass surgery or a hip replacement and being sent an invoice? Remember that, in addition to these procedures, the patient would need a preoperative physical examination, blood work, and perhaps an X-ray, magnetic resonance imaging (MRI), an arteriogram, or a computed tomography (CT) scan. He or she would have to pay for the hospital stay, tests, nursing care, and supportive care (e.g., physiotherapy, respiratory therapy)—and would even be charged for the use of the equipment to remove the sutures and the bandages covering the wound. What would you do if you needed such a procedure and knew it would cost you thousands of dollars?

Despite issues of resource availability and wait times, the majority of Canadians have a great deal of pride in their health care system. When they are sick, they seek care, present their health card, and ultimately receive the medical attention they need. If their case proves urgent, the appropriate care is almost always provided immediately. Most of the time, no money comes out of their pockets. Many Canadians believe, though, that because they do not have to shell out money at the point of service or pay a medical bill at the end of the month or upon discharge from a hospital, health care is free. The reality is that Canadians do pay for their **publicly funded health care** services. The money comes from the taxes they pay to all levels of government. Residents of Ontario and British Columbia may also pay health care premiums.

In 2013, an estimated $211 billion was spent on health care. That is an average cost of about $5988 for each Canadian (Canadian Institute for Health Information, 2013a). This chapter examines the actual cost of health care and how health care is funded. The numerous statistics and dollar values presented are approximate because costs change yearly, monthly, and sometimes even daily.

> **Publicly funded health care**
> Health care services whose finances are managed by the government or a government agency for the good of the entire population.

FUNDING VERSUS THE DELIVERY OF HEALTH CARE

The funding and delivery of Canada's health care are accomplished through a mix of public and private—both for-profit and nonprofit—businesses and organizations. *Funding* refers to how health care is paid for, and *delivery* refers to how health care services are managed, structured, and distributed.

In Canada, all medically necessary physician and hospital services are publicly funded but are, for the most part, delivered by either private for-profit or private not-for-profit businesses or organizations. For example, doctors (unless salaried) operate as private for-profit businesses. They deliver health care services and are paid, using varying payment formulas, by the government.

Although hospitals are primarily private, not-for-profit organizations, the majority of services in a hospital—food and meal preparation, maintenance, cleaning, security, and laundry—are delivered by private, for-profit businesses. The hospital negotiates for cost-effective services and pays for them out of the funds allotted them by the government. The majority of laboratory and diagnostic services are other examples of private, for-profit services. Some nonessential services within a hospital—for example, a semi-private or private room, television, or telephone—must be paid for directly by the patient or by a third party, such as through private insurance. Patients can also pay for medical enhancements, such as a fibreglass cast, instead of getting the publicly funded plaster cast. A patient must also pay for any services or treatment not deemed medically necessary—from an MRI scan to knee or cataract surgery. Any cosmetic surgery not deemed medically necessary is not covered by insurance (either public or private).

LEVELS OF HEALTH CARE FUNDING

Canada's public health insurance is funded, for the most part, by the federal, provincial, territorial, and municipal governments through a blend of personal and corporate taxes, and by workers' compensation boards. Some provinces also use revenue from sales taxes and lotteries for health care. Although not mandated by the *Canada Health Act*, British Columbia and Ontario require eligible residents to pay health care premiums (see Chapter 7). At the community level, many volunteer organizations (e.g., hospital auxiliaries, service clubs) also raise money for local hospitals to support such initiatives as expansion, updating of facilities, and purchasing of new equipment. Often the provincial, territorial, or municipal government will match funds raised or a portion thereof.

A portion of health care is funded privately, through households and private insurance. The CIHI (2012) estimates that 30% of health care spending comes out of consumers' pockets or from private insurance, and the remaining 70% is covered by public health plans.

FEDERAL HEALTH TRANSFER PAYMENTS

In 2012, the Government of Canada, through the Canada Health Transfer, paid approximately $27.2 billion for health programs, representing 10 cents of each tax dollar spent and approximately 20% of total health expenditures (Matier, 2012). The government claims this figure will reach $38 billion by 2018 (Department of Finance Canada, 2011c).

The exact dollar figure that the federal government transfers to the provinces and territories is almost impossible to calculate, with figures given continually debated among the jurisdictions. With the federal government's 2014 funding formula (the 2004 Health Accord renegotiation, discussed in Chapter 1), which ties federal to provincial and territorial transfers to the gross domestic product (GDP), the transfer totals will be even more challenging to determine. The government claims the revised formula will bring the federal government's share of health care spending to historic lows, warning that provinces and territories must curb spending and find ways to save money. Provinces and territories have implemented a number of cost-saving strategies, including one called Lean (discussed in Chapter 10). Lean operates on the principle of finding more efficient ways to deliver all levels of health care by eliminating wasteful practices. To date, efficiencies have been found by merging some services, cutting others, and requiring Canadians to pay for services formerly covered by their provincial or territorial plan. Each jurisdiction manages how it spends—and saves—health care dollars.

The exact amount of money spent on health care at the provincial and territorial level is also difficult to determine because of the complexity of the various formulas used to calculate the federal government's transfer payments to each jurisdiction, which are made in the form of both cash and tax points (see Chapter 1). Federal health transfer payment amounts are calculated using a complex formula and are distributed through the following four main transfer models:

1. **Territorial Formula Financing.** The federal government uses the Territorial Formula Financing (TFF) to calculate money given to the territorial governments for public services. This money—allotted to these jurisdictions because of their unique geography, population distribution, and related high cost of delivering health care and other public services—constitutes over 60% of the total monetary resources in Yukon and the Northwest Territories and over 85% in Nunavut.

2. **Equalization payments.** Some provinces and territories have more money than others and thus can provide more public services to their residents. Provinces and territories with less money receive equalization payments from the federal government to allow them to offer their residents services similar to those available in richer jurisdictions. A needy jurisdiction will receive the difference between its *fiscal capacity* (i.e., its ability to generate income) and the *10-province standard* (i.e., the national average). Without equalization payments, these provinces and territories would have to raise their taxes significantly to generate revenue.

In 2012–2013, British Columbia, Alberta, Saskatchewan, and Newfoundland and Labrador did not receive equalization payments. In 2013, Quebec received the largest payment of $7.833 billion; Ontario was next, with $3.169 billion; and Prince Edward Island. received the least, $340 million (Department of Finance Canada, 2011b). These subsidies are distributed in 12 payments over the fiscal year. Nunavut, Yukon, and the Northwest Territories are excluded from equalization payments since the federal government deals with the fiscal needs of the territories through the TFF (Isfeld, 2013).

The concept of equalization payments was established in the Constitution in 1982 (Box 8.1). The provinces and territories are free to determine how they will spend their equalization payments; many use this money, at least in part, for health care.

Box 8.1   Equalization Payments Embedded in the Canadian Constitution

Parliament and the Government of Canada are committed to the principle of making equalization payments to ensure that provincial governments have sufficient revenues to provide reasonably comparable levels of public services at reasonably comparable levels of taxation.

Source: *Constitution Act, 1982*, being Schedule B to the *Canada Act 1982 (UK)*, ss. 36(2).

3. **Canada Health Transfer.** The Canada Health Transfer (CHT) (introduced in Chapter 1), from the federal to the provincial and territorial governments, consists of tax points and cash. Unlike equalization payments, this money has to be used on health care and is subject to other stipulations. However, the 2014 Health Accord, which was a renegotiation of the 2004 accord unilaterally imposed on all jurisdictions (see Chapter 1), removes some stipulations, such as the requirement to reduce wait times for certain hospital procedures. The remaining conditions require the jurisdictions to abide by the rules and regulations outlined in the *Canada Health Act*. The 2014 accord also outlines the government's intentions for federal support until the year 2024. The federal government has guaranteed the provinces and territories 6% health care funding increases until the fiscal year 2016–2017. After that time, the annual funding will be tied to the GDP, with a base guarantee of 3%.

4. **Canada Social Transfer.** The Canada Social Transfer (CST) provides funding to the provinces and territories through cash and tax points for social programs, child care, early childhood development and learning programs, and postsecondary education. The money must be applied to these designated areas. Under the renewal plan (the ending of the 2004 accord), the CST will continue to grow at a rate of 3% per year until 2024 (Department of Finance Canada, 2011a).

Negotiating Funds: Health Accords

Bargaining for health care funding is ongoing among the provinces, territories, and federal government. Needs are studied and analyzed, proposals are made, and agreements, often referred to as *accords*, are signed. The latest accord, which came into effect in 2014 and will expire in 2024, affects funding to the CHT and the CST, as discussed above. The federal government more or less imposed this agreement on the provinces and territories, outlining the government's terms well before negotiations were to begin. Jurisdictions were ultimately told it was a "take it or leave it" offer, effectively eliminating negotiations.

Federal Government Costs for Direct Health Care

As discussed in Chapter 6, under the Canadian Constitution, the federal government is responsible for direct health care services for Canada's Inuit population, First Nations people living on reserves, serving Canadian Forces personnel, inmates in federal prisons, and specified groups of refugee claimants. In 2012, the federal government spent an estimated $6.38 billion on direct health care, and an estimated $6.21 billion in 2013 (Canadian Institute for Health Information, 2013a). The federal departments that have the highest direct health expenditures are Health Canada, followed by the Department of Veterans Affairs, Solicitor General of Canada, and the Department of National Defence (Canadian Institute for Health Information, 2013a).

Provincial and Territorial Costs for Direct Health Care

Canada's total health care spending was an estimated $207 billion in 2012. This figure marked a slight decline of the proportion of Canada's GDP spent on health care to 11.6%, compared with the all-time high of 11.9% in 2010. Though the decline is slight, it may indicate that provinces and territories are making viable efforts in reducing the costs of health care (Canadian Institute for Health Information, 2013a). The provinces and territories spent $130.7 billion on direct health care in 2011 and was forecasting expenditures of $134.7 billion in 2012 and $138.3 billion in 2013 (Canadian Institute for Health Information, 2013a).

A number of things influence the per capita spending among the provinces and territories, including the services paid for by the public plan (i.e., what is considered medically necessary), the type and extent of social programs, the mix of health care providers delivering health care, the relative age of the population, the number of individuals in institutions and long-term care facilities, and the population density of the jurisdiction versus its geographic profile. Note in Table 8.1 that per capita health spending in the Northwest Territories, Yukon, and especially Nunavut is considerably higher than in other jurisdictions. These regions have a lower population base, but their large geographic area and distance between communities make the delivery of health care more complicated and more expensive. For example, population health initiatives such as doing routine screening for colon and breast cancer and educating people on disease prevention are more difficult, as is managing diagnosed chronic health problems.

Table 8.1 Provincial and Territorial Health Spending per Capita: 2013 (estimated)

Province/Territory	Amount	Province/Territory	Amount
Alberta	$6787	Nova Scotia	$6514
British Columbia	$5775	Nunavut	$13,513
Manitoba	$6633	Ontario	$5835
New Brunswick	$6474	Prince Edward Island	$6354
Newfoundland and Labrador	$7132	Quebec	$5531
Northwest Territories	$10,686	Saskatchewan	$6626
		Yukon	$9979

Source: Canadian Institute for Health Information. (2013). Health expenditure summary, by province/territory and Canada [Table 5]. *National health expenditure trends, 1975–2013*, p. 44. Ottawa: Author. Retrieved from https://secure.cihi.ca/free_products/4.0_TotalHealthExpenditureProvTerrEN.pdf.

The provinces and territories spent an estimated $135 billion on health care in the 2012 fiscal year, representing 65% of total health expenditures by government bodies (Canadian Institute for Health Information, 2013a), and yet the prevailing thought is that Canada's government needs to spend more money on health care.

INDIRECT COSTS OF POOR HEALTH

We often think about the cost of poor health relating to what Canada pays directly for health care in terms of treatments and services—nurses' salaries, doctor visits, surgery, rehabilitation, long-term care. However, the cost of illness, injury, and premature mortality to the general Canadian economy, as well as to individuals, is staggering. These indirect costs of poor health include costs associated with loss of productivity and earnings while workers are incapacitated because of a disability or illness.

Unsurprisingly, governments at all levels want to find ways to reduce health care costs while still providing high-quality health care. Disease prevention and health promotion, early diagnosis, and prompt intervention are deemed some of the most effective approaches to achieve this goal. Financial investments in such initiatives (e.g., the focus in primary care models on educating individuals about how to live a healthy lifestyle, reducing the incidence of diabetes, heart disease, and obesity) are believed to be effective upstream strategies with long-term cost-saving benefits.

A 2012 study by Queen's University entitled *Applied Physiology, Nutrition and Metabolism* indicates that chronic diseases that can result from inactivity alone resulted in billions of dollars in both direct and indirect health care costs.

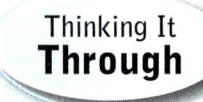

The seasonal flu vaccine and childhood vaccinations are examples of strategies that are believed to have contributed greatly to saving lives and reducing both direct and indirect health care costs. However, in early 2014, there was a resurgence of measles among children who had not been vaccinated against the disease.

1. How do you think vaccinations contribute to a reduction in indirect health care cost?

2. What effect, if any, do you think a resurgence of measles, if not contained, will have on both direct and indirect health care costs?

EXPENDITURES FOR HOSPITALS

As mentioned previously, most Canadian hospitals are not-for-profit facilities. Community-based not-for-profit corporations, religious organizations, and sometimes universities or municipal governments "own" and run these facilities. The province or territory is the main source of revenue for hospitals. Hospitals are, by far, the leading health care expenditure in Canada, as evident in Figure 8.1.

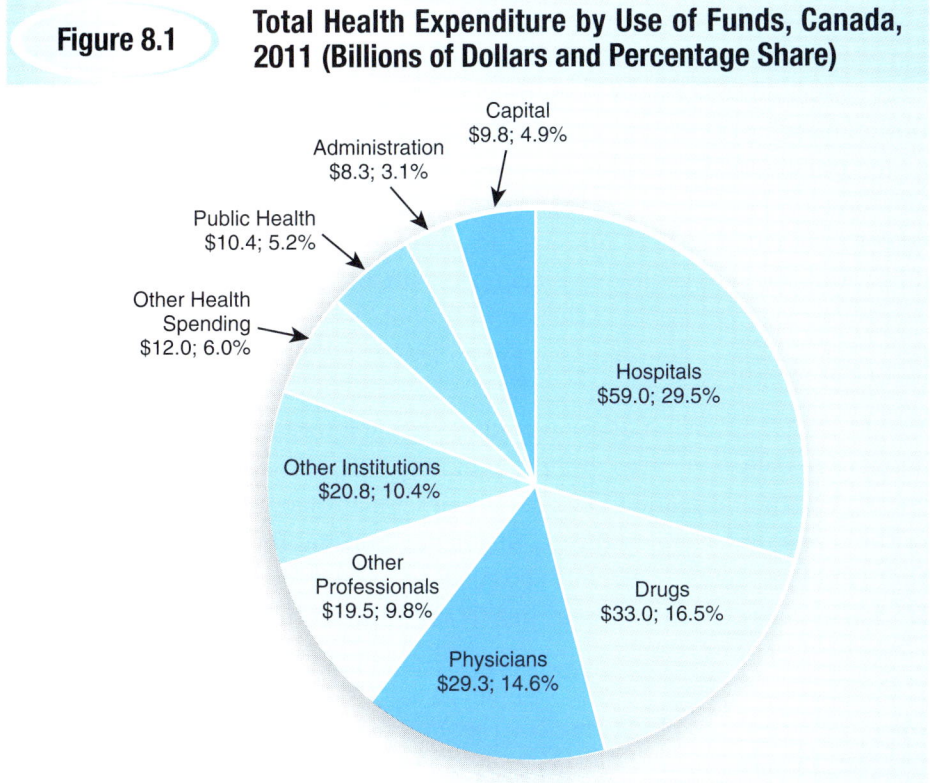

Figure 8.1 **Total Health Expenditure by Use of Funds, Canada, 2011 (Billions of Dollars and Percentage Share)**

Source: Canadian Institute for Health Information. (n.d). *National health expenditure trends, 1975–2013* [Figure 15], p. 22. Retrieved from https://secure.cihi.ca/free_products/3.0_TotalHealthExpenditureFunds EN.pdf.

Hospitals do collect a significant amount of revenue from the private sector through chargeable services (e.g., parking, food services), investments, real estate, rentals, bequeathment, and donations. The rising price of parking at hospitals is a contentious issue. In some cities across Canada, parking fees top $16 per hour (convenient spots, usually metred, cost more), potentially a huge burden for those requiring repeated and lengthy visits to the hospital for treatment, as well as for family members and caregivers visiting inpatients.

Many different types of health care facilities exist, including general and acute care facilities, nursing homes, chronic care facilities, rehabilitation centres, and psychiatric hospitals. All are publicly funded, in part or in whole. Some hospitals treat certain conditions (e.g., Princess Margaret Hospital in Toronto specializes in cancer treatment) or specific age groups (e.g., Vancouver's B.C. Children's Hospital). Other hospitals (e.g., long-term care facilities) may be covered only in part by provincial or territorial insurance, in which case, patients pay a portion of the services they use. Psychiatric hospitals, as well as the services of psychiatrists, however, are fully covered in all provinces.

Problems facing hospitals, communities, and individuals include cuts to services, reductions in hospital beds, closures or merging of hospitals, **rationalization of services** (i.e., improving efficiency by relegating certain types of care to one facility—pediatrics, for example), insufficient and demoralized staff, and long wait lists for surgery, related tests, and admission to hospitals. The following sections will examine how hospitals are funded, how they operate, why operational costs are high, and what is being done to lower costs.

> **Rationalization of services**
> Any changes that increase the effectiveness and efficiency of health care services—clinical, administrative, or financial.

Hospital Funding Mechanisms

The provincial or territorial ministry or department of health provides funds to hospitals to deliver services to the community. The hospital is then expected to operate as a business, ending the fiscal year with a balanced budget.

The terms under which this money depend on the funding model the hospital functions under. Currently, hospitals in several provinces and territories are working closely with regional health authorities to revise funding models to increase efficiencies.

In the case of *block funding*, popular since the 1970s, a hospital's funding amount is determined by its previous year's expenditures. Block funding is still relatively prevalent across Canada.

Line-by-line funding, still popular in British Columbia and New Brunswick, itemizes the costs of specific services and equipment within a hospital, referred to as *line items* or *inputs*, and the hospital receives the amount of money needed for each service.

Ontario hospitals are reviewing the model of *service-based funding* (also called the *case-mix approach*), which is gaining popularity. The types of cases treated and the volume of patients seen provide the foundation for an analysis of expenditure needs. Patients who have similar types of medical problems and undergo similar treatments are grouped using a formula; the cost of their treatments and services is estimated; and the amount of funding the hospital receives relates to how many patients it treats requiring each combination of services. The funding is then provided in the form of a global budget (i.e., an annual lump sum of money). Many hospitals adopting this funding approach also use line-by-line funding. For example, a hospital would receive money to complete a designated number of hip or knee replacements.

Activity-based funding pays hospitals in accordance with the number and types of services the facility provides to each patient. The goal of this model is to make the facility more efficient and reduce wait times. Implemented first in Ontario, the model was used to reduce wait times for selected services such as cataract surgery, cardiac bypass surgery, and joint replacement. Alberta implemented activity-based funding in 2010 for selected services, and British Columbia has dramatically reduced wait times for selected services (e.g., shoulder surgery, MRIs, and emergency care) in facilities where this model has been applied. New Brunswick and Quebec are also testing this payment model (Mickleburgh, 2012; Canadian Agency for Drugs and Technologies in Health, n.d.).

The *population-based funding model* (sometimes called *capitated funding*), used by Alberta and Saskatchewan for several years, grants hospitals money based on demographics (e.g., patients' ages, gender, socioeconomic status). In all, more than 100 different individual prototypes exist based on these criteria, with varying amounts awarded depending on location and on how many patients fall into certain categories. For example, a hospital in an area with a large population of older adults may receive more money than one with a mainly younger clientele, and since lower socioeconomic groups require more health care services, hospitals catering to patients in that category receive more funding. The hospital's size and location, as well as the services it offers, are also factored into the budget.

Requirements for Funding

Every hospital must be accountable for the funds it requests. After completing its budget, the hospital assesses its financial needs, prepares documentation, and negotiates with the minister of health for appropriate funding. To facilitate these activities, the hospital must track the expenses of all departments and services.

At the end of the fiscal year, a hospital must report on its financial status—whether it is in the black (i.e., posting a surplus) or in the red (i.e., posting a deficit). A hospital in the red must look for ways either to reduce costs or to be approved for extra funding—not an easy feat. It must critically examine the services it offers and the cost of each and determine where cuts can be made.

A hospital may have to reduce services and staff, close beds, decrease operating time, or do all of these things to keep within its budget. Under certain circumstances, the ministry or department of health may grant extra money to hospitals with budget shortfalls.

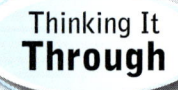 

Thinking It Through

Not realizing that they pay for health care services with their tax dollars, many Canadians believe health care is free, leading to misuse and abuse of the system.

1. If people were given a receipt showing the cost of each doctor's visit, hospital stay, and services received, do you think they might use health care services more prudently?

2. Do you think that lack of awareness of the costs of services contributes to the attitude that health care is free?

3. Two provinces pay health care premiums. Do you think these extra charges void the concept that health care is free?

The Cost of Hospital Care

Hospitals offer diagnostic tests, treatment, and patient care for most serious illnesses and diseases. The cost for caring for patients in hospital in Canada topped $24 billion in 2012–2013, not including physicians' fees. When grouped by general categories, the most expensive hospitalizations were for cardiovascular conditions, followed by mental health disorders, diseases of the digestive system, and then diseases of the respiratory system. However, when broken down by diagnosis, diseases of the respiratory system (i.e., COPD, followed by pneumonia) cost hospitals the most. In terms of hospitalization for interventions, hip and knee replacements were the costliest (Canadian Institute for Health Information, n.d.b). Pregnancy and childbirth, the leading cause of hospital admissions for women of childbearing age, costs $2500 per person on average, although the cost varies with the nature of the delivery—an uncomplicated vaginal delivery costs just under $2285 while a Caesarean section costs just over $5085 (Canadian Institute for Health Information, n.d.b).

The majority of Canadians remain unaware of how much the government pays for various procedures. Table 8.2 provides a list of the costs of some of the more common procedures and conditions for which individuals are admitted to hospital. Imagine having to pay to have a baby and then your two-year-old

Table 8.2 Average Cost of Procedures and Conditions for Inpatients, 2010–2011

Procedure/Condition	Average Cost per Hospitalization* ($)	Average Length of Stay (days)
Lung or heart transplant	98,051	33
Liver transplant	67,958	26.6
Heart valve replacement	30,008	10
Surgery resulting in a colostomy (e.g., due to cancer)	18,158	14
Hip replacement (one hip)	9284	4
Palliative care	9090	9.7
Knee replacement (one knee)	8855	4.4
Open cholecystectomy, uncomplicated	8623	7.6
Heart attack (plus angiogram)	7944	4.5
Hysterectomy (diagnosis of cancer)	7368	3.4
Depressive episode	6753	10
Stroke	6552	8
Chronic obstructive pulmonary disease (COPD)	6335	5.3
Chemotherapy/radiotherapy session (neoplasm)	5125	3.9
Hysterectomy (no diagnosis of cancer)	4556	2.6
Caesarean section (no induction)	4079	3.2
Diabetes	3965	4
Laparoscopic cholecystectomy (gallbladder removal)	3471	2.2
Influenza/acute upper respiratory infection	3341	3
Appendectomy	3251	1.6
Symptom of digestive system	2539	3
Croup (child 1–7 years)	1505	1

* Costs exclude physicians' fees for procedures or in-hospital visits; they bill the jurisdiction for services rendered.

Source: Canadian Institute for Health Information. (n.d.). *Patient cost estimator*. Retrieved from http://www.cihi.ca/cihi-ext-portal/internet/en/documentfull/spending+and+health+workforce/spending/pce_application.

needing admission to the hospital for croup and your dependant father needing a hip replacement because of a fall. How would you handle the costs if you had to pay out of pocket?

The Cost of Hospital Services

The staff and infrastructure needed to provide hospital care incur significant costs. In 2012, staffing took up over 50% of the hospital's budget. Diagnostic and therapeutic services are the next largest expenditure, accounting for approximately 24% of a hospital's budget in 2010–2011 (Canadian Institute for Health Information, 2011). Administrative costs can also be significant.

Administration and Support Services

Every hospital has administrative expenses, such as human resources (e.g., clinical secretaries, admission clerks), information technology (e.g., communication, systems support), and finance. Support services include materials management, security, housekeeping, volunteer services, health records, registration, food services, and laundry. According to the CIHI (2012b), in 2011, total costs for administration in health care were $6.27 billion, meaning the administration costs of hospitals and health care facilities accounted for 3.1% of total health spending in Canada. Ontario has the highest administrative costs, at close to 6%. Many regions have consolidated their hospitals under one CEO and one board to reduce administrative costs (Ogilvie & Poisson, 2012).

Nursing Services

Registered nurses (RNs), practical nurses (called *registered practical nurses* [RPN] in Ontario and *licensed practical nurses* [LPN] in all other provinces and territories), nurses' aides, orderlies, and personal support workers make up the nursing staff within health care facilities. The particular mix of regulated and nonregulated health care providers used will vary with each facility. Typically, acute care hospitals rely on regulated professionals to deliver nursing care, but, again, the mix may vary, depending on the level of care patients require. Nursing staff work in most departments that interact with inpatients or outpatients.

In analyzing their costs, most hospitals exclude the cost of nursing services for inpatient care. Expenditures for other nursing staff may be accounted for in the costs of specialized departments (e.g., outpatient clinic, **renal dialysis**, cancer day treatments).

> **Renal dialysis**
> A process that filters waste and fluid from the blood similar to the way kidneys do. Individuals whose kidneys are not functioning must undergo this procedure several times a week to stay alive while waiting for a kidney transplant.

Medical Staff

You might think that medical staff—doctors, residents, interns—would represent the highest costs, but most of these individuals operate independently of the hospital, although some medical staff members may be on contract or in salaried positions (e.g., the chief of a department, a hospitalist, or an emergentologist). Other physicians may assume teaching responsibilities for interns and residents. Doctors who admit, visit, and treat inpatients are usually not paid by the hospital. Rather, they bill their provincial plan for services or receive payment in other ways.

Other Departments

Other hospital departments usually have their own budget and are expected to function in a cost-effective manner within that budget. The operating room, for example, has specific expenses, including costs for its use; supplies, instruments, and other equipment (e.g., devices implanted into a patient, such as an artificial hip); and staff with specialized skills (e.g., nurses with specialized training). Likewise, those managing an emergency department (ED) must do so with their budget in mind. Some EDs (also called *emergency rooms* [*ER*s]) employ nurse practitioners to see patients with less serious conditions so as to offset the costs of an employed emergentologist. Some hospitals restrict the hours of operation of their ED; some have closed their emergency departments altogether.

COST-REDUCTION STRATEGIES

As mentioned, hospitals use a variety of methods to reduce their overall costs. The most commonly applied strategies include decreasing patients' length of stay and rationalizing services.

Length of Stay

Decreasing the length of hospital stays is an important way to reduce costs and to make beds available for those who need them. Over the past ten years, great strides have been made toward this goal.

The province or territory determines the cost of an insured bed to a hospital (paid for out of the allotted budget) by estimating the services required by the person occupying the bed. For example, a patient in an acute care bed recovering from hip surgery would be deemed more expensive than one recovering from an appendectomy. A long-term care bed typically costs the hospital less than beds in other wards because the person occupying the bed usually requires less care. Interestingly, the use of semi-private and private rooms generates income for a hospital (Case Example 8.1).

The following strategies have helped to reduce the length of stays in hospitals across Canada.

Case Example 8.1

Margaretha, a 65-year-old woman who will be admitted to hospital for knee replacement next week, is wondering whether she can afford private accommodation. A semi-private room (i.e., a room containing two beds) would cost approximately $220 more per person per day than would a ward or standard bed, and a private room would cost a further $220 per person per day above that. So, if Margaretha had regular provincial or territorial health insurance and wanted a private room, she would pay $440 per day out of her own pocket. However, if she had semi-private coverage through a private insurance or group benefits plan and wanted to have a private room, she would pay $220 per day out of her own pocket.

Same-Day Admissions

In the past, individuals scheduled for major surgery were admitted one or two days prior to their operation for tests and what was called *preop preparation*, which consisted of a medical history, a physical, bowel cleansing, shave if needed, preoperative instruction, and nighttime sedation to ensure a sound sleep.

Today, for many surgeries, this preparation is done on an outpatient basis. The family doctor typically performs the physical and takes a preoperative history a week or so prior. Tests, such as blood work and an electrocardiogram, are done several days before the surgery. Pre- and postoperative instruction are given on an outpatient basis: the patient makes an appointment at the hospital, watches a video, and has an opportunity to have questions answered, usually by a surgical nurse or nurse educator. Any necessary preparation (e.g., not eating or drinking for eight hours before the operation) is done at home by the patient (shave preps are frequently omitted). On the morning of the surgery, the individual is admitted, preoperative information not already obtained is gathered, and the preoperative sedation, if any, is administered. Considering the large number of surgeries that take place within each province or territory each day, omitting one night in hospital for every patient results in a significant savings.

Technology and Day Surgery

Because of technological advances in many fields, particularly in **laparoscopic surgery**, many surgeries are now done on an outpatient basis. For example, the routine removal of the gallbladder (called a *cholecystectomy*) once required a large abdominal incision but now requires only a small incision using a laparoscope. The patient, admitted as an outpatient, goes home the same day. When

---

Laparoscopic surgery
A type of surgical procedure in which a small incision is made in the body, through which a viewing tube (laparoscope) is inserted. A small camera in the laparoscope allows the doctor to examine internal organs. Other small incisions may be made to insert instruments to perform surgery.

the surgery required a larger incision, the patient would stay in hospital for seven days or more. However, even when larger incisions are done today, the patient seldom remains in hospital longer than two or three days. Many other procedures are also performed on an outpatient basis, including cataract surgery, tubal ligations, and hernia repairs.

Services Within the Community

Gaining support in all jurisdictions, community-based care offers patients a variety of services delivered within their own community or at home. Often accessed through a central body, such as Community Care Access Centres in Ontario (CCAC), these services support patients through illness, providing medical care, supportive and rehabilitative care as necessary, long-term support, and palliative care. A significant number of people with health problems now receive care at home instead of in the hospital. Patients are first accepted into a home care program, their health and care needs are assessed, and care is provided.

Community-based care reduces both hospital admissions and the length of stay for individuals who do become hospitalized. The Canadian Home Care Association, the Victorian Order of Nurses, and Meals on Wheels are just three organizations that offer community-based care services. Home care services are not always fully covered by provincial or territorial insurance plans, but these organizations themselves often provide coverage in whole or in part; any residual uninsured costs remain the responsibility of users. Various levels of government, regional health authorities, insurance companies, or private corporations may hire an organization to provide a specific service.

Timely Discharge

Hospitals endeavour to discharge inpatients by 10:00 or 11:00 A.M. Depending on the policies of the jurisdiction, the province or territory will charge the hospital for an additional 24-hour period if a patient is not discharged by a certain time, often noon. If a discharged patient cannot arrange to leave before the discharge time, the nurses will, if possible, have the patient vacate his or her bed and perhaps wait in a lounge so that the room can be cleaned and readied for an admission. Individuals undergoing day procedures such as surgery are likewise kept only until they are deemed stable, and then they are discharged.

Discharge of Postoperative Patients

Even those undergoing major surgeries may receive early discharge. Several years ago, a person having a hip replacement would be in an acute care hospital bed for up to 10 days and then moved to a rehabilitation bed for several weeks. Today, hip replacement patients are often discharged within a week; a visiting nurse will follow up with them at home to assess their progress, to dress the incision, and to provide any other necessary medical care. Afterward, a physiotherapist will make home visits to help the patient become mobile again. In addition, an occupational therapist will often assess the home to make recommendations for creating a safe environment and prescribe the appropriate assistive devices to ensure a safe recovery.

Palliative Care Patients

Palliative care is care provided to individuals with terminal illnesses. In the past, when people became too ill to be cared for at home, they were admitted to hospital to die. Many still are, especially if their need for pain control cannot be met at home or if family members simply cannot emotionally or physically manage without the intervention of community services. However, many terminally ill people prefer to spend their remaining time at home. A visiting nurse and other community support services then provide the necessary care, supporting both the family and the patient. Palliative care facilities (hospices) are becoming more popular across the country. Many are funded largely through local organizations, with some funding from the government or **nonprofit organizations** or both. The Canadian Hospice Palliative Care Association states that 16% to 36% of Canadians have access to hospice palliative care and end-of-life services. As our population continues to age, the urgency for more hospice beds increases, as well as for more specially trained health care providers and volunteers.

Other Conditions Managed at Home

Many other medical conditions, including cancer, can now be managed on an outpatient basis. In the past, a patient receiving chemotherapy following cancer surgery was admitted to hospital for a day or more to receive treatment. Today, oncology outpatient clinics provide this treatment. The patient comes in at a designated time, receives his or her treatment, and goes home. Outpatient cancer treatments are made possible, in part, because of improved chemotherapy drugs. Whereas, in the past, many chemotherapy drugs caused severe nausea and vomiting, today's have fewer adverse effects.

A variety of other medical problems can also be managed at home. Patients receiving fluids through an intravenous (IV) needle used to be hospitalized. However, advances in IV equipment and monitoring mean IVs can be used safely at home. A visiting nurse comes several times a day, if needed, to assess the infusion (called *parenteral therapy*) and to provide IV antibiotics or other medications as necessary. Individuals needing parenteral pain management may also use "pain pumps" (electronic infusion pumps that deliver a prescribed amount of painkillers intravenously), which come in various types.

> **Nonprofit organizations (NPOs)**
> Organizations that return surplus revenue (profits) back to the facility for purposes of maintaining or improving the facility and its operations; usually managed by a board as opposed to private owners.

People with multiple chronic diseases may also remain at home and manage their illnesses with support from organizations or individuals, such as family doctors, outpatient clinics, community nurses, and community health centres.

Community Health Centres

Fairly similar in structure across the country, community health centres (CHCs) offer the services of a health care team that includes doctors, nurse practitioners, counsellors, community workers, and dietitians. CHCs provide support, treatment, and preventive care services to Canadians who have difficulty accessing health care because of language or cultural barriers, disabilities, poverty, or homelessness. These nonprofit centres also are pivotal in keeping individuals out of hospital by supporting them within the community setting.

Rationalization and Mergers

Governments have also cut costs by rationalizing hospital services (e.g., restructuring, downsizing, merging care or administrative services, decentralizing, and closing) in an effort to prevent the duplication of services, to provide care at the necessary level within a community, and to better use resources. For example, in Kitchener, Ontario, cardiac and cancer services are centralized—St. Mary's Hospital has become the cardiac centre, and Grand River Hospital, the cancer centre. Government funds were invested in both hospitals to update, upgrade, and expand services in these specialty areas. Obstetrical services are offered only at Grand River Hospital, although both hospitals maintain a viable emergency department. Eliminating the duplication of services saves money, and, ultimately, a higher level of care results because more sophisticated and technologically advanced equipment can be purchased and operated by highly skilled health care providers.

Rationalization also involves delivering the right kind of care at the right level to the right person. Adopting regional health authorities and similar organizations across the country has contributed to supplying appropriate health care for individual communities.

Hospital mergers occur in two main ways:

1. The *horizontal model* merges several hospitals under one administration—one board, one CEO, one budget—but maintains several sites.

2. The *vertical model* merges specific programs within a single organization; however, the administration of various programs may remain independent of one another, thus not be under the direction of one board.

The advantages of merging are broad: reduced duplication of services, higher levels of efficiency, lower administration and management costs, and the ability to offer more services with better results for patient care and recovery. Larger institutions are also believed to attract more staff. However, studies have shown some negative outcomes when larger hospitals merge, one of the greatest being the effects on staff. Mergers often result in a disruption in a hospital's culture, lost seniority, and displacement of staff members, either through a reorganization of positions or layoffs. Mergers of smaller hospitals appear to be more successful because the resulting facility broadens its service base while retaining staff and improving care. How successful mergers are in reducing costs remains controversial.

LONG-TERM CARE ACCOMMODATION

> **Alternate levels of care (ALC)**
> Inpatient care in a facility or part of a facility in which the level of care provided meets the physical, mental, and emotional needs of the patient.

As the Canadian population ages, the number of individuals requiring **alternate levels of care (ALC)** will continue to increase. Patients in acute care beds in hospitals waiting to be discharged either home or to some form of residential care are among those needing ALC. In Canada, various terms apply to facilities caring for individuals (mostly older adults) who have more complex health issues and require different levels of support. The needs of these individuals are varied and complex and often include both physical and mental infirmities (e.g., dementia). Residential care, in general, includes lodges, assisted living, nursing, long-term care, and special care and personal care homes. In Ontario alone, the number of people requiring ALC is expected to rise by 32% over the next 10 years.

> **Nursing home**
> A facility or part of a facility that provides accommodation to persons usually over the age of 16 requiring intensive personal care under the supervision of a registered nurse.

In 2012, over $20.77 billion was spent on long-term care and other institutions, the fifth largest health care spending category. The estimated cost for 2013 was $22.28 billion (Canadian Institute for Health Information, 2012a). The number of older Canadians living in nursing homes and similar dwellings has risen by 38% in the past decade (De Souza, 2012). **Nursing homes**, also called *long-term care* or *personal care facilities*, provide varying levels of care—from care for those who require minimal support but are unable to live on their own to care for those who require total care and supervision for physical or mental reasons—24 hours a day, seven days a week. Levels of care are classified as independent, semi-independent, and dependent (Case Example 8.2).

Provincial and territorial governments oversee long-term care for all Canadians, with the exception of those individuals eligible for federal care through Veterans Affairs Canada, workers' compensation boards, federal government acts, and medical health insurance. Licensed by the provincial and territorial ministries of health, long-term care facilities (often privately owned) must meet standards regarding staffing levels, training, food preparation, pricing, and medical care, including the administration of medications. Unsubsidized and unlicensed residences also exist, but they offer limited or no nursing care and are usually regulated by municipal bylaws, which do not control the quality of care.

The provincial or territorial government controls the number of long-term beds in the province or territory, so all beds must be approved by the government.

Case Example 8.2

Seventy-two-year-old Olivia has had a stroke. She is fully cognizant and can manage some activities of daily living but needs assistance with dressing, eating, and moving about. Because she was unable to manage at home despite home care support, she is now in a nursing home, semi-dependent, and receiving a moderate level of nursing supervision and supportive care.

However, if Olivia had severe Alzheimer's disease (i.e., had no memory, wandered, and could not feed herself) and fell and broke her hip, she would be placed in a secure unit with maximum nursing supervision and be almost completely dependent.

Governments at this level also subsidize public nursing home beds; however, in most provinces and territories, the patient must pay a flat rate for basic accommodation, a fee called a copayment. This copayment covers the cost of room and board and possibly some operational costs, such as laundry services, administrative services, equipment costs, and mortgage expenses. The portion of costs a resident must pay may depend on his or her financial circumstances (Case Example 8.3) and whether he or she has a spouse living in the community, in which case, payment would be adjusted so that the spouse can retain enough money to remain in his or her home. All jurisdictions have alternative funding options for those unable to pay, and no one can be denied accommodation or care.

Case Example 8.3

After falling and breaking her hip, 80-year-old Ibia can no longer live independently at home. Arrangements have been made for her to move to Happy Meadows, a nursing home close by. Ibia has concerns about being able to afford nursing home care and is even more worried about what will happen to her life's savings and her house. "They will take all of my money," she laments. "What will happen to my house? I heard they take everything to pay for staying there!" What might happen to Ibia?

The answer depends on what province or territory Ibia lives in and what type of nursing home Happy Meadows is. In most jurisdictions, the patient's monthly income must be used toward payment of his or her accommodation. Ibia need not worry about her house and savings,

Continued on next page

however. These assets are protected (although the amount of protection varies across jurisdictions) and will not be accounted for in the assessment of her ability to pay. If Ibia's monthly income from her pensions is $2000 and the copayment is $3000 per month, Ibia will have to surrender the bulk of her income for her accommodation but will not be required to make the full copayment. The government will cover the balance, leaving her with enough money for personal expenses, and Ibia would be eligible only for basic accommodation. Depending on the minimum accommodations available at Happy Meadows, she may be in a ward with several beds (up to six) or in a semi-private room with only one other person.

If Ibia's monthly income were $3000 and the cost of her standard accommodation were $2500 monthly, Ibia would be required to pay the full amount, leaving her with $500 left over to spend as she pleases.

In Newfoundland and Labrador, the approximate cost of a basic long-term care bed in the public system is $2800 per month, which the resident is asked to pay. If the resident cannot afford this fee, the regional health authority will perform a financial assessment to determine how much the patient can afford. In Saskatchewan, the monthly cost ranges from $1025 to $1951, depending on income, because the Ministry of Health pays about 80% of the province's long-term care costs.

Generally, government subsidies covering the cost of a nursing home bed apply only to basic (or ward) accommodation. As in hospitals, ward accommodation can mean a four- or even six-bed room. Many newer or renovated facilities, however, offer only semi-private and private accommodation. In these facilities, a semi-private room would qualify as basic accommodation. Some facilities include "preferred" semi-private rooms, which are divided by a partial wall, affording a greater level of privacy and dignity to each resident.

Across Canada, the aging population poses a challenge to governments and private nursing home facilities to ensure that an adequate number of long-term beds are available. The quality of long-term care is also an ongoing concern, with horror stories about the abuse of residents surfacing nationwide. In 2013, a man hid a video camera in his mother's room and caught on tape outright abuse (Leung, 2013). As well, there have been multiple reports of residents abusing and, in some cases, killing other residents. Staff members are also sometimes at risk for injury from residents. Another continuing challenge is the question of housing potentially combative individuals with mental health issues including dementia in long-term care facilities, but often there is no other place for them to go. Staff shortages related to inadequate financing are most often cited as the cause of many of these problems.

THE RISING COST OF DRUGS

Next to hospital services, drugs represent the second largest health care expense (see Figure 8.1). According to the CIHI (2013a), drug spending continues to increase, but not as rapidly as in previous years. In total, including public and private insurance and out-of-pocket expenditures, spending on drugs in 2012 was $33 billion. The largest portion (45% paid for with public funds) was for prescription drugs. Averaged, nearly $1000 was spent on each Canadian—the least in British Columbia, with Nova Scotia having the highest per capita expenditure. Spending on drugs by hospitals was $2.4 billion, including $800 million for cancer drugs.

Major Cost Drivers for Drug Expenditures

Increased drug expenditures can be attributed to several factors, including the facts that more people are taking medications and more people are taking multiple medications. Drugs used for high blood pressure, high cholesterol, and gastrointestinal disorders are most common. It is worth noting that although older Canadians have a significantly higher per capita spending related to drugs, compared to other cost drivers (volume increase and drug mix), drug expenditure for older Canadians is and will remain modest.

Newer drugs' being brought to market increases the cost of drugs. Many pharmaceutical companies are researching and producing more specialized medications, which are more expensive. A class of drugs called *biologics* (e.g., immunosuppressants and cancer drugs), which are derived from living material, are growing in popularity. Added to the expense are "targeted drugs" that require biomarker testing to ensure they are right for the patient. For example, one course of trastuzumab (Herceptin), a cancer drug, can cost up to $40,000. Coverage under provincial- and territorial-funded plans for this and similar drugs is variable across the country (Reinberg, 2005; CBC News, 2011).

Over the next few years, patents on a large number of brand-name drugs will expire; generic equivalents will then be available, bringing down the cost of prescription drugs. Most provincial and territorial formularies use generic drugs, although brand-name drugs are allowed by special permission if there is not a generic equivalent to effectively treat a specific condition (Canadian Institute for Health Information, n.d.d; University of British Columbia, 2012; Law, Cheng, Dhalla, et al., 2012).

Drug Insurance

All provinces and territories provide some kind of drug insurance to certain groups, such as older Canadians, people with disabilities, and individuals who earn low incomes or are on social assistance. A copayment or deductible may apply (see Chapter 5), but some pharmacies will waive deductibles and copayments in certain circumstances.

Canada is one of only a few developed countries without a national drug plan. However, most provinces and territories have some form of catastrophic drug coverage, meaning they will assume the cost of very expensive drugs for specific health conditions when the family is unable to cover the expense. Quebec has had a provincial drug plan since 1997 for those who do not have private drug insurance.

A drug's accessibility and coverage through an insurance plan are determined by its category: over-the-counter (OTC) medications can be purchased without a prescription and are rarely covered by public or private health plans; prescription medications can be purchased only with a prescription from a health care provider (e.g., family doctor or specialist; in some jurisdictions, nurse practitioner or midwife) and may be covered in part or in full by insurance.

Occasionally, a province or territory will remove a drug from the list of drugs that may be obtained only with a prescription. Once removed, however, insurance will no longer cover the drug.

BRAND-NAME AND GENERIC DRUGS

Brand-name drugs—those that are owned and sold by the company that developed them—cost more than generic drugs. They are protected under a piece of legislation called the *Patent Act*. Currently, patents last 20 years from the time the pharmaceutical company applies to the board for approval to sell the drug in Canada. Once a patent expires, any drug company can produce the drug (called a *generic drug*) and sell it at a lower cost (a quarter to a half of the brand-name counterpart). Brand-name drug names are always capitalized; generic drug names are not (e.g., *ibuprofen* is a generic drug; *Advil* is a brand-name drug).

Because they do not have to spend money on research and development, companies producing generic drugs can do so at a greatly reduced cost. Generic drugs contain the same **active ingredients**, although the other ingredients (called *nonmedicinal ingredients*) vary. All generic drugs go through an approval process and analysis similar to those of brand-name drugs. Some claim that brand-name drugs are of a higher quality and that different nonmedicinal ingredients can alter the action and efficacy of the drug. Unless a doctor specifically indicates on a prescription "no substitution," pharmacists may substitute a generic drug for a brand-name one.

Active ingredients
Those ingredients in a drug that have therapeutic value meant to cure, palliate, or otherwise treat a health problem.

Controlling the Cost of Patented Drugs

An independent government agency, the Patented Medicine Prices Review Board (PMPRB), regulates the price at which patentees—pharmaceutical companies—sell their patented medicines in Canada to wholesalers, hospitals, pharmacies, and others (e.g., clinics), called the *factory-gate price*. Although the PMPRB can ensure that drug companies themselves do not charge excessive prices, the board does not have jurisdiction over the prices retailers charge customers or over pharmacists' dispensing fees. For the duration of the patent, the PMPRB regulates the prices of all *patented* products, including those available only through prescription, those sold over the counter, and those available through Health Canada's Special Access Program, a program that provides physicians access to existing drugs not currently on the market that might prove effective for treating serious or life-threatening conditions when mainstream medications have proven ineffective, are not readily available, or cannot be tolerated by a specific patient. Importantly, the PMPRB has no authority to regulate the prices of nonpatented drug products (i.e., drug products that were never patented or for which the patent has expired).

HUMAN HEALTH RESOURCES

The term *human health resources* (HHR) refers to all people who work in the health care field, ranging from doctors and nurses to laboratory technologists, respiratory therapists, and chiropodists. Estimates suggest that more than 1.197 million people work in the health care field in Canada (Statistics Canada, 2014). The largest of the regulated professions is nursing, followed by medicine (i.e., physicians). Currently, postsecondary institutions offer more than 150 different health care programs across the country, with more emerging (Canadian Institute for Health Information, n.d.a).

In recent years, several new related professions have been introduced, including hospitalist, emergentologist, physician's assistant, nurse practitioner, nurse endoscopist, clinical specialist radiation therapist, and anaesthesia assistant.

Over the past decade, Canada has endured a shortage of many health care providers, particularly doctors and nurses—the two largest cost drivers of HHR—but the numbers are slowly beginning to recover. In 2012, Canada had more doctors per capita than ever before, with the highest growth in rural areas. Manitoba had the lowest physician growth rate, while British Columbia and Newfoundland and Labrador reported the largest increases. Surprisingly, although physician shortages in all sectors persist, a large number of specialists (e.g., general surgeons, orthopedic surgeons, oncologists, critical care specialists, and urologists)—about 16%—cannot find jobs in Canada. Several reasons are cited, including too many doctors in relation to resources such as operating rooms and hospital beds. Many hospitals, clinics, and other facilities simply cannot afford to hire them. Numerous specialists are deferring their retirement, making opportunities for others scarce. An overabundance of physicians in some specialties and poor geographic distribution of specialties are other reasons given (Di Matteo, 2013). In 2011–2012, doctors were paid $22 billion for clinical services, up almost 8% over the previous year. Physician services account for about 15% of overall health care spending (Canadian Institute for Health Information, 2013b).

The number of nurses in the workforce also has increased significantly—by 8% within five years—with more than 408,000 RNs in Canada. While the numbers of those entering the field are up, the increase can also be attributed to nurses staying in the profession longer. The number of RNs has grown by only 15%; LPNs and RPNs, by approximately 50%; and NPs, also by 50% (Canadian Institute for Health Information, 2014). Many facilities, however, employ nurses on only a part-time basis. It can take licensed or registered practical nurses up to ten years to find a full-time position, and registered nurses or registered psychiatric nurses, up to five years (Canadian Institute for Health Information, 2014). Nevertheless, nursing remains the largest expenditure in acute care hospitals (Canadian Institute for Health Information, 2013a).

Despite the growing numbers of doctors, nurses, and other health care providers, disparities in the availability and access to health professionals still exist from one region to another. Compared with other countries in the **Organisation for Economic Co-operation and Development (OECD)**, Canada spends significantly more on health care but has fewer physicians and nurses than do other countries. According to 2013 OECD health statistics, Canada ranked twenty-eighth out of 34 countries in the ratio of patients to doctors, with 2.4 practising physicians per 1000 people. Greece had the most, and Chili the fewest. There were 9.3 qualified nurses per 1000 people, slightly higher than the OECD average of 8.7 (Organisation for Economic Co-operation and Development, 2014).

Organisation for Economic Co-operation and Development (OECD)
Established in 1961 and now representing 30 countries, the OECD provides a setting in which member governments compare policy experiences, seek answers to common problems, identify best practices, and coordinate domestic and international policies.

How Physicians Are Paid: Billing Options

Most physicians, an estimated 71% in 2011–2012, are paid through the fee-for-service method, but that trend is changing, with more doctors opting for alternative modes of payments. The following sections summarize the most common payment options for doctors in Canada.

Fee-for-Service

Fee-for-service (FFS) is the oldest and, for the moment, most widely accepted method of physician payment in Canada. Using this method, doctors charge the provincial or territorial plan for every service they perform. Each province or territory has slightly different parameters for FFS billing. Invariably, though, the amount the doctor bills relates to the complexity and length of the patient visit.

Within the FFS model, doctors can also bill for things other than the actual office visit. For example, doctors who make house calls can charge more to ensure they are compensated for travel, for seeing a patient away from the office, for the time of day or night the house call is made, and for the patient visits cancelled if making a house call during office hours. Doctors may also bill for procedures such as giving an injection or suturing a wound or for visiting a patient in hospital. Amounts billed also vary depending on whether the doctor is the most responsible physician (MRP) or is only providing a consultation. (In the hospital, the MRP is the physician with the primary responsibility for caring for the patient; the MRP may be the patient's family doctor but is usually a specialist.) Many doctors prefer to hang on to FFS, at least in part. Some of the primary health care reform models blend capitation-based funding (described below) with FFS.

Capitation- or Population-Based Funding

Capitation-based funding (also called *population-based funding*) pays the doctor for each rostered patient in his or her practice. This funding format is often used by doctors in private practice who also operate under the umbrella of an alternative health care delivery format, such as a primary health care reform group. Rostered patients of a primary health care network are asked to sign a form to say that they will seek medical nonemergent care only from their family doctor or members of that particular health care group. (For more details, see Chapter 9.) Physicians must receive approval from their provincial or territorial government to form such a group. Once physicians begin working in their selected primary care model, they are usually paid monthly. With capitation-based funding, doctors receive for each patient a set amount that is determined by the patient's age, health care needs, or both. A doctor, therefore, would be paid more per year for an 89-year-old patient with multiple health problems than for a 22-year-old healthy patient. Whether the patient visits the doctor once or 30 times in that year, the doctor receives the same amount of money. Additionally, doctors are paid extra for achieving certain milestones, such as immunizing a given portion of eligible patients and doing routine Pap smears and Pap smears for women in high-risk groups. (Physicians must track women in their practice and put procedures in place to do Pap smears in accordance with the criteria of the jurisdiction.) Setting such goals encourages doctors to be actively involved in disease prevention and health promotion.

Capitation-based funding
A funding formula to pay physicians who participate in some type of primary health care reform group (see Chapter 9). The doctor receives a set amount (determined by the age and health status of each patient) for each rostered patient per year.

The fundamental components of capitation-based funding are summarized as follows:

- Physician payment is based on a given group of patients who are rostered, thus forming the foundation of the doctor's practice.
- The physician receives a guaranteed income based on the defined population base of his or her practice.
- The physician may enter into other compensation schemes; for example, a portion of his or her practice may still be FFS.
- Incentives provided to the physician incorporate a strong element of disease prevention and health promotion to result in better health outcomes for patients of the practice.

Indirect Capitation

Indirect capitation is a funding model through which an organization such as a regional health authority receives a set amount of money to manage health care—including staff, services, administrative costs, and capital expenditures—for a population base. Employees within the organization may be compensated in various ways.

Global Budget

Doctors practising in underserviced areas are paid a certain fee for maintaining these practices. The global budget plan also usually includes ample vacation time and educational leave.

Salary

Doctors on salary receive a negotiated amount of money per time frame (usually a month). Larger hospitals, medical centres, clinics, and some nonprofit clinics often employ this model.

Blended Funding

Most physicians in Canada who engage in a form of funding other than FFS also partake in another method of payment. For example, a physician in a primary health care network group can have a certain portion of his or her practice nonrostered and on an FFS funding scheme and another portion calculated on capitation-based funding.

Specialists' Compensation

At teaching hospitals, specialists may have teaching responsibilities and receive a salary. Most specialists, even if on salary, maintain a private practice as well.

In their private practice, they see a patient upon referral from a family doctor until the problem for which the patient was referred is resolved.

Specialists not employed by a hospital or other organization rely on fee-for-service and, therefore, bill the province or territory for services rendered. Specialists belonging to a primary health care reform group may receive other forms of compensation reflective of the payment formula for that particular group.

In most jurisdictions, after a certain period of time (often one year), if a patient's health problem recurs, the patient may call the specialist's office directly and return for another evaluation (called a *repeat consultation*). If a new problem occurs, or if the same problem returns *after* the designated time period, the patient will need another referral (called a *consultation request*) from his or her family doctor. In most jurisdictions, a person cannot call a specialist's office and simply make an appointment. Channelling specialist visits through a primary care provider results in specialists' seeing only those patients who have legitimate problems and, thereby, creates cost savings (Canadian Institute for Health Information, 2013).

OTHER HEALTH CARE COST DRIVERS

Technology

The impact of technological change as a cost driver in health care is significant but difficult to put a dollar value to. Technology includes information technology (electronic health records and electronic medical records); medical devices, particularly those used for imaging; and tools and procedures to carry out new surgical techniques, such as bariatric (weight loss) surgery, an expensive and high-demand surgery.

CT and PET Scanners and MRIs

Although offering improved diagnostic outcomes, imaging options such as computed tomography (CT) scanners, magnetic resonance imaging (MRI), and PET scanners are expensive to purchase, maintain, and operate. Canada has fewer machines per capita than other developed countries do, and waiting lists for access can be long. For example, in 2011–2012, 1.7 million MRI exams and 4.4 million CT scans were performed, representing increases in these tests of 8.7% and 2.7%, respectively, over 2003–2004. The highest number were in Ontario, and the lowest in Prince Edward Island (Canadian Institute for Health Information, n.d.c; Canadian Institute for Health Information, 2012c).

The cost of an MRI machine depends on if it is purchased new or refurbished and on the size and functionality of the scanner. Other costs include things like room shielding, which can run upwards of $35,000/machine; construction to make a room ready; installation costs; and freight. Ongoing costs are those for training and employing individuals to operate the machine and are between $2 million and $3 million annually (Liewicki, 2014).

A new CT scanner costs about $750,000, depending as well on if it is new and the size (i.e., the number of slices it has). Overall costs include the same elements as those to set up and run an MRI scanner.

A **positron emission tomography (PET) scanner** will run approximately $1.5 million to $1.8 million. Canada had 29 publicly funded PET scanners in 2012. Twelve of those are in Quebec and nine in Ontario (combined PET/CT scanners are also available in some regions) (Canadian Press, 2012). Most jurisdictions cover the cost of PET scans only for specific conditions such as selected cancer and cardiac conditions. Scans are also covered for people who are part of a Health Canada clinical trial. The cost of a single PET scan varies from $956 (in Quebec—possibly because of the large number of scans done there) to $1800 (in Manitoba). The efficacy of a PET scan is not well established by Health Canada.

> **Positron emission tomography (PET) scanner**
> A scanning device that uses nuclear imaging techniques to obtain 3-D images of parts of the body.

Outsourcing

In many jurisdictions, health care services are contracted out to independent facilities. In Ontario, for example, some independent health care facilities have been licensed to perform MRI and CT scans for medically necessary procedures. To prevent queue jumping, patients must be referred to the facility for these procedures. The provincial government claims that contracting out these services costs 36% less than operating the same services within the hospital setting (Government of Ontario, 2003). These independent facilities may offer uninsured MRI and CT scans (e.g., to athletes or corporate executives whose firms cover such costs) only if they have signed a contract with the government to offer a designated number of insured scans per month as well. Not until the insured scans have been completed can the company offer remaining spaces to the private sector.

Electronic Health Records

The amount of health information to be managed has increased dramatically over the past few years, but the ability to process, analyze, and use this information has not kept pace. The implementation of an electronic health record (EHR) network carries a high price tag but is essential to a modern health care system that is accessible, productive, and high quality. All levels of government in Canada are involved in creating an EHR network. The Canada Health Infoway, a federally funded, independent nonprofit organization, is responsible for its implementation. Since its inception, the Canada Health Infoway has received $2.1 billion in funding from the federal government for an estimated 370 e-health projects Canada-wide. Funding for projects is received as block payments every few years. For example, the agency received $400 million in 2007 and $500 million in 2010. In 2010, a funding agreement was signed between the Canada Health Infoway and the Minister of Health, who governs the allocation of funds. The agency works with provinces and territories to determine what projects the money will support. The cost of each project is shared with the respective jurisdiction and sometimes with partners in the jurisdiction in which the money is spent. At the end of 2012, according to the Canadian Health Infoway, 52.2% of Canadians had EHRs.

The benefits of the EHR are significant. For patients, it offers improved safety, coordination of personal health information, and improved continuity of care. For the health care system, there are substantial cost savings and a high return on investment. The plan for the Canadian Health Infoway includes a system to monitor wait times, manage chronic diseases, and add EMR systems to physicians' offices and an interoperable order-entry system in hospitals. Completion of the system will cost $10 billion, and the annual operating costs are an estimated $1.5 billion (Canada Health Infoway, n.d.). Chapters 4 and 10 offer more information about EHRs.

CONCLUSION

Have you found the answers to the questions you were asked at the beginning of the chapter? How close were your estimates? To summarize, an intermediate assessment by a doctor will cost an uninsured patient about $40. A knee replacement could cost as much as $10,281; a hip replacement, $12,802; and having an appendix removed, $3251 for a simple procedure, and $5146 for a complicated removal (e.g. if the appendix had ruptured).

Now, consider your health card—just identification you must show when you seek health care services, right? Not really. Your health card is similar to a credit card but for health care services.

What does the future of health care in Canada hold? It is near impossible to know, although change is a certainty. Resources are limited, and services may need to be rationed—an alien concept to Canadians. Excluding people from the treatment they need (or want) based on factors such as age, health status, or type of disease seems unthinkable, but it may become a reality. We must use health care resources wisely and continue to promote healthy lifestyles and disease prevention.

Summary

8.1 Although health care in Canada is for the most part publicly funded, delivery of health care services is accomplished through a mix of private for-profit and not-for profit organizations. For example, most hospitals are private nonprofit facilities, and although funded by the government, many of the services they deliver are done so by private businesses. Doctors, although paid for with public funds, can be considered small business owners.

8.2 Public funding for health care in Canada is provided by the federal, provincial/territorial, and municipal governments through a blend of taxes and tax points as well as by workers' compensation boards. Some jurisdictions also use revenue from sales taxes and lotteries for health care—with two provinces charging their residents health premiums. Presently, the federal government uses four models to make transfer payments to the provinces and territories.

8.3 Hospitals, drugs, and human health resources represent the three top health care expenditures in Canada. Most hospitals are nonprofit facilities and, although almost entirely government funded, use an array of private businesses and organizations to deliver their services. Human health resources account for most of hospital spending.

8.4 Long-term care facilities in Canada are primarily publicly funded and regulated by the provincial and territorial governments. Private facilities do exist, offering varying levels of care. In most jurisdictions, the patient is required to make a copayment for room and board, food, and other services. The amount the patient is required to pay is related to his or her monthly income.

8.5 The cost of drugs in Canada continues to rise, but at a lower pace than in previous years. Reasons include the fact that there are more people using medications and more people using several medications. In addition, newer drugs, especially a class called *biologics*, are very expensive. Canada does not have a national drug-funding program, but all jurisdictions cover the cost of most drugs for certain groups, including seniors, disabled persons, and those on assisted income.

8.6 Human health resources (HHR) are a significant expense to the health care system. Physicians and nurses are the largest of the regulated professions and account for the largest financial output for the HHR sector. Physicians are paid through a number of funding formulas, with the majority still billing fee-for-service. The shortage of physicians and nurses, although improving, still persists.

8.7 Technological advances in health care include everything from surgical procedures to diagnostic equipment and both the establishment and maintenance of electronic health records and electronic medical records. New technologies related to medical imaging promote early diagnosis, prompt treatment, and improved treatment outcomes but come at a price. Electronic health records, as well, are expensive to implement. Putting an actual value to these cost drivers is difficult, and it is thought that, in time, many of these advances will actually save the health care system money.

Review Questions

1. Why do some Canadians regard health care as "free"? Do you feel that way? Why or why not?
2. Explain the concept of equalization payments, including why they are given and how they are calculated.
3. What types of services are covered by provincial and territorial insurance both in and out of hospitals?
4. What are the three largest expenditures for provincial and territorial health plans?
5. List five strategies for reducing the length of hospital stays and, thus, hospital expenses.
6. What are the key differences between prescription drugs and over-the-counter drugs?
7. How has advanced technology contributed to rising health care costs?

References

Canada Health Infoway. (n.d.). *What we do*. Retrieved from https://www.infoway-inforoute.ca/index.php/about-infoway/what-we-do.

Canadian Agency for Drugs and Technologies in Health. (n.d.). *Activity-based funding models in Canadian hospitals*. Retrieved from http://www.cadth.ca/products/environmental-scanning/health-technology-update/ht-update-12/activity-based-funding-models-in-canadian-hospitals.

Canadian Institute for Health Information. (n.d.a). *Canada's health care providers*. Retrieved from https://secure.cihi.ca/free_products/hctenglish.pdf.

Canadian Institute for Health Information. (n.d.b). *Leading hospitalization costs in acute inpatient facilities in 2012–2013*. Retrieved from http://www.cihi.ca/CIHI-ext-portal/pdf/internet/CAD_COSTINGDATA_INFOSHEET14_en.

Canadian Institute for Health Information. (n.d.c). Medical imaging. Retrieved from www.cihi.ca/CIHI-ext-portal/internet/en/tabbedcontent/types+of+care/specialized+services/medical+imaging/cihi010642.

Canadian Institute for Health Information. (n.d.d). *National prescription drug utilization information system database*. Retrieved from http://www.cihi.ca/cihi-ext-portal/internet/en/document/types+of+care/pharmaceutical/services_drug.

Canadian Institute for Health Information. (2011). *Health care cost drivers: The facts*. Ottawa: Author. Retrieved from https://secure.cihi.ca/free_products/health_care_cost_drivers_the_facts_en.pdf.

Canadian Institute for Health Information. (2012a, October 30) *Canada's health care spending growth slows*. Retrieved from http://www.cihi.ca/cihi-ext-portal/internet/en/document/spending+and+health+workforce/spending/release_30oct12.

Canadian Institute for Health Information. (2012b). *Hospital cost drivers technical report—What factors have determined hospital expenditure trends in Canada?* Ottawa: Author. Retrieved from http://www.cihi.ca/CIHI-ext-portal/pdf/internet/HOSPITAL_COSTDRIVER_TECH_EN.

Canadian Institute for Health Information. (2012c). *Medical imaging in Canada 2012*. Retrieved from http://www.cihi.ca/CIHI-ext-portal/pdf/internet/MIT_SUMMARY_2012_en.

Canadian Institute for Health Information. (2013a). *National health expenditure trends, 1975 to 2013—Executive summary*. Ottawa: Author. Retrieved from http://www.cihi.ca/CIHI-ext-portal/pdf/internet/NHEX_EXEC_SUM_2013_EN.

Canadian Institute for Health Information. (2013b, September 26). *Number of doctors in Canada rising, as are payments for their services*. Retrieved from http://www.cihi.ca/cihi-ext-portal/internet/en/document/spending+and+health+workforce/workforce/physicians/release_26sep13.

Canadian Institute for Health Information. (2014, July 8). *Canada's nursing workforce continues to grow*. Retrieved from http://www.cihi.ca/cihi-ext-portal/internet/en/document/spending+and+health+workforce/workforce/nurses/release_8july14.

References

Canadian Press. (2012, February 27). PET scans underused, national strategy needed: Report. *CTV News*. Retrieved from http://www.ctvnews.ca/pet-scans-underused-national-strategy-needed-report-1.774472#ixzz2W8H4a7Mq.

CBC News. (2011, March 21). The promise of Herceptin. *CBC*. Retrieved from http://www.cbc.ca/news/health/the-promise-of-herceptin-1.1017139.

Department of Finance Canada. (2011a). *Canada social transfer*. Retrieved from http://www.fin.gc.ca/fedprov/cst-eng.asp.

Department of Finance Canada. (2011b). *Equalization program*. Retrieved from http://www.fin.gc.ca/fedprov/eqp-eng.asp.

Department of Finance Canada. (2011c). *Making a major new investment in health care and putting transfers on a long-term, sustainable growth track*. Retrieved from http://www.fin.gc.ca/n11/data/11-141_1-eng.asp.

De Souza, M. (2012, September 19). Census: Aging population fuels retirement residence, nursing-home boom. *Canada.com*. Retrieved from http://www.canada.com/Census+Aging+population+fuels+retirement+residence+nursing+home+boom/7265408/story.html.

Di Matteo, L. (2013, July 30). Trouble ahead for health costs: Doctors working less, making more. *The Globe and Mail*. Retrieved from http://www.theglobeandmail.com/globe-debate/trouble-ahead-for-health-costs-doctors-working-less-making-more/article13497288/.

Government of Ontario. (2003). *Ministry of Community and Social Services*. Retrieved from http://ogov.newswire.ca/ontario/!GPOE/2003/02/21/c2902.html?lmatch=%3C=_e.html.

Health Council of Canada. (2007). *Health care renewal in Canada: Measuring up? Annual report to Canadians, 2006*. Toronto: Author.

Isfeld, G. (2013, November 4). Equalization payments make for unequal services: Study. *Financial Post*. Retrieved from http://business.financialpost.com/2013/11/04/equalization-payments-make-for-unequal-services-study/.

Law, M. R., Cheng, L., Dhalla, I. A., et al. (2012, January 16). The effect of cost on adherence to prescription medications. *Canadian Medical Association Journal*. Retrieved from http://dx.doi.org/10.1503/cmaj.111270.

Leung, M. (2013, May 19). Nursing home workers suspended after son turns over hidden camera video. *CTV News*. Retrieved from http://www.ctvnews.ca/canada/nursing-home-workers-suspended-after-son-turns-over-hidden-camera-video-1.1288544.

Liewicki, N. (2014, May 30). MRI for Moose Jaw. *Moose Jaw Times Herald*. Retrieved from http://www.mjtimes.sk.ca/News/Local/2014-05-30/article-3744550/MRI-for-Moose-Jaw/1.

Matier, C. (2012). *Renewing the Canada health transfer: Implications for federal and provincial–territorial fiscal sustainability*. Ottawa: Office of the Parliamentary Budget Officer.

Mickleburgh, R. (2012, September 6). Patient-based funding breathes new life into hospitals. *The Globe and Mail*. Retrieved from http://www.cadth.ca/products/environmental-scanning/health-technology-update/ht-update-12/activity-based-funding-models-in-canadian-hospitals.

Ogilvie, M., & Poisson, J. (2012, April 5). Ontario hospitals spend more on administration. *Toronto Star* Retrieved from http://www.thestar.com/news/gta/2012/04/05/ontario_hospitals_spend_more_on_administration.html.

Organisation for Economic Co-operation and Development. (2014). *OECD health statistics 2014: How does Canada compare?* Retrieved from http://www.oecd.org/els/health-systems/Briefing-Note-CANADA-2014.pdf.

Reinberg, S. (2005, November 29). Powerful breast cancer drug carries high price. *HealthDay*. Retrieved from http://consumer.healthday.com/cancer-information-5/breast-cancer-news-94/powerful-breast-cancer-drug-carries-high-price-529378.html.

Statistics Canada. (2014). *Labour force survey estimates (LFS), by national occupational classification for statistics (NOC-S) and sex* [Table 282-0010]. Retrieved from http://www5.statcan.gc.ca/cansim/a05?lang=eng&id=2820010.

University of British Columbia. (2012, January 16). One in ten Canadians cannot afford prescription drugs: UBC study. *Public Affairs*. Retrieved from http://www.publicaffairs.ubc.ca/2012/01/16/one-in-ten-canadians-cannot-afford-prescription-drugs-ubc-study/.

Chapter Nine

Practitioners and Practice Settings

 Learning Outcomes

9.1 Understand or outline the different categories of health care practitioners.

9.2 Discuss the regulation of health care providers in Canada.

9.3 List and describe the roles of conventional health care providers.

9.4 Describe the various practice settings that exist across the country.

9.5 Summarize the concept of primary health care reform.

KEY TERMS

Accredited program, p. 313
Affiliating body, p. 321
Allied health professional p. 291
Clinic, p. 290
Community-based care, p. 291
Controlled act, p. 301
Delegated act, p. 302
Evidence-informed, p. 293
Geriatrics, p. 307
Health care provider, p. 291
Hospice, p. 290
Interprofessional collaboration, p. 291

Intubate, p. 318
Modalities, p. 291
Practice setting, p. 290
Primary care setting, p. 290
Refraction, p. 308
Rostering, p. 326
Scope of practice, p. 300
Specialist, p. 306
Telehealth, p. 327
Title protection, p. 300
Urodynamic, p. 323

Health care in Canada is provided by a wide variety of health care providers—from conventional (or mainstream) medical practitioners to those who practice complementary and alternative medicine. Also integral in delivering care are informal workers: volunteers of community organizations and friends and family members who care for loved ones at home.

Practice settings include the community, hospitals, long-term care facilities, rehabilitation centres, **hospices**, and a variety of **clinics**, offices, and family practice, and **primary care settings**. Who delivers health care and where it is delivered are undergoing continual change, largely in an attempt to provide Canadians with timely, cost-effective access to primary care, accommodate the health needs of an aging population, and reduce wait times.

All jurisdictions have experimented with different ways to deliver primary care. In 2013, Statistics Canada reported that 4.6 million Canadians did not have a family doctor (Statistics Canada, 2014). To address the issue, a recent proposal, called the Patient's Medical Home (PMH), initiated by the College of Family Physicians of Canada builds on existing concepts of family practice and primary care models such as Alberta's Primary Care Networks, Saskatchewan's

---

Practice setting
The context and environment in which health care is delivered.

Hospice
A facility that provides supportive and compassionate care to individuals who are in the final stages of a terminal illness and their loved ones.

new Collaborative Emergency Centres, Ontario's Family Health Teams, and the Family Medicine Groups in Quebec. The goal is to ensure that every Canadian has a primary care provider who is the hub of a *team* of health professionals. Added to the original concept is providing a stable medical environment where the patient feels comfortable and can access any health care required. **Interprofessional collaboration** and the changing roles of health care providers strengthen the team approach to primary health care. For example, many nurses function in expanded roles as nurse practitioners; physician assistants perform many physician functions, freeing up the doctor; and respiratory therapists also assume many functions previously done by a physician. An individual entering the health care profession can look forward to being part of a team cooperatively sharing information, advice, support, and expertise to provide comprehensive, high-quality care to patients.

Over the past decade, much of the care a patient would have once received in hospital has moved into the community. This shift to **community-based care** has been made, in part, to reduce health care costs by shortening hospital stays, to enhance patient recovery, and to minimize the risk for hospital-based infections. New procedures, increased community support for home-based recovery, and multidisciplinary teams in primary care settings have facilitated this change.

This chapter will look at some of the different health care workers in Canada—who they are, what they do, and where, with an emphasis on primary care settings. It will briefly examine some of the professional organizations that support these people and the mechanisms in place to ensure that care is given by individuals qualified in their field. This chapter focuses mainly on primary care renewal.

CATEGORIES OF HEALTH CARE PROVIDERS

Health care providers have been commonly divided into three categories: *core health professionals* (e.g., doctors, nurses, ophthalmologists, psychiatrists), **allied health professionals** (e.g., osteopaths, personal support workers, optometrists, psychologists), and complementary and alternative practitioners (e.g., Aboriginal healers, naturopathic doctors, massage therapists). With the current focus on interprofessional collaborative care and practice, the label *allied health professional* is losing popularity; those professionals are now being classified along with core health professionals in one overarching group: *conventional health professionals*. Complementary and alternative health practitioners are also health care providers but are categorized separately largely because of the **modalities** used to treat

Clinic
A setting in which multiple health care providers work collaboratively, usually in a similar field, to provide cost-effective, patient-centred health care.

Primary care setting
The organizational and physical environment in which a person receives point-of-entry care (e.g., a doctor's office, walk-in clinic).

Interprofessional collaboration
Multiple health care workers from a variety of professions working together to deliver evidence-informed, patient-centred health care.

Community-based care
Care provided for the patient in the home (e.g., incorporating visits from nurses or physiotherapists) or on an outpatient basis rather than in the hospital or another health care facility.

patients. See Table 9.1 for a categorization of *some* of Canada's many health care providers.

Health care provider
A person who has graduated from a health-related college or university program and is accredited by a professional or regulating body. Often, the person must be licensed by a provincial or territorial government.

Allied health professional
A health care provider other than a doctor, nurse, or, according to some sources, pharmacist or dentist who provides supportive health care, including direct patient care, technical care, therapeutic care, and support services.

Modalities
Prescribed methods or techniques.

Table 9.1 Canada's Health Care Providers

Conventional Health Care Providers	Alternative and Complementary Health Care Providers
Chiropodists (podiatrists)	Aboriginal healers
Dental assistants	Acupuncture practitioners
Dental hygienists	Aromatherapists
Dentists	Chiropractors
Licensed practical nurses	Homeopathic doctors
Medical laboratory technologists	Massage therapists
Medical radiation technologists	Naturopathic doctors
Midwives	Reflexologists
Nurse practitioners	Reiki practitioners
Occupational therapists	Therapeutic touch practitioners
Opticians	Traditional Chinese medicine practitioners
Optometrists	Yoga practitioners
Osteopaths	
Personal support workers (health care aides)	
Pharmacists	
Physician assistants	
Physicians	
Physiotherapists	
Psychologists	
Registered nurses	
Registered psychiatric nurses	
Respiratory therapists	
Social workers	
Speech-language pathologists and audiologists	

Note: This list is neither exclusive nor definitive. Titles, roles, and categorization vary by region. For example, chiropractors and acupuncture practitioners may well be considered conventional health care providers by some.

Conventional Medicine

Conventional medicine is frequently referred to as *mainstream*, *traditional*, or *Western* medicine. Conventional health care providers typically encompass all those not considered alternative practitioners. They diagnose health problems; treat prediagnosed health problems; and render technical, therapeutic, or supportive care with scientifically proven therapies, medication, and surgery.

Complementary and Alternative Medicine (CAM)

Complementary and alternative medicine are practised by all health care providers not considered mainstream or conventional. Note, however, that although the terms are sometimes used interchangeably, strictly speaking, a difference exists between alternative and complementary medicine. As their names suggests, *complementary medicine* (meaning "in addition to") supports, or complements, conventional medicine, while *alternative medicine* typically provides an option—an alternative—often to the exclusion of conventional medicine. What is considered alternative and what is considered complementary are somewhat fluid and subjective.

Moreover, what is considered standard treatment in one country or even in one province or territory may not be in another. Acupuncture is standard medical care in China but considered by many to be part of CAM in Canada. In Canada, although private insurance plans may cover some complementary or alternative therapies, most provincial and territorial insurance plans do not, and, as a rule, these therapies are not used in hospitals. Many of these techniques originate from spiritual, cultural, or religious beliefs and remain unproven by scientific standards.

Some critics of alternative medicine believe that treatment should be **evidence-informed**—that is, proven to work—before it is used. Therapeutic touch, for example, claims to use balance and energy coupled with the healing force of the practitioner's hands to facilitate a patient's recovery; however, no scientific evidence exists to prove it alters the course of a disease. That is not to say that therapeutic touch does not benefit the patient in terms of reducing stress and promoting relaxation, though. An alternative or complementary modality that is scientifically proven to work becomes accepted medical practice.

A significant number of Canadians use CAM at some point in their lives, possibly because disillusionment with conventional treatment, difficulty getting appointments with their doctor, cultural influences, information available on the Internet, and simply that many more people are actively participating in their own health care and treatment options. As long as an alternative therapy is safe and results in some benefits for the patient, many medical practitioners welcome it as a complementary option.

> **Evidence-informed**
> Proven, through high-quality scientific studies, to be effective.

Opposition to alternative medicine usually arises when people use it in place of scientifically proven treatments. Occasionally, a person will seek alternative treatment when conventional medicine has nothing more to offer—for example, in the case of terminal cancer. If the treatment does no harm, it may provide optimism and comfort and perhaps prolong life and ease suffering. Individuals may disregard conventional medicine for several reasons, including the following:

- At some point during an illness, mainstream medicine may have nothing left to offer.
- The patient may have suffered a bad experience with conventional practice.
- A patient may hold a health belief system that contradicts mainstream medicine.

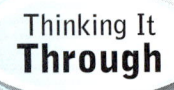

A patient who was treated for breast cancer two years ago has just been diagnosed with metastases (the spread of cancerous cells from their original site). The doctor has recommended chemotherapy and radiation therapy, followed by surgery. Hopes for a cure are guarded. The patient, based on her former unpleasant experience with the side effects of these treatments, has decided to seek a homeopathic remedy. Considering these alternatives, what would you do if you were this patient?

When a patient is using CAM, it is essential that the patient, CAM practitioner, and medical practitioner work together to ensure no dangerous overlaps result. For example, herbal medicine can interfere with prescribed medications. St. John's wort, a common herbal supplement taken to ward off depression, and prescription antidepressant drugs used together can result in an overdose. Many people use herbal medications (available over the counter at health stores and pharmacies) but fail to inform their doctor of such. They may believe that herbal medications are harmless, or they may be embarrassed or fearful to admit to taking such medications, believing their physician will disapprove. Health care providers' embracing both conventional and complementary medicine can medically and psychologically benefit patients and help them be open with and trusting of the professionals who provide their health care.

Chiropractic: Conventional, Complementary, or Alternative?

Chiropractors (doctors of chiropractic medicine) form the largest group of CAM practitioners. To obtain a degree to qualify for clinical practice, chiropractors complete four to five years of postsecondary education. Working in solo or group practices, they diagnose and treat a wide range of conditions that deal primarily with disorders of the spine, pelvis, extremities, and joints and the resulting effects on the central nervous system. Taking a relatively holistic approach to patient care, chiropractors use various types of noninvasive therapies, such as exercise routines and spinal adjustments. Chiropractors are not licensed to prescribe medicine or to do surgery, and chiropractic care is not covered by most provincial or territorial plans, but most private insurance plans will pay for a specified number of visits and treatments.

Chiropractic medicine is still considered by many to be on the cusp of alternative and complementary medicine, and the relationship between chiropractors and physicians is variable, some sharing a mutual respect, while others prefer to keep their professional distance: some chiropractors retain negative views of conventional medicine and of physicians' acceptance of chiropractic care, and vice versa. In general, the farther apart the philosophies of the practitioners, the less likely they are to understand and work with one another (In the News: Treatment Versus Risk: What Are the Facts?).

In the News — Treatment Versus Risk: What Are the Facts?

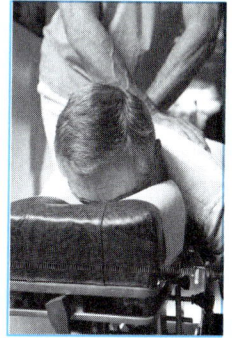

Several cases in the news over the past years have implicated chiropractic neck adjustments in strokes. In a 2004 case in which the stroke victim died, a jury ruled the death an accident but recommended that all chiropractors make patients aware of the potential risk for stroke and require patients to sign informed consent documents prior to neck manipulation. In September 2007, an Edmonton woman suffered a stroke following a neck adjustment performed by chiropractor for a shoulder problem. She claimed that she was not informed of the risks associated with the procedure and had not signed a consent form. The ensuing lawsuit was settled out of court. It was proven, however, that the chiropractor had forged the woman's signature on a consent form.

In 2012, a group of stroke survivors in Manitoba asked the provincial government to ban chiropractic high-neck manipulation. They also requested a public inquiry into the injurious effects of the procedure.

Despite ongoing public concerns, a Canadian study done in 2008 concluded that no increased risk for stroke exists with chiropractic neck adjustments. While the researchers found an increased association between

Continued on next page

chiropractic care and stroke, they discovered the same association between a visit to the family doctor and stroke—an association likely explained by patients' seeking help from a chiropractor or medical doctor for neck pain (caused by an already damaged artery), rather than by the care itself.

Sources: CBC News. (2012, October 4). Chiropractic neck procedures cause strokes, say survivors. *CBC*. Retrieved from http://www.cbc.ca/news/canada/manitoba/story/2012/10/03/mb-chiropractic-neck-adjustments-stroke.html; CTVNews.ca Staff. (2012, October 3). Chiropractor forged consent form after patient's stroke. *CTV News*. Retrieved from http://www.ctvnews.ca/health/health-headlines/chiropractor-forged-consent-form-after-patient-s-stroke-1.982655; Barrett, S. (2004). Coroner's jury concludes that neck manipulation killed Canadian woman. *Chirobase*. Retrieved from http://www.chirobase.org/15News/lewis.html; Cassidy, J. D., Boyle, E., Côté, P., et al. (2008). Risk of vertebrobasilar stroke and chiropractic care: Results of a population-based case-control and case-crossover study. *Spine, 33*(4 Suppl), S176–183; Alphonso, C. (2008, January 19). Chiropractors don't raise stroke risk, study says. *The Globe and Mail*. Retrieved from http://www.theglobeandmail.com/life/chiropractors-dont-raise-stroke-risk-study-says/article18442351/.

Photo Credit: © iStock.com/LattaPictures.

REGULATION OF HEALTH CARE PROFESSIONS

The majority of health care professions are self-regulated, meaning that a professional body enters into an agreement with the government to exercise control over and set standards for its members. Others are regulated by the government, meaning that legislation controls the conduct and practice of the profession and its members. Regulatory authority is granted through legislation, such as an act or statute that outlines the framework for behaviour and values for a given profession. In Canada, provincial and territorial legislation (e.g., British Columbia's *Health Professions Act*, Ontario's *Regulated Health Professions Act*) provides the legal framework for regulating most health care professions.

Nursing and medicine make up the largest groups of regulated health care providers. The nursing profession includes registered nurses (RNs), registered psychiatric nurses (RPNs), and licensed practical nurses (LPNs) (called registered practical nurses [RPNs] in Ontario). Regulated professions have self-governing bodies called colleges (e.g., College of Registered Nurses of Nova Scotia, College of Massage Therapists of Newfoundland and Labrador), which regulate the conduct and practice of their members. Each province and territory has 20 to 30 regulated health care professions, but professions regulated in some provinces and territories may not be regulated in all (Table 9.2). For example, psychiatric nurses in British Columbia are regulated by a college unique to their specialty—the College of Registered Psychiatric Nurses of British Columbia—while in Ontario, psychiatric nurses are under the umbrella of the College of Nurses of Ontario.

Table 9.2 Regulated Health Care Professions in Each Province and Territory

Profession	AB	BC	MB	NB	NL	NS	NT	NU	ON	PEI	QC	SK	YT
Cardiology technologists	•										•		•
Chiropodists (podiatrists)	•								•		•	•	•
Chiropractors	•	•	•	•	•	•			•	•	•	•	
Combined certified lab/X-ray technicians	•		*										
Counsellors (guidance counsellors, psychoeducators, and marital and family therapists)											•		
Dental assistants	•	•	•	•	•				•		•	•	•
Dental hygienists		•	•	•	•	•			•	•	•	•	•
Dental technicians/technologists	•	•		•		•			•	•	•	•	•
Dental therapists							•	•				•	
Dentists	•	•	•	•	•	•	•	•	•	•	•	•	•
Denturists	•	•	•	•	•	•	•	•	•	•	•	•	•
Dietitians/nutritionists	•	•	•	•	•	•	•	•	•	•	•	•	•
Hearing aid practitioners	•			•							•		
Kinesiologists									•		•		
Licensed practical nurses/registered practical nurses	•			•		•			•				
Massage therapists		•											
Medical diagnosticians and therapeutic technicians	•												

Continued

Table 9.2 Regulated Health Care Professions in Each Province and Territory—cont'd

Profession	AB	BC	MB	NB	NL	NS	NT	NU	ON	PEI	QC	SK	YT
Medical laboratory technologists	•											•	
Medical radiation technicians	•	•							•		•	•	
Midwives	*	•	•	•	•	•			•		•	•	
Naturopathic physicians	•	•	•									•	
Nurse practitioners (included as registered nurses in some provinces)	•	•		•	•							•	
Occupational therapists	•	•	•	•	•	•			•	•	•	•	•
Ophthalmic medical assistants													
Ophthalmologists													
Opticians	•	•	•	•	•	•	•	•	•		•	•	
Optometrists	•	•	•	•	•	•	•	•	•	•	•	•	•
Paramedics, ambulance/emergency medical attendants	*	*					•	•				•	
Pharmacists	•	•	•	•	•	•	•	•	•	•	•	•	•
Physicians	•	•	•	•	•	•	•	•	•	•	•	•	•
Physiotherapists	•	•	•	•	•	•	•	•	•	•	•	•	•
Psychiatric nurses	•	•	•				•	•	•			•	•
Psychologists	•	•	•	•	•	•	•	•	•	•	•	•	•
Psychotherapists									•				

Registered nurses	•	•	•	•	•	•	•	•	•	•	•	•
Respiratory therapists		•				•	•	•			•	•
Social workers	•	•	•	•	•	•	•	•	•		•	*
Speech language pathologists and audiologists	•					•	•	•	•		•	
Traditional Chinese medicine and acupuncture practitioners	*					•	•					

• self-regulated   * government regulated

Sources: Alberta Health. (n.d.). *Regulated health professions*. Retrieved from http://www.health.alberta.ca/professionals/regulated-professions.html; British Columbia Ministry of Health. (n.d.). *Professional regulation*. Retrieved from http://www.health.gov.bc.ca/professional-regulation/; Manitoba. (n.d.). The Regulated Health Professions Act (RHPA). Retrieved from http://www.gov.mb.ca/health/rhpa/; Manitoba. (n.d.). *Legislation—Manitoba health, healthy living and seniors*. Retrieved from http://www.gov.mb.ca/health/legislation/contact.html; New Brunswick. (n.d.). *Health-related regulated occupations*. Retrieved from http://www.welcomenb.ca/content/wel-bien/en/immigrating_and_settling/working/foreign_qualification_recognition/health-related_regulatedoccupations.html; Newfoundland and Labrador Council of Health Professionals. (n.d.). Retrieved from http://www.nlchp.ca/; Nova Scotia Department of Health and Wellness. (n.d.). Retrieved from http://www.gov.ns.ca/health; Northwest Territories Health and Social Services. (n.d.). *Professional licensing*. Retrieved from http://www.hss.gov.nt.ca/professional-licensing; Nunavut Department of Health. (n.d.). Retrieved from http://www.hss.gov.nu.ca/en/About Us Legislation.aspx; Ontario Ministry of Health and Long-Term Care. (2012, June 25). *Legislation*: Regulated Health Professions Statute Law Amendment Act, 2009. Retrieved from http://www.health.gov.on.ca/en/common/legislation/bill179/default.aspx; Prince Edward Island Department of Health and Wellness. (2014). Regulated Health Professions Act. Retrieved from http://www.gov.pe.ca/law/statutes/pdf/r-10_1.pdf; Santé et Services sociaux Québec. (2014). *Réseau: Annuaire des associations et ordres professionels du secteur de la santé et des service sociaux*. Retrieved from http://msssa4.msss.gouv.qc.ca/fr/organisa/AnnAsSec.nsf/Tous?OpenView&Start=1; Conseil interprofessionnel du Québec. (2014). *Regulated professions*. Retrieved from http://www.professions-quebec.org/index.php/en/element/visualiser/id/62; Saskatchewan Ministry of Health. (2011). *Saskatchewan's health human resources plan*. Retrieved from http://www.health.gov.sk.ca/adv/aspx/adxGetMedia.aspx?DocID=f9a8ff18-7963-48c2-acd3-946e10f13e35&MediaID=5580&Filename=sask-health-human-resources-plan-appendices.pdf&I=English; Government of Saskatchewan. (2012). *Self-regulating health professional associations*. Retrieved from http://www.health.gov.sk.ca/professional-associations; Yukon Health and Social Services. (2009). *Yukon regulates psychiatric nurses under Health Professions Act*. Retrieved from http://www.hss.gov.yk.ca/news/09-195.php; Yukon Health and Social Services. (2007). *Yukon regulates physiotherapists under Health Professions Act*. Retrieved from http://www.hss.gov.yk.ca/news/07-018.php; Yukon Health and Social Services. (n.d.). *So you want to make a difference.... Your health care career in Yukon*. Retrieved from http://www.hss.gov.yk.ca/pdf/recruitment_booklet.pdf.

TITLE PROTECTION

Regulated professionals—those who belong to a professional body—are licensed to practise their profession and are legally entitled to use a specific designation such as registered massage therapist (RMT). These professions receive **title protection**, meaning only properly trained persons can legally use that title. For example, people who have cared for loved ones at home but have no formal training cannot call themselves licensed or registered practical nurses. Likewise, someone who dropped out of college halfway through a respiratory therapy program cannot call himself a respiratory therapist. Nor can health care aides call themselves nurses. Fully trained nurses registered in other countries cannot call themselves registered nurses here until they have met the standards set by the college of nurses in the province or territory they want to practise in. Along with title protection, regulated professions share other collective elements (Box 9.1).

Title protection
Legal restrictions around and guidelines for the use of a professional title.

Scope of practice
A range of skills, learned in school or through on-the-job training, that a practitioner can perform competently and safely. From a professional perspective, legal parameters usually, but not always, dictate what a practitioner may or may not do, based on the profession's education, training, and licensure.

Box 9.1   Regulated Professions: Common Elements

- Educational standards
- Provincial and territorial examinations
- Practitioner's **scope of practice,** which outlines skills, acts, and services the practitioner is able to perform competently and safely
- Curbing of individual's practice if standards are not met
- Formal complaints process for the public
- Complaints investigation and follow-up
- Title protection
- Competence and quality assurance

Any health care profession can apply to the government to become regulated, but it must meet strict criteria. The minister of health and some type of advisory body within the province or territory usually oversee the lengthy and often arduous application process.

Regulation protects both the profession and the public by ensuring that those within a given profession are who they claim to be and do what they claim to do in a competent and safe manner. Just as the possession of a legitimate driver's licence promises that a person knows how to drive and has passed a driving test, regulation proves a person has undergone training and gained a predetermined degree of knowledge, skill, or ability. Mind you, possession of a driver's licence does not guarantee driving excellence: even in regulated professions, some health care providers offer substandard services.

All regulated professionals must practise within a framework of skills and services defined by their governing body. Nurses have certain skills and acts they have been trained to do; doctors have a range of skills and services they have been trained to offer; and medical laboratory technologists and other health care practitioners, likewise, have a defined scope of practice. Even within a single profession, different levels of practice exist. For example, registered nurses with special training may perform acts that those without this training cannot, such as starting an intravenous line, working strictly with patients receiving chemotherapy, or managing wound care. Similarly, a medical doctor in family practice is not qualified to remove a gallbladder or do a hip replacement; a licensed practical nurse is not qualified to do a complete physical, but a nurse practitioner is; and a massage therapist is not qualified to deliver a baby, but a midwife, nurse practitioner, or obstetrician is. In health care, many of these skilled procedures, some specific to certain professions, are called *controlled acts*.

Controlled Acts

As previously noted, each profession has a scope of practice statement that describes what the profession does and the methods it uses. Within some professions' scopes of practice are procedures or interventions called **controlled acts** (referred to as *reserved acts* in British Columbia), which only certain health care providers may be allowed to perform. Considered potentially harmful if executed by an untrained individual, controlled acts vary slightly from one jurisdiction to another. Ontario's *Regulated Health Professions Act (RHPA)*, for example, has identified 13 controlled acts (College of Physicians and Surgeons of Ontario, 2008). Specific acts may be within the scope of practice of any one (or more) profession, while other acts may not be within the scope of that same profession. Examples of controlled acts include giving an injection, setting or casting a fracture, passing a nasogastric tube, and prescribing a medication.

Controlled act
An act that, as specified in the *Regulated Health Professions Act*, may be performed only by authorized regulated health care providers.

Exceptions to Controlled Acts

Most provinces and territories allow controlled acts to be performed in certain situations by competent yet nonregulated individuals, including the following:

- Someone with appropriate training providing first aid or assistance in an emergency
- Students learning to perform an act under the supervision of a qualified person, as long as that act is within the scope of practice of graduates of the student's professional program

- A person, such as a caregiver, trained to perform an act (e.g., giving injections to a person with diabetes)
- An appropriate person designated to perform an act in accordance with a religion—for example, a rabbi may circumcise a male child

Exclusions also apply in the case of body piercing for the purpose of jewellery, electrolysis, tattooing, and ear piercing.

Thinking It Through

Miranda, a personal support worker working for a home care agency is looking after an older woman, Ibia. Ibia has not gone to the bathroom for several hours and is very uncomfortable. Ibia's visiting RN occasionally has to catheterize her; however, the nurse is unavailable for several hours. Miranda, who had done the procedure in her country of origin, successfully inserts the urinary catheter, drains off 800 cc of urine, and makes the patient comfortable. Clearly, Miranda was performing a controlled act that she was not qualified to do in Canada.

1. Would you have done the same thing?
2. What alternatives did Miranda have?
3. Do you think that because Miranda, a nurse in her own country, had done the procedure many times before her actions are somewhat justifiable?

DELEGATED ACTS

As our health care system continues to evolve, so, too, do health care providers' scopes of practice. Reforms in the health care system, in methods of delivery, and in health care providers' responsibilities have affected the traditional roles of health care providers. The needs of patients also continue to evolve—more complex care is required more frequently. For patient needs to be met, occasionally the acts, procedures, and treatments rendered by health care providers must go beyond standard boundaries. To this end, health care providers sometimes receive special training and share responsibilities. Under specific conditions, a health care provider who is not a physician may perform an act, treatment, or intervention that is typically outside of his or her scope of practice—that is, a **delegated act.**

Guidelines and protocol for delegation of medical acts vary across Canada. For example, in some jurisdictions, controlled acts can be delegated only to a person who is a member of a regulated profession, but in others, certain acts may be delegated to a nonregulated health care provider. Generally, the delegated act must

Delegated act
A controlled act that a physician authorizes another health care provider, either regulated or unregulated, to do in his or her stead and under supervision.

be clearly defined and supervised accordingly. Supervision can be direct (i.e., the delegating physician is physically present) or indirect (i.e., the delegating physician is available for consultation by phone). In health care organizations, the board of directors and the medical advisory committee or their equivalents must agree to the rules and procedures for delegated acts. A physician with expert knowledge has a commitment to his or her patient to ensure that the person performing the act—called the *delegate*—is properly trained and demonstrates competence in completing the act. In many cases, written rules dictate that the delegating physician must remain either within the room or close by (e.g., same office or clinic) during the procedure.

The delegating physician, the delegate, and the facility in which the act is performed share responsibility for the act. The physician who teaches or assesses the delegate's initial performance of the delegated act (and certifies the delegate as competent) is accountable for ensuring the act is, in fact, carried out competently. The person carrying out the act is liable if he or she performs the act ineffectually. Lastly, if the delegated act is carried out in a hospital or an equivalent facility, the board of directors is responsible for ensuring the availability of training for persons performing the act (Canadian Medical Association, 1988).

Usually, the patient must give informed consent to allow someone other than a physician to perform a procedure. In most cases, delegation will occur only with the patient's consent and only after the physician has assessed the patient, discussed the procedure, and answered any outstanding questions. The Web link for the Canadian Medical Association's *Guidelines for the Delegation of a Medical Act*, along with other resources pertaining to controlled acts, can be found in Web Resources on Evolve.

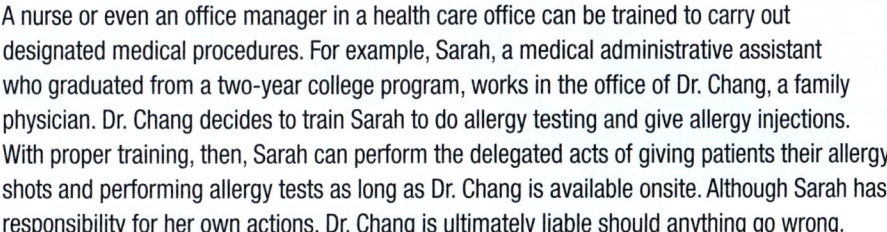

Thinking It Through

A nurse or even an office manager in a health care office can be trained to carry out designated medical procedures. For example, Sarah, a medical administrative assistant who graduated from a two-year college program, works in the office of Dr. Chang, a family physician. Dr. Chang decides to train Sarah to do allergy testing and give allergy injections. With proper training, then, Sarah can perform the delegated acts of giving patients their allergy shots and performing allergy tests as long as Dr. Chang is available onsite. Although Sarah has responsibility for her own actions, Dr. Chang is ultimately liable should anything go wrong.

1. Do you think the delegation of acts should be allowed? Under what circumstances?

2. As a health care patient, what type of assurance would you like that the person performing the procedure has received adequate training?

Complaint Process

Regulated professions have a system in place whereby the public can launch complaints against a health care provider. A designated committee investigates all complaints, protecting both the public, who can rest assured that legitimate complaints will be looked into and appropriate action taken, and health care providers, who will have illegitimate or unfounded complaints against them dismissed. Health care providers found to be at fault may face suspension, an order for additional training, the loss of their licence to practise, or even legal proceedings, such as a criminal investigation.

Educational Standards

A regulator of a profession has the authority to set educational standards for the training of its professional members, including theoretical and practical components of their education as well as examinations for entry to practice. The educational process both prepares professional members and provides assurance to the public that the health care provider is competent to practise.

Professional bodies often use competency-based assessment programs to ensure the continued maintenance of practice standards, protecting both the health care provider and the public. The requirements may include self-assessment tools, continuing education programs, keeping a record of professional activities, or a combination of these. Often, proof that these standards have been met is a requirement for renewal of a professional's licence to practise.

Licence to Practise

In each province and territory, regulators of professions, in conjunction with educational facilities and in keeping with provincial and territorial requirements, oversee the licensing of their members. Regulated professions almost always require licence renewal annually. Many now have other criteria that must be met, such as peer reviews or other proof of ongoing education.

Moving from one province or territory to another can cause issues for some professionals since not all regulated professions have agreements and standards in place for members to practise in other jurisdictions (Case Example 9.1).

Nonregulated Professions and Occupations

Only about 20% of Canada's workforce works in regulated professions (Canadian Institute for Health Information, n.d.). All others work in the many

Case Example 9.1

Because physicians write a national examination, they are qualified to practise anywhere in Canada, but each jurisdiction must license physicians to practise. Dr. Hiraki, a licensed general surgeon in Newfoundland and Labrador, wants to practise medicine in British Columbia, so she must apply to the College of Physicians and Surgeons of British Columbia and follow its protocol before working in the province. While the standards of practice for doctors are the same across the country, medical and legal issues are often different, and every physician practising in a particular jurisdiction must be aware of guidelines that pertain in that region. Once licensed in British Columbia, Dr. Hiraki will be assigned a billing number, which she must use to bill the provincial plan for services rendered.

professions and occupations that remain nonregulated across Canada, ranging from jobs that require university degrees and in-depth, specialized training (e.g., computer scientists, botanists) to those requiring very little education or training.

People who work within nonregulated occupations do not have federal or provincial legislation governing their occupations, although, in several provinces and territories, some professionals, such as electricians and plumbers, must complete strict examinations, both practical and written, to obtain a licence.

Like regulated professions, many nonregulated occupations have professional organizations or bodies that award certification when a person completes a set of written or practical examinations or both. To work as a medical secretary or administrator in a doctor's office or as a clinical secretary or ward clerk in a hospital, a person requires a specialized knowledge base; however, an employer may hire someone with or without certification. A doctor, for example, could choose to hire a person with no experience as a medical secretary and provide on-the-job training, or he or she can hire someone who has graduated from a one-year certificate or two-year diploma program in medical office administration. A hospital may require a clinical secretary to have a grade 12 diploma with some secretarial experience or, alternatively, a diploma from a two-year health administration program. The person or organization doing the hiring sets the requirements when a profession is nonregulated (Case Example 9.2).

Many nonregulated disciplines have no specific standards to meet. For example, anyone can learn how to do ear candling or aromatherapy and put out a sign inviting the public to seek treatment.

Case Example 9.2

A doctor in Nova Scotia decides that the person he hires as office nurse must be an RN (as opposed to a graduate nurse). One applicant, Marika Smith, has written her certification examinations and can use the designation RN. Because Marika has this designation, the doctor knows she has met minimal standards of competence.

CONVENTIONAL HEALTH CARE PROVIDERS

Health care traditionally has been dominated by physicians—from family doctors to specialists. However, a shift toward a team approach to health care is taking place, bringing to the fore the skills and expertise of many other health care providers, particularly in the primary care setting. The Canadian Interprofessional Health Collaborative (CIHC) provides a nucleus for health professions to work together to improve patient care and promote, among other things, interdisciplinary education.

Following are brief descriptions of only some of the physician specialties and the functions of other members of the health care team, including those with multiple titles, newer specialties, changing scopes of practice, or obscure job descriptions.

Physicians

> **Specialist**
> A physician trained in a specific field, usually concerning body systems or organs—for example, cardiology, internal medicine, orthopedic surgery—although some specialties (e.g., geriatrics) have a socioeconomic focus.

Entrance requirements for medical school vary across Canada, but most universities require the applicant to complete two to four years of undergraduate work, usually obtaining a bachelor's degree, and then write an entrance examination, called the Medical College Admission Test (MCAT), before applying for placement in one of Canada's medical schools. Medical school consists of three to four years of study, followed by a residency in the person's area of specialty (e.g., family medicine, internal medicine, general surgery).

A doctor with specialized training in one area, called a **specialist**, usually sees patients only upon request from a family doctor or another specialist. In fact, most provincial or territorial insurance plans will not cover the cost of a patient visiting a specialist without such a referral. A family doctor will refer a patient to a specialist (also called a *consultant*) when the patient requires assessment and treatment outside the family doctor's scope of practice. Many specialists work in solo practice; others work in private or public organizations or are employed by hospitals.

Family Physicians

Family doctors are also called *general practitioners* or *primary care physicians*. With a wide knowledge base not limited to any specific disease or system or to any particular sex or age group, the family doctor provides ongoing care that includes the diagnosis and treatment of conditions and diseases not requiring the care of a specialist, counselling, health promotion and disease prevention, and primary maternity and mental health care. Most family doctors work in primary care team settings (discussed later). A few remain in solo practice, and some in various types of clinics or health centres, especially in more remote regions of the country. Many family doctors also oversee the medical care of patients in health care facilities such as long-term care residences. Some still make house calls, for which the patient must pay out of pocket, but that service is not as prevalent as in the past. As well, many family doctors now choose to give up their hospital privileges, temporarily turning over the care of their hospitalized patients to a hospitalist or other specialist.

Emergentologists

Some physicians, called emergentologists, have chosen careers practising full-time emergency medicine. This specialty has developed because many emergency departments (EDs), also often referred to as emergency rooms (ERs), are choosing to hire full-time physicians rather than staffing the ED with on-call physicians, as in the past.

Geriatricians

Geriatrics focuses on the care of older people, typically those over 65. A geriatrician is usually an internist who has additional training in caring for older adults.

Geriatrics does not attract a large number of physicians: the assessment and treatment of an individual with complex medical conditions is time-consuming. Additionally, geriatricians are typically paid less than other specialists. Most work in private practice, team-oriented practices, or health care facilities.

Geriatrics
The branch of medicine dealing with the physiological characteristics of aging and the diagnosis and treatment of diseases affecting the aged.

Cardiologists

Cardiologists specialize in conditions and diseases of the heart, ranging from abnormal rhythms and heart attacks to related vascular problems. The cardiologist treats patients from a medical perspective but does not do surgery. If surgery is required, the patient may be referred to a cardiac surgeon. Aside from seeing patients in the office setting, cardiologists, with special training, may carry out diagnostic procedures such as cardiac catheterizations in a hospital or private diagnostic facility.

Gynecologists and Obstetricians

Specializing in women's health, gynecologists diagnose and treat disorders of the gynecological and reproductive systems. Obstetricians focus on the care of pregnant women and the delivery of their babies in both normal and high-risk situations. Closely related, these two specialties are usually undertaken together (resulting in the abbreviation OB/GYN).

Internists and Hospitalists

An internist typically diagnoses and renders nonsurgical treatment for diseases of a person's internal organs (e.g., problems of the digestive tract, liver, or kidneys). An internist often refers patients to other specialists who deal with specific organs.

A hospitalist is a physician—usually an internist—who oversees the medical care of patients in the hospital, usually those who do not have a family doctor with admitting privileges to that hospital. As well, a hospitalist will collaborate with specialists as required. Usually employed by the hospital, a hospitalist may or may not have a private practice.

Neurologists

A neurologist treats conditions of the nervous system, including chronic and potentially fatal conditions such as Parkinson's disease and multiple sclerosis, sleep disorders, headaches, peripheral vascular disease, brain tumours, and spinal cord injuries. Neurologists do not perform surgery. Patients requiring surgery would be referred to a neurosurgeon.

Ophthalmologists

Ophthalmologists, medical doctors who specialize in diseases of the eye, can carry out both medical and surgical procedures, such as cataract removal and ocular emergencies (e.g., glaucoma, eye trauma). Although ophthalmologists can perform **refractions** and prescribe glasses, these functions have largely been taken over by optometrists (who are not medical doctors). Cataract surgery is done either in hospital or in free-standing medical facilities, such as Lasik MD clinics or the Canadian Centre for Advanced Eye Therapeutics Inc.

> **Refraction**
> Testing of the eyes to evaluate their ability to see. An ophthalmologist or optometrist does a refraction to determine the type of lens a patient needs in his or her glasses to maximize vision.

Oncologists

Oncology is the branch of medicine that deals with all forms and stages of cancerous tumours—development, diagnosis, treatment, and prevention. An oncologist specializes in the care and treatment of people with cancer. Because cancer treatment has become so highly specialized, oncologists may specialize in only certain areas, such as radiation therapy, chemotherapy, gynecological oncology, or surgery. Oncologists usually practise in large hospitals or medical centres specializing in cancer treatment. They also provide ongoing treatment for patients in hospices and related facilities.

Psychiatrists

Psychiatrists specialize in mental illness and emotional disorders, including depression, bipolar disorder, schizophrenia, obsessive compulsive disorder (OCD), borderline personality disorder, bulimia, anorexia nervosa, and personal stress issues. As medical doctors, psychiatrists can order laboratory and diagnostic tests and prescribe medicine. Psychiatrists do not perform surgical procedures. Geriatric psychiatry is an emerging field. (Note that psychiatrists differ from psychologists, who are not medical doctors.)

Physiatrists

Physiatrists, medical doctors specializing in physical and rehabilitative medicine, work closely with other health care providers, such as physiotherapists, occupational therapists, and geriatricians. Stroke and accident victims and postsurgical patients are among the types of patients that a physiatrist would see. Comprehensive care aims to restore the patient to his or her maximum level of function. The family almost always plays a role in the restorative and rehabilitative process, as treatment is usually long and arduous. For this reason, social workers, psychologists, or psychiatrists may also participate on the health care team.

Radiologists

A radiologist is a physician with additional training in the use and interpretation of imaging techniques to diagnose and treat disease. The radiologist is primarily a consultant to other physicians but may also be involved in the planning of patient care. The work is tedious, and any misinterpretation of the scans can have devastating effects on patients. Radiologists are primarily found in large diagnostic centres, either hospital- or community-based, private or publicly funded.

Respirologists

Respirologists, sometimes referred to as *pulmonologists*, are medical doctors who further specialize in the diagnosis and treatment of lung disease, such as asthma, emphysema, or pneumonia. Respirologists perform tests to check how well a person is breathing and may use procedures such as bronchoscopy to diagnose a breathing problem.

Surgeons

Surgeons complete their surgery residency in their field of choice, usually over a period of four years or more, after completing medical school. A general surgeon completes a number of rotations through various specialties. General surgeons are qualified to perform a wide range of procedures, mostly involving the gastrointestinal tract. Their scope of practice may be limited, however, by the presence of other surgeons with specific specialties at the same hospital or in the community (Case Example 9.3).

Case Example 9.3

Robert presents in the ED with a blockage in his bowel. Dr. Xiong, a general surgeon, is qualified to assess and operate on Robert, but if Dr. Silanka, a gastric surgeon, is available, the emergentologist may call on Dr. Silanka instead.

NURSES

Many agree that the nurse, with skills across several disciplines, is the backbone of the health care system. For example, when a respiratory therapist is not available, the nurse may do the inhalation treatments or set up oxygen for a patient. When the chaplain is not available, the nurse counsels and comforts the patient and loved ones. When the clinical secretary is ill, the nurse assumes administrative responsibilities for the patient care unit.

Registered Nurses

All Canadian jurisdictions except Quebec now require bachelor degrees in nursing (BN or BScN) to enter the profession. Degrees in nursing can be completed in two, three, or four years. Accelerated (two-year) programs are available across Canada. In the Northwest Territories, Aurora College graduates now hold a bachelor of science degree in nursing, obtained through linkage with the University of Victoria in British Columbia. The related regulatory body in each province or territory must ensure that the individuals seeking to practise as nurses meet designated levels of competence. To that end, program graduates in all jurisdictions except Quebec must write a national examination (the Canadian Registered Nurse Examination, or CRNE), which further assesses their competencies. The provincial and territorial regulatory bodies administer the examination and decide who is eligible to write it.

Previously diploma-prepared RNs may obtain a bachelor's degree in nursing by completing a two- or three-year program that, in many regions, can be taken on a part-time basis. Several universities offer a postdiploma degree program via teleconference, correspondence, and satellite classes held in various communities. Additional educational opportunities for RNs vary among provinces and territories. Some specialties include critical care, emergency nursing, community health nursing, hospice and palliative care, and perinatal and woman's health.

The RN usually assumes the most complex components of nursing care as well as administrative and case management responsibilities. Many hospitals and other facilities employ RNs only in specific areas, such as intensive care units, where most of the nursing care demands skills only the RN is licensed to practice.

Nurse Practitioners

Nurse practitioners (NPs) are registered nurses with extended training and skills (RN Extended Class), authorizing them to independently carry out specified controlled acts and activities that other nurses, by law, cannot do. To become an NP, an RN must earn either a postbaccalaureate certificate or a graduate degree for the designation and then pass an entry-to-practice examination that, in some jurisdictions, may be specific to the person's chosen area of specialty (there is no national examination). Licensed nurse practitioners, like registered nurses, must renew their licence yearly. Requirements for licence renewal vary among the jurisdictions but usually include a minimum number of practice hours and participation in designated quality-assurance programs, ongoing education, or both.

An NP's competencies vary among jurisdictions, and all jurisdictions have NP legislation (In the News: Yukon Finally Licenses Nurse Practitioners). Practising independently of but collaboratively with physicians and other members of the health care team, NPs diagnose and treat a wide range of health problems. Likewise, they can order specific lab and diagnostic tests and prescribe a wide range of medications. A significant number of NPs work in primary care settings and clinics (some independently led by NPs). They may also practise in hospitals under specialty designations (e.g., pediatrics, cardiology) and in emergency departments.

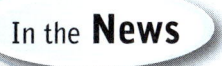 **Yukon Finally Licenses Nurse Practitioners**

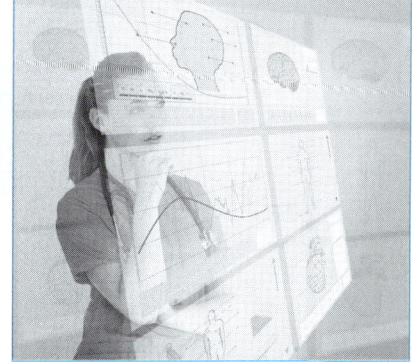

Legislation to regulate nurse practitioners was passed in Yukon on November 23, 2012, making Yukon the last jurisdiction in Canada to do so. Early in April 2013, the territory licensed its first nurse practitioner. Territory-specific legislation allows NPs to diagnose health problems, order and interpret diagnostic tests, prescribe medications, and perform designated procedures. The Yukon Medical Association supports this legislation despite its earlier reservations. The integration of NPs means more comprehensive, accessible care for Yukon residents.

Sources: Gillmore, M. (2013, April 26). Yukon licenses first nurse practitioner. *Yukon News*. Retrieved from http://yukon-news.com/news/yukon-licenses-first-nurse-practitioner/; Yukon Registered Nurses Association. (n.d.). *NP licensure information*. Retrieved from http://yrna.ca/np-licensure-information/.

Photo Credit: © Can Stock Photo Inc./4774344sean.

Registered Psychiatric Nurses (RPNs)

Registered psychiatric nurses (RPNs)—not to be confused with registered practical nurses (RPNs) in Ontario—are recognized as a separate regulated health profession in Western Canada (Manitoba, Saskatchewan, Alberta, and British Columbia) and Yukon. They form the largest body of mental health professionals providing services in Western Canada. Registered psychiatric nurses focus on the mental and developmental as well as the physical components of health of individuals within the context of their overall health and life situations.

RPNs work with a variety of other health care providers and mental health and community organizations. Practice settings are diverse and can include crisis stabilization and forensic assessment units, hospitals, the community, and academic facilities. Unique and separate from BN or BScN programs, education for RPNs (available only in Western Canada) is offered at both the diploma and the degree level and incorporate medical and surgical nursing skills with those specific to the area of mental health. Their national organization, the Registered Psychiatric Nurses of Canada (RPNC) is an incorporated body in Canada.

Licensed Practical Nurses

To become a licensed practical nurse (LPN), called a registered practical nurse (RPN) in Ontario, a person must complete high school (or the equivalent) and a two-year diploma program at a community or private college. All jurisdictions require graduates to write the Canadian Practical Nurse Registration Examination (CPNRE) for provincial or territorial registration and to use the professional designation.

The skill set and scope of practice of licensed practical nurses have expanded dramatically over the past few years, with practical nurses now assuming many of the skills and responsibilities formerly limited to registered nurses. Their skill set includes doing dressings, dispensing medications, and, in some facilities, taking charge of units. The practical nurse collaborates with registered nurses and other members of the health care team to render patient care. Practical nurses can be found in almost all practice settings and in the community.

Physician Assistants

Physician assistants (PAs) are academically prepared health care providers who work directly with or under the direction of a physician. Their responsibilities are usually outlined in a formal contract between the PA and the physician(s) and may sometimes include the facility in which they work. The PA's scope of practice ranges from interviewing patients and health teaching to performing physical examinations and selected diagnostic tests.

Certification is awarded upon successful completion of an entry-to-practice examination, after completion of a two-year Canadian Medical Association–**accredited program**. A PA program offered by the Canadian Armed Forces Medical Services School in Borden, Ontario, provides training for the military; civilian programs are limited, offered only in selected jurisdictions, including Ontario and Manitoba.

> **Accredited program**
> A program that meets standards requisite for its graduates; usually, the standards are set by the profession's governing body, which may be national or provincial or territorial.

PHARMACISTS

A licensed pharmacist, among other things, dispenses medications in response to prescriptions. Experts in their field, pharmacists provide other members of the health care team with valuable information about medications. The physician looks to the pharmacist for advice about current prescription drugs and interactions between them. The patient looks to the pharmacist for direction and advice about taking medications, their risks, and their potential adverse effects. In most jurisdictions, the provincial or territorial plan will pay pharmacists to periodically review a person's medication profile with him or her, offering advice and counselling or referring the person to his or her physician if need be.

To practise pharmacy, a person must earn a bachelor's degree in pharmacy, complete an internship, and successfully pass a national board examination through the Pharmacy Examining Board of Canada. Many jurisdictions, including B.C., Alberta, Saskatchewan, Manitoba, New Brunswick, Nova Scotia, and Prince Edward Island, allow pharmacists to write prescriptions under designated guidelines. Ontario pharmacists can prescribe smoking-cessation drugs and give flu shots. Since September 2013, Quebec pharmacists have been authorized to write prescriptions, give extensions on existing prescriptions, adjust medication doses, and order and interpret laboratory tests (Plante, 2013). The goal of adding new responsibilities to the scope of practice for the pharmacist is to reduce the volume of work for doctors, clinics, and emergency departments and to provide Canadians with easier access to some front-line services.

MIDWIVES

Depending on the jurisdiction, women experiencing normal pregnancies may choose to see a midwife. Midwives provide prenatal care before the baby's birth, deliver the baby (either at the patient's home or in the hospital), and provide postpartum and newborn care for up to six weeks after the birth. Strict guidelines dictate that the care of a pregnant woman must be turned over to a physician if her pregnancy becomes high-risk or shows signs of other problems during any phase of the pregnancy, labour, or delivery.

Midwifery is licensed in most jurisdictions in Canada. New Brunswick moved to license midwives, but by 2012, there were still no practising midwives, so the licensing body was disbanded as a cost-cutting measure (Picard, 2013). Yukon, Prince Edward Island, and Newfoundland and Labrador have not licensed midwives (Canadian Midwifery Regulators Consortium, 2013).

Optometrists and Opticians

Most optometrists obtain an undergraduate degree, often in mathematics or science, before completing a four-year university program in optometry at one of Canada's two schools of optometry (in Waterloo, Ontario, and in Montreal, Quebec). The minimum requirement for entry to these programs is three years in a university science program with good academic standing. Graduates of a school of optometry are awarded a doctor of optometry degree. To practise, optometrists must be licensed by their province or territory. Skilled in assessing eye function and conditions, they may prescribe selected medications (topical and oral) to treat a variety of eye conditions (e.g., bacterial or viral eye infections, allergic conjunctivitis, glaucoma, and eye drops to dilate the eyes for examination). Optometrists also prescribe glasses and contact lenses to patients who need them. Most optometrists work in group or solo practices.

An optician completes a two- or three-year college program, sometimes followed by a practical component. Opticians can fill prescriptions for eyeglasses or contact lenses, fit glasses, help patients select frames, organize the grinding and polishing of lenses, and cut and edge lenses so they fit selected frames. They also do a considerable amount of health instruction related to contact lenses and glasses, including providing information about options such as lens coating and bifocal lenses. They may work independently or in a larger centre with other eye-care specialists. Opticians are regulated in nine jurisdictions across Canada.

Osteopathic Physicians

As a natural medicine, osteopathy applies the knowledge of anatomy and physiology to all diseases, disorders, and dysfunctions. Osteopathic physicians, or *osteopaths*, use a holistic and hands-on or manual approach to identify and correct problems. It is worth noting that there are unregulated practitioners in Canada sometimes called *osteopathic manual practitioners* or *manual therapists* with limited training in the field. By law, they cannot call themselves *osteopaths*.

In Canada, osteopaths are licensed physicians with specialized training in osteopathic medicine. Many are internists, anaesthesiologists, pediatricians, family doctors, and psychiatrists; thus, they can order all imaging studies, laboratory tests, and pharmaceuticals. Coverage for osteopathic treatment varies among jurisdictions. Many insurance companies cover the services of osteopaths who are licensed, registered, or certified by a government-recognized regulatory body for osteopathic physicians.

PODIATRISTS (CHIROPODISTS)

The term *podiatrist* is used internationally as the name for a foot specialist. In Canada, only Ontario uses the term *chiropodist*. Podiatrists specialize in the diagnosis, assessment, and treatment of foot disorders. They treat sports injuries, foot deformities (related to the aging process as well as misalignments), infections, and general foot conditions, including calluses, corns, ingrown toenails, and warts. Included in their scope of practice is performing specified foot-related surgical procedures, administering injections to the feet, and prescribing medications (e.g., nonsteroidal anti-inflammatory drugs and antibiotics, depending on the jurisdiction). Podiatrists refer patients to surgeons or other doctors when necessary.

In Canada, the chiropody/podiatry program is offered only at the Michener Institute in Toronto. Although Quebec offers a podiatry program for residents of the province, students are required to do a year of training in New York. Individuals can also be trained in the United States, the United Kingdom, and Australia. Practice requirements and scope of practice vary from one jurisdiction to another. In jurisdictions with no regulatory body, there are no standards of practice; essentially anyone can call him- or herself a podiatrist and treat patients.

Practice settings include health care facilities, clinics, the community, primary care reform groups, and private practice. Some podiatrists specialize in such areas as biomechanics, diabetic foot care, or foot care in long-term care facilities.

PERSONAL SUPPORT WORKERS

Most jurisdictions recognize a category of health care worker who provides basic care and carries out auxiliary duties for patients. The title varies: personal support worker (PSW), health care aide, health care assistant (commonly used in B.C.), home care support worker, resident care aide, orderly, health care attendant, patient service associate. This category of worker is not considered a health professional as such and is not regulated, and the training varies. Some facilities still train individuals informally or on the job. More often, though, this type of position requires formal training that may take three months to a full academic year to complete. These care providers work closely with their patients, providing personal care, psychological comfort, and assistance with daily activities. Primarily used in long-term care facilities and by home care organizations, this care provider works with and under the direction of other members of the health care team. Practice settings include hospitals, long-term care facilities, clinics, industry, the community, interdisciplinary primary care practices, and private practice.

Psychologists

Psychologists graduate from university programs at the bachelor's, master's, or doctoral level. To practise psychology in Canada, psychologists must be licensed by the regulatory body in the province or territory where they work.

Psychologists work primarily as clinicians in hospitals, academic facilities, clinics, primary care facilities, correctional facilities, and private practice. Psychologists work with individuals and families to treat emotional and mental disorders, mainly through counselling. They administer noninvasive written and practical tests such as personality tests, intelligence tests, assessment tests for attention deficit disorder (ADD), and diagnostic tests for the early stages of Alzheimer's disease or dementia. Since psychologists are not medical doctors, they do not have the authority to prescribe medications, perform medical procedures, or order lab or diagnostic tests. Often, a psychiatrist and a psychologist will work as a team for more effective and ongoing patient treatment. Private insurance usually covers a specified number of visits to a psychologist. but for the most part, provincial and territorial plans do not.

Speech-Language Pathologists and Audiologists

Speech-language pathologists are experts in disorders of human communication. They assess and manage persons with a wide variety of related conditions, including problems with swallowing and feeding, stuttering, and delays in speaking, as well as social communication and literacy issues. Practice settings include hospitals, long-term care and mental health facilities, research and academic facilities (schools and universities), group homes, the community, and private practice.

Audiologists work with patients with problems related to such things as sound, hearing, deafness, and balance. They provide ongoing education and diagnostic services, as well as create and manage treatment plans for all age groups. In most jurisdictions, audiologists can prescribe and fit hearing aids and other hearing devices. Practice settings are similar to those of the speech-language pathologist, with the addition of industrial settings.

In Canada, the minimal requirement to be a speech-language pathologist or an audiologist is a master's degree in the relevant course of study.

Communications Disorders Assistant

Communications disorders assistants (CDAs) work with or under the direction of both speech-language pathologists and audiologists. They assist clients to communicate effectively or to use alternative forms of communication, among other things. Their scope of practice includes initiating and carrying out diagnostic tests (e.g., audiology screening), assisting with treatments, and health teaching. CDAs require a graduate certificate along with an undergraduate degree or diploma in a related field such as linguistics, early childhood education, social work, or educational assistants.

Respiratory Therapists

To become a respiratory therapist (RT), one must successfully complete an RT program from a college or university that has been accredited by the Council on Accreditation of Respiratory Therapy Education. College programs are three years in length, and university programs, four. The Canadian Society for Respiratory Therapists (CSRT) is the national professional association for respiratory therapists and the certifying body for RTs who practise in nonregulated jurisdictions. In regulated provinces, provincial regulatory bodies provide the certification for RTs. To obtain the RRT designation and be licensed to practise in Canada, graduates of accredited programs in respiratory therapy must write the national certification examination and meet designated registration criteria from CSRT and their respective regulatory bodies.

Respiratory therapists have expertise in several areas of respiratory care and perform cardiorespiratory health-related functions—both in and out of hospital settings. In the hospital setting, they are available to evaluate, treat, and support inpatients and outpatients throughout the facility; however, they are especially vital within critical care areas such as the ED and intensive care units, where they manage advanced life support for patients with cardiopulmonary problems (e.g., persons on respirators). With their advanced skills, RTs respond to emergencies (such as heart attacks) and are able to **intubate** patients as well as initiate the use of respirators. RTs are often required in the transfer of critically ill patients from one facility to another or from an accident scene to a hospital. They are also required in the delivery room when doctors suspect the baby has or may develop respiratory problems. RTs perform diagnostic testing, including arterial blood gases and pulmonary function tests. In the hospital setting, the RT is often responsible for setting up oxygen therapy or inhalation treatments. Other facilities RTs work in include medical centres, clinics, and complex continuing care and rehab facilities; many also work in the community.

> **Intubate**
> The passing of a tube into a person's trachea to facilitate breathing.

Physiotherapists

Physiotherapists graduate from university at the master's level and must pass a national exam to enter professional practice. An essential part of the primary care team, physiotherapists work with individual patients to limit and improve upon physical impairments and disabilities and to prevent and manage pain. They work in a variety of settings such as health care facilities and clinics, as part of a primary care team, in the community (home care), and in private practice. Some physiotherapists specialize in such areas as geriatrics, sports medicine, or pediatrics. Most jurisdictions cover physiotherapy services under specific conditions and for limited time frames. Many private insurance plans also offer some coverage.

Occupational Therapists

Occupational therapists (OTs) are health care providers who help people learn or relearn to manage important everyday activities, including caring for themselves or others, maintaining their home, participating in paid and unpaid work, and engaging in leisure activities. Occupational therapists work with patients who have difficulties as the result of an accident, disability, disease, emotional or developmental problems, or aging. In most jurisdictions, individuals can visit occupational therapists without a referral, although the decision to see an OT is usually made jointly with a primary care provider. Occupational therapists work in hospitals, private homes (usually through provincial or territorial home care programs), schools, long-term care facilities, mental health facilities, rehabilitation clinics, community agencies, public or private health care offices, and employment evaluation and training centres.

To practise as an occupational therapist in Canada, the minimal educational requirement is a baccalaureate degree in occupational therapy. All OTs must be registered with their provincial or territorial college. Upon passing the national certification exam, OTs can practise anywhere in Canada.

Physiotherapy Assistants and Occupational Therapy Assistants

Physiotherapy assistant (PTA) and occupational therapy assistant (OTA) programs are offered at many community and private colleges in Canada. Most are two years and combine the two disciplines. A number of private colleges have single-discipline programs, usually for PTAs. Program names vary. For example, the Southern Alberta Institute of Technology offers a two-year diploma program called Rehabilitation Therapy Assistant and graduates students with both OTA and PTA skills. All programs are in the process of becoming accredited through the Occupational Therapist Assistant and Physiotherapist Assistant Education Accreditation Program.

OTAs and PTAs work collaboratively with and under the direction of physiotherapists or occupational therapists to administer rehabilitation treatments to individuals who are experiencing physical, emotional, or developmental problems. Work settings include rehabilitation centres, long-term care facilities, the community (e.g., home care), physiotherapy clinics, and sports and medical clinics. Some jurisdictions, such as Alberta, have a professional therapy assistant association for PTAs, OTAs, speech-language pathologist therapy assistants, and recreation therapy assistants.

ADMINISTRATIVE ROLES

Health Information Management

Health Information Management (HIM®) professionals hold the designation of CHIM—Certified in Health Information Management. They provide leadership and expertise in the management of clinical, administrative, and financial health information in all formats and in a variety of settings (e.g., hospitals, community care, long-term care and nursing homes, physician offices, clinics, research facilities, insurance companies, and pharmaceutical companies).

The Canadian College of Health Information Management (CCHIM) administers the National Certification Examination (NCE) on behalf of the Canadian Health Information Management Association (CHIMA), the national body representing approximately 5000 HIM® professionals. To become a CHIM, one must graduate from a CHIMA accredited diploma or degree program, offered at colleges and universities across the country, and successfully challenge the NCE. Certified members of CHIMA are required to participate in earning continuing professional education (CPE) credits to maintain their certification. Conestoga

College in Ontario offers a Bachelor of Health Information Sciences (BAHIS) degree and will also consider graduates of CHIMA accredited HIM® diploma programs for advanced standing opportunities. Detailed contact information on current CHIMA accredited programs, including those offered through distance education, can be found on the CHIMA Web site.

The HIM® profession has four domains of practice: *data quality* (the collection and analysis of health information, the coding of clinical information, and quality assurance); *e-HIM®—electronic health information management* (the physical to digital conversion of health records, digital cloud storage and distribution of health information, and the management of complex communications systems); *privacy* (keeping health information confidential and secure and enforcing privacy legislation as it pertains to the information for which they are responsible); and *HIM® standards* (records management standards, documentation standards, terminology standards, etc.).

Health information managers are involved with almost every aspect of health information throughout its lifecycle, from data and information collection, analysis, and retrieval, to the destruction of information once it is no longer needed. For example, when working with health records, HIMs facilitate the collection of health information and oversee proper access to and use of the information. They ensure that data are stored properly and safely and, when no longer needed, are disseminated and destroyed according to facility and legal guidelines. HIMs also conduct quantitative analysis of health records, ensuring they are accurate and complete, and statistical analysis used for identifying trends, such as births, deaths, diseases, and health care costs.

In Canada, HIM® professionals are trained in six core competency areas that include biomedical sciences; health care systems in Canada; health information, including the HIM® lifecycle; information systems and technology; management aspects; and ethics and professional practice. The HIM® professional is playing a pivotal role as Canada continues to work toward the implementation of integrated electronic health information systems at local, provincial and territorial, and national levels. They will be instrumental in directing and reshaping how health care is delivered.

Health Services or Health Office Administration

Every aspect of health care requires some level of administrative support. Being responsible for the day-to-day administrative management of a hospital unit, a clinic, or a physician's office requires skill, knowledge, patience, commitment, and a high level of professionalism. The name for individuals working in these roles varies from medical secretary or medical office assistant to unit clerk, clinical secretary, or administrative coordinator. Demands require people in this role to have a sound knowledge base in several areas, including pharmacology, diagnostic and laboratory testing, medical terminology, anatomy and physiology, disease pathophysiology, and the principles of triage. Those working in a doctor's office must have both clinical and administrative capabilities to manage electronic health records, schedule and triage patients, and be able to do provincial or territorial billing. In the hospital setting, administrative staff have to navigate complex computer software systems (e.g., Meditec) for data-entry responsibilities and understand hospital policies and procedures. All must have the ability to multitask and to work efficiently under pressure and must be flexible, friendly, empathetic, supportive, and comfortable around individuals experiencing health problems.

Practice settings include doctors' offices and group practices, specialists' offices, all hospital units, and long-term care facilities. Health services or health office administrators are not regulated, so there are no provincial or territorial standards to meet. In addition, no jurisdictions other than British Columbia have a professional organization. The Medical Office Assistants' Association of British Columbia is an **affiliating body** specifically for administrative health care providers. The International Association of Administrative Professionals (IAAP) welcomes members from any administrative discipline and has chapters across Canada.

Affiliating body
An association that provides, among other things, direction, support, continuing education, and networking opportunities for its professional members (who may be regulated or nonregulated).

Laboratory and Diagnostic Services

The field of medicine depends greatly on laboratory and diagnostic services. Many diagnoses cannot be confirmed without a lab or diagnostic test of some sort. Even to prescribe the appropriate antibiotic, doctors rely on laboratory tests. Highly qualified individuals, including physician specialists and laboratory technologists and technicians, populate this field. As well, many specialties exist within this area (e.g., pathology, hematology), most of which are regulated in each province and territory.

Volunteer Caregivers

It is only appropriate to note the tremendous support that friends and family and organized volunteers provide to those who are ill. With current shortages in all categories of health care providers, many patients depend on this group of people to fill in the gaps in their care that cannot otherwise be filled. The hours of care provided by these individuals are uncountable, the output unequalled, and the stress phenomenal. Many ill people could not manage without this supportive network. Volunteer caregivers work in partnership with professional caregivers.

PRACTICE SETTINGS

The practice settings described here provide a cross-section of where health care is delivered. Included in some detail are practice settings that physicians and interdisciplinary teams work in. Several types of clinic settings are also described.

A patient's home is fast becoming a place of health care delivery by a variety of health care providers, with patients recovering at home from surgical procedures and illness or being cared for at home as an alternative to long-term care. Across the country, however, providing sustainable, affordable, and high-quality home care remains a challenge for reasons that include the expense, the difficulty of organizing the delivery of effective care, and, in some jurisdictions, a lack of human resources.

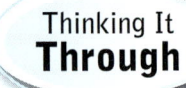

Thinking It Through

An older family member falls ill and requires constant supervision at home for a period of time. Home care options are limited.

Assuming that you work full-time and have a family of your own, what would you do to ensure your family member receives the care he or she needs?

CLINICS

Urgent Care and Walk-in Clinics

Canadian residents who do not have a family doctor, are away from home, or cannot get an appointment with their primary care physician can seek medical care from an urgent care or walk-in clinic. These clinics reduce the burden on emergency departments by providing nonemergency care to patients who would otherwise clog the ED. Clinic visits also usually cost the health care system less than visits to the ED do. Some urgent care clinics offer more immediate access to diagnostic testing, such as ultrasound, and to minor procedures, such as suturing, whereas walk-in clinics often refer the patient elsewhere for these procedures.

Ambulatory Care Clinics

In the most literal interpretation, ambulatory care clinics have traditionally encompassed any clinic—for example, a walk-in, urgent care, or private clinic—that offers services and discharges the patient immediately thereafter—that is, a clinic in which a patient does not spend the night. Ambulatory care, therefore, may include day surgeries, visits to emergency rooms, cast changes, postsurgical assessments (perhaps after hip or knee surgery), and cancer treatment. Within the past five years, the term has referred more specifically to facilities that offer groups of services in one location—often, a hospital.

Outpatient Clinics

Outpatient clinics offer services that vary from hospital to hospital and community to community in an effort to meet the unique needs of a particular area.

An outpatient clinic can operate under the umbrella of an ambulatory care clinic—a clinic within a clinic. Services may include family doctor care, minor surgery, screening procedures (e.g., vascular screening), laboratory and diagnostic procedures, and foot care. Outpatient clinics in large hospitals offer an even wider range of services. Some hospitals divide clinics into areas of specialty and related services; others offer many disciplines within one clinic. For example, in Moncton, New Brunswick, the hospital has divided its ambulatory care clinics into five specialized areas: healthy living, which includes services to assess and treat ongoing conditions, such as asthma, diabetes, and chronic obstructive pulmonary disease; specialty procedures clinics, which include **urodynamic** and eye clinics; treatments and orthopedics; diagnostic clinics, which includes pulmonary assessment and electrocardiograms; and endoscopy and minor surgery.

Urodynamic

Referring to tests and assessments done to measure the function of the bladder and urinary tract.

Nurse Practitioner–Led Clinics

Nurse practitioners in some jurisdictions have taken the lead role in seeing patients in a clinic setting much like a walk-in clinic. The NP sees patients in the same manner that a physician would and will refer the patient to a physician—usually a member of the same interdisciplinary—if he or she encounters something a doctor should diagnose or treat. The NP-led clinic provides an option for patients who do not have access to traditional walk-in clinics and for regions with a shortage of physicians. The clinic may also be used for routine checkups, prenatal or well-baby care, or managing a chronic disease.

Why Clinics Make Sense

Clinics have gained prominence for a number of reasons, including the following:

- Cost-effectiveness: The past few years have yielded a shift toward community-based care. New technologies have shortened surgeries and made them less invasive, allowing for earlier discharges and follow-up in clinics. It costs less to care for patients at home than to maintain them as inpatients. Many tests formerly done in a hospital are now done in a clinic on an outpatient basis. Having patients see a specialist or other health care provider in the clinic setting on a first-come, first-served basis usually costs less than having them make an appointment with a specialist or other health care provider. Organizations can staff clinics more efficiently according to perceived need. As well, equipment booking, if handled centrally, can result in available equipment being maximized.
- Timely access, fewer patient visits, convenience: With proper organization, patients can access more services faster, possibly in one clinic visit. The move toward multidisciplinary health teams has enabled clinics to readily provide the

patient with a variety of services (Case Example 9.4). With centralized resources, the patient should have to make fewer visits, a result that is especially beneficial to patients with multiple health problems or mobility or transportation issues.

- Patient focus: Specialized clinics are usually better prepared to work with patients, to consider their individual needs, and to offer streamlined and patient-friendly health education. Clinic staff members typically have experience dealing with a specific condition and take the opportunity to learn from their patients, which increases the professionals' overall effectiveness in meeting patients' health care needs.

Case Example 9.4

Diagnosed with diabetes six months ago, Jim is still learning how to live with the disease. He visits the ambulatory care clinic at 7:00 Monday morning. First, he goes to the lab and has blood work done. The nurse reviews with him his blood sugar levels for the past two weeks and how much insulin he is taking each day. He then sees the dietitian at 8:20 to discuss changes to his diet. At 9:30, he sees the doctor, who checks his blood pressure and general health and does an eye examination. The doctor reviews his insulin intake and diet, as well as his blood work—which is back from the lab and shows slightly elevated levels—and recommends some changes. Jim then returns to the nurse to discuss some of his personal concerns. He is finished at noon. At 12:20, he goes for a cardiac stress test, as he has been experiencing chest pains, which may or may not be related to his diabetes.

PRIMARY HEALTH CARE REFORM

The need for primary care reform arose in the late 1990s, when it became evident that there was a shortage of family doctors in Canada. To address the problem, Canada began investing millions of dollars to improve how primary health care was delivered. Initial funding was provided through the Primary Health Care Transition Fund, a financial agreement reached by the provincial and territorial and federal governments. That funding ended in 2011, and since then, monetary contributions from the federal government for primary care reform and other health renewal initiatives have been included as part of the overall federal transfer of funds to the provinces and territories for health care.

To meet their goals, the provincial and territorial governments began experimenting with various models for delivering primary care. Since 2009, significant gains have been made, despite thousands of Canadians' still having only limited access to primary care providers. Even for people who do have a family doctor, getting an appointment can take days or even weeks, unless the condition is acute.

It became apparent early on that the most effective way to deliver high-quality primary care to the greatest number of people was through aligning health care providers from varying disciplines into some sort of group practice. It also soon was realized that no one particular model would meet everyone's needs. The structure and function of these groups had to be flexible to meet the needs of the population in the geographic area it served. The primary objective of primary care renewal, however, has remained consistent: to deliver patient-centred, comprehensive care that is affordable, assessable, coordinated, and tailored to the needs of the population.

Primary Health Care Groups

A number of family doctors can unite to create a primary health care group. They first need to choose what particular model they want to use (it must be an acceptable model within their province or territory). In most jurisdictions, the physicians must apply to the provincial or territorial government or the appropriate body for permission to form the group. Once approved, the physicians enter into a formal contract with their provincial or territorial government, which details the organizational structure, funding mechanisms, and the doctors' professional obligations to the group and patients (e.g., hours of availability, clinic hours, telephone availability).

Structure and Function of the Groups

Each province and territory is likely to have more than one model from which the group can choose to follow. The location, structure, organization, number of physicians, the number and mix of other health care providers, services offered, and payment arrangements within a group vary, as does the name of the group. All such groups are composed of a number of physicians. Other health care providers within the group vary and may include, for example, registered nurses, nurse practitioners, pharmacists, chiropodists, dietitians, counsellors, and physiotherapists. The responsibilities of most group members are fairly straightforward but, for physicians, may be more complex, (e.g., on-call hours, clinic availability, Telehealth access, and expectations related to other services offered and patient care).

In Ontario, a model called the Family Health Team (FHT) has emerged as the most comprehensive interdisciplinary prototype. Patients can be enrolled or rostered (discussed below) to a single physician or to a group of physicians. Service offerings, other than core services, vary from one team to another (e.g., chronic disease management and rehabilitation, specialist services). FHTs are the only model that receives funding for an executive director and for electronic medical records.

Alberta's Family Care Clinics (FCCs) are the newest and most comprehensive primary care model in that province. They are meant to complement the existing Primary Care Networks, which are currently considered the basic building block for delivering front-line care. Alberta also recently introduced two additional organizations: Strategic Clinical Networks (SCNs) focus on improving health outcomes in the fields of mental health, respiratory and heart health, emergency, and critical care, and Operational Clinical Networks (OCNs) work to improve general health outcomes for Albertans by, for example, improving patients' experiences with the health care system, shortening wait times, and ensuring care availability. Both networks work collaboratively with each other and with other primary care organizations and health care providers.

In 2012, the Saskatchewan government invested $3.6 million to improve primary care services. The government has established eight "innovative learning sites" to test models for primary care delivery built on partnerships between health regions, communities, and health care providers. The government of Saskatchewan has committed to several milestones, including the elimination of ED wait times by 2017.

Primary care in British Columbia is delivered through Divisions of Family Practice, community-based groups of family physicians working collaboratively to deliver health care. Each division works with its respective health authority.

Payment Mechanisms for Primary Care Groups

Fee-for-service was the most prevalent payment mechanism for physicians prior to the formation of primary care groups. Within the groups, capitation-based funding and blended funding (Chapter 8) are most popular. Included also in many primary care models are billing opportunities for milestones reached for certain services so as to encourage health care providers to improve patient care outcomes and lower costs. Incentive billing encourages preventive care within a practice. For example, to be paid, a physician must ensure that a given percentage of applicable patients have the suggested immunizations, colorectal screening, Pap smears, and mammograms. The higher the percentage of patients who receive the recommended services, the more the doctor is paid. Bonus payments may also be made when a doctor provides additional services such as diabetic management, smoking cessation counselling, insulin therapy support, and fibromyalgia or chronic fatigue syndrome management.

Patient Enrollment and Primary Care Models (Rostering)

Many primary health care groups (including all groups in Ontario) require that a certain percentage of patients formalize their relationships with the group by signing a form agreeing to become part of the doctors' practice, a process called **rostering**, *patient attachment*, or *formal registration*. The idea is that the physician and patient establish a mutual commitment for care.

Rostering
The registering of a patient in a primary health care reform group. Patients sign a nonbinding form stating that they will seek care only from a specific doctor or primary care group. Also called *patient attachment* or *formal registration*.

Signing the form is purely voluntary and not binding; a patient may leave the agreement at any time, or become unrostered. But being rostered entitles the patient to all of the services and benefits offered by that particular primary health care reform group, such as access to after-hours clinics and a telephone helpline (see Chapter 8). If a rostered patient visits another medical doctor for a routine health problem (i.e., not an emergency), the government may deduct from the family doctor's monthly stipend the fee for that visit (Case Example 9.5). Being rostered is probably not appropriate for a person living in a temporary residence (e.g., a college student living away from home to attend school) because he or she may need to seek health care elsewhere.

Case Example 9.5

Although rostered with Dr. Gregory, Nathan, who is experiencing extreme stress, goes to see Dr. Gresham, a family physician who exclusively offers counselling services and psychotherapy. Dr. Gresham bills the provincial plan $100 for Nathan's visit.

At the end of the month, Dr. Gregory gets a notice from his provincial health ministry stating that $100 has been deducted from his monthly payment to compensate the ministry for the amount it was charged for Nathan's visit to Dr. Gresham.

Thinking It Through

You move to a new town and set out to find a family doctor. You find one physician in solo practice who agrees to take you as a patient because he cares for friends of yours. However, you also find a newly formed primary health care reform group with two physicians taking new patients.

Consider the benefits the primary health care reform group offers versus the close relationship you would be likely to develop with the physician in solo practice. Which would you choose?

TELEPHONE HELPLINES

Because telephone services are considered an important element in primary care, the government has invested significant funds into this initiative. Often called **Telehealth** or Teletriage, these helplines offer callers advice from health care providers (usually RNs) 24 hours a day, 7 days a week.

Telehealth

A telephone help system, usually available 24/7 and funded by the provincial or territorial government, used to provide professional health care advice to Canadians who cannot readily access a doctor or other primary care provider.

Telephone helplines differ across the country in the type and scope of service they offer. Some offer only telephone advice, whereas others refer the patient to another resource (e.g., a clinic, a nurse practitioner, a doctor, the ED). Some will forward the call to the physician on call for the group or ensure that the patient's physician receives information about any care or advice the patient received (Case Example 9.6).

Although most helplines have follow-up procedures, these are not always foolproof. If a helpline attendant does not diligently obey such rules, using telephone helplines can be dangerous, as demonstrated in a rather extreme but not entirely unheard-of circumstance in Case Example 9.7.

Case Example 9.6

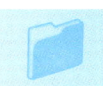

Helena lives in British Columbia and has a 3-year-old daughter, Gillian. Gillian wakes up at 2:00 A.M. She is warm, crying, and has diarrhea. Helena is not sure what to do. Should she take Gillian to the emergency department, or is it something that can wait until morning? Helena calls HealthLink B.C., which offers British Columbians health information and advice from a registered nurse around the clock. The nurse tells Helena to sponge the baby, to try to give her some clear fluids, and to monitor her until the morning, at which time she can call her family doctor—which Helena does. In the meantime, HealthLink B.C. transmits an electronic report of the occurrence to the family doctor's office.

Case Example 9.7

Theo called a telephone helpline at 2:00 A.M. Monday. He said he'd tried to kill himself by taking a bottle of Aspirin and half a bottle of sleeping pills. The pills had only made him slightly drowsy. With a change of heart, he wondered what he should do. The nurse advised him to go to the nearest emergency department and offered to call an ambulance for him. He responded that he would go but that he had someone to drive him.

The helpline did not follow up with Theo's family doctor about this call, which is not unusual in some circumstances. At 3:00 P.M. on Wednesday, a family friend found Theo semiconscious and dehydrated on the floor in his kitchen and called 911. Theo's kidneys had failed. Today he is alive but on dialysis. If Theo's doctor had been notified of the event Tuesday morning, he could have arranged for follow-up immediately and perhaps minimized the kidney damage.

COMMUNITY HEALTH CENTRES

Community health centres (CHCs) are staffed by interdisciplinary teams to provide medical care in communities that have limited access to health care (known as *hard-to-serve communities and populations*). CHCs also focus on disease prevention and related health teaching and look at underlying social and physical conditions that may affect a community (e.g., poor diet, housing issues, drug and alcohol addiction). Hours in these health centres are usually extended and include evenings and weekends. Physicians and other health care providers are most often salaried and paid by the provincial or territorial or federal government.

HEALTH SERVICE ORGANIZATIONS

The concept behind health service organizations (HSOs), also called *health care organizations*, *comprehensive care organizations*, or *group health centres*, is similar to that of primary health care reform groups. Providers may be paid per enrolled patient or salaried (Ronson, 2011). HSOs can be private/public partnerships. Health care providers operate within an organization and more or less ration care to their rostered patients, with the goal of rendering high-quality care while containing costs. For example, physicians may be expected to adhere to a protocol for ordering tests based on best practices guidelines. Integrated health organizations (IHOs) are another model that combines multiple services (e.g., acute care, hospital corporations, primary care, and home care).

A successful incorporated HSO in Sault Ste. Marie, Ontario, called the Group Health Centre, is a nonprofit, alternatively funded ambulatory health organization constructed from a partnership between the Sault Ste. Marie and District Health Group and the Algoma District Medical Group (Group Health Centre, 2009). The Algoma group comprises approximately 74 physicians with varying specialties. A corporation, it is governed by a board of directors from the community, owns its building, equipment, and furniture, and hires the staff (excluding physicians). The centre serves a population of 75,000 and has an estimated 66,000 patients (G. B. Walsh, personal communication, August 22, 2013).

Across Canada, trials of various models for delivering health care continue, with governments recognizing that different regions and different populations have different needs.

Summary

9.1 Conventional medicine is frequently referred to as *mainstream*, traditional, or *Western medicine*. Conventional health care providers (i.e., doctors, nurses, nurse practitioners, midwives, dentists, pharmacists, etc.) diagnose health problems; treat prediagnosed health problems; render technical, therapeutic, or supportive care with evidence-informed therapies, medication, and surgery. Complementary or alternative medicine includes all health care practitioners not considered conventional. Although the terms are sometimes used interchangeably, a difference exists between alternative and complementary medicine: complementary medicine supports, or complements, conventional medicine, while alternative medicine typically provides an option, or alternative, often to the exclusion of conventional medicine.

9.2 Regulation provides the public with a wider choice of health care providers, with the assurances that the professional they choose meets legislated standards of practice. Some nonregulated professions are in the process of seeking regulation. As well, health care providers—regulated and nonregulated alike—have support from a wide range of professional organizations, many of which offer education and certification to their members. A designation ensures a high standard of performance.

9.3 The list of conventional health care providers is long and includes such roles as physicians with a wide variety of specialties, nurses, pharmacists, midwives, optometrists, personal support workers, psychologists, administrative workers, and laboratory workers.

9.4 Practice settings include primarily hospitals and doctors' offices—either in solo practice or in a group or clinic setting. Several types of clinics act as practice settings: urgent care, walk-in, ambulatory care, outpatient, and nurse practitioner–led. Patients' homes are also becoming a place to deliver health care by a variety of health care providers.

9.5 A nationwide initiative of primary health care reform probably holds the answer to providing effective point-of-contact care to all Canadians. Interdisciplinary collaborative teams are better able to meet the health needs of Canadians, applying knowledge and expertise from a variety of health care providers to individualize patient care, thus achieving better health outcomes. Because telephone services are considered an important element in primary care, the government has invested significant funds into this initiative. Community health centres, which provide medical care in communities that have limited access to health care, focus on disease prevention and related health teaching. Health service organizations are similar to primary health care reform groups, except that a third party receives and manages their funding.

Review Questions

1. Explain the difference between a conventional health care provider and a complementary or alternative health care practitioner. Provide examples.
2. Outline the benefits that a regulated profession offers to the public.
3. Differentiate between a controlled act and a delegated act, giving an example of each.
4. Discuss why there is some dispute over whether a chiropractor is an alternative health care practitioner or a conventional health care provider.
5. Explain why some complementary or alternative health care practitioners in Canada may be considered conventional health care providers in other countries.
6. Explain the purpose of primary health care reform.
7. Describe the structure and function of primary health care groups.
8. State the purpose of telephone helpline services. Explain how some differ in the services they offer.

References

Canadian Institute for Health Information. (n.d.). *Canada's health care providers.* Retrieved from https://secure.cihi.ca/free_products/hctenglish.pdf.

Canadian Medical Association. (1988). A CMA position. Guidelines for the delegation of a medical act. *Canadian Medical Association Journal, 138.* Retrieved from http://www.ncbi.nlm.nih.gov/pmc/articles/pmc1267562/pdf/cmaj00159-0083.pdf.

Canadian Midwifery Regulators Consortium. (2013). *Legal status of midwifery in Canada.* Retrieved from http://cmrc-ccosf.ca/node/19.

College of Physicians and Surgeons of Ontario. (2008). *Delegation of controlled acts.* Retrieved from http://www.cpso.on.ca/policies/policies/default.aspx?ID=1554.

Group Health Centre. (2009). *Algoma District Medical Group.* Retrieved from http://www.ghc.on.ca/admg/content.html?sID=15.

Picard, A. (2013, July 10). Midwives: Underused and misused assets in Canada. *The Globe and Mail.* Retrieved from http://www.theglobeandmail.com/life/health-and-fitness/health/midwives-underused-and-misused-assets/article13133123/.

Plante, C. (2013, January 23). Bill 41 bringing changes for Quebec pharmacists. *Global News.* Retrieved from http://globalnews.ca/news/382606/bill-41-bringing-changes-for-quebec-pharmacists/.

Ronson, J. (2011). Are integrated healthcare organizations right for Ontario? *Essays.* Retrieved from http://www.longwoods.com/content/22607.

Statistics, Canada (2014, June 12). *Access to a regular medical doctor, 2013.* Retrieved from http://www.statcan.gc.ca/pub/82-625-x/2014001/article/14013-eng.htm.

CHAPTER TEN

Current Issues and Future Trends in Health Care in Canada

Learning Outcomes

10.1 Discuss the state of mental health and mental health services in Canada.

10.2 Summarize the challenges in managing health care for Canada's aging population.

10.3 Discuss how Canada is dealing with the current shortage of human health resources.

10.4 Explain the problems facing home care services in Canada.

10.5 Describe the drug funding situation in Canada.

10.6 Summarize the main barriers to accessing health care services.

10.7 Outline the major health care issues and related concerns Aboriginal Canadians face.

10.8 Understand the impact electronic health records will have on health care.

10.9 Discuss future initiatives for primary health care.

Key Terms

Disease burden, p. 337

Food insecurity, p. 359

Forensic psychiatric hospitals, p. 335

Interoperable EHR, p. 367

Non-status Indians, p. 356

Orphan patient, p. 354

Reserve, p. 356

Status Indians, p. 356

Consider the following stories. What do they suggest about the current state of health care in Canada?

> *Lucy, an Aboriginal woman, suffers from mental illness. She often does not take her medications, causing her to be in and out of psychotic episodes. She has little medical support and is incapable of caring for herself. She often steals or begs for money and sleeps on the street or in shelters. She frequents the emergency department (ED), brought in by police, especially after a drinking binge.*
>
> *At 78 years of age, Merle is legally blind, has congestive heart failure, debilitating osteoarthritis, hypertension, diabetes, and chronic pain. She qualifies for some home care, but an inadequate amount. Without home care, it is likely she will have to go into a nursing home.*
>
> *Hakeem, a new immigrant to Canada, is 23, works part-time, and needs medication for asthma. Although he can access clinics, he has no family doctor, so his care and medical records are fragmented. He has no drug plan and does not qualify for provincial drug coverage. As a result, he goes without his medication most of the time.*
>
> *Experiencing chest pain, Helga went to Emergency. She waited two hours to be seen, despite being evaluated as urgent. She had had a cardiac arrest and was told that she would require surgery to clear a blockage in her heart. Several months passed between her doctor making an appointment with a cardiac surgeon and Helga having surgery.*

These stories illustrate some of the major issues the Canadian health care system faces:

- Although care for mentally ill people is improving, it is still underfunded and often poorly coordinated.
- Canada's Aboriginal population faces disparities with respect to socioeconomic conditions and health care.

- Home care remains underfunded—many Canadians cannot pay for the services they need; others end up in long-term care facilities because home care is inadequate.
- Thousands of Canadians have no drug benefits and do not qualify for government assistance; others cannot afford the cost of some drugs not covered by private or public insurance (e.g., chemotherapeutic agents). A national catastrophic drug plan does not exist although nearly all jurisdictions have some form of catastrophic coverage.
- Wait times for emergency departments and for some medical and surgical services are excessive.

Despite numerous positive things about Canadian health care, there are many inadequacies as well. Health care in Canada is in transition, struggling to adapt to changing demographics and economic realities. This chapter will discuss some of the current issues in health care, their probable causes, and the measures that have been taken to deal with them. It will also look briefly at future trends.

MENTAL HEALTH

The overall annual cost of treating mentally ill Canadians is more than $50 billion (Mental Health Commission of Canada, n.d.a). According to a 2012 Statistics Canada survey, approximately 6.7 million people in Canada are living with a mental illness—approximately 20% of Canada's population (Canadian Mental Health Association, n.d.). As a result, mental illness is considered a significant public health problem. Timely access to appropriate care remains a central issue for these people. Other concerns include underfunding, the stigma attached to having a mental illness, and the related socioeconomic consequences.

STRUCTURE AND IMPLEMENTATION OF SERVICES

In Canada, mental health falls under the jurisdiction of the provincial and territorial governments, which collaborate with agencies such as Health Canada and the Public Health Agency of Canada to plan strategies and interventions aimed at caring for mentally ill people.

Mental health care is offered in tertiary care psychiatric hospitals, **forensic psychiatric hospitals** and clinics, community mental health centres and related agencies, some correctional facilities, adolescent assessment and treatment facilities, alcohol and drug treatment programs, and long-term care facilities. In most jurisdictions, acute care hospitals offer mental health care to varying degrees, usually through outpatient clinics or in specialized inpatient units.

Forensic psychiatric hospitals
Hospitals that assess and treat individuals referred by the Canadian courts and those requiring a secure inpatient facility due to a risk for harm to self or others.

Community-based mental health care is provided in a variety of ways:

- Many jurisdictions offer a centralized point of contact to help people navigate the mental health care system and to provide them direction regarding their legal rights (e.g., Alberta's Access Mental Health initiative).
- In every province and territory, health organizations provide care and public education. For example, the Canadian Mental Health Association and its nationwide branches deliver services and support to those with mental health and addiction challenges. This organization depends heavily on a dedicated team of volunteers to deliver and maintain its community programs. Other organizations, such as the United Way, fund some uninsured services for those unable to pay, although many services remain accessible only to people who can afford them.
- Some health care providers (e.g., registered psychiatric nurses, found primarily in Western Canada) give private care for people with mental illness. These practitioners operate, for the most part, outside of provincial and territorial health insurance plans.

THE STIGMA OF MENTAL ILLNESS

According to the Mental Health Commission of Canada (MHCC), 60% of people with mental health issues will not seek help because they are afraid of being stigmatized—and with good reason (Mental Health Commission of Canada, n.d.b). Despite improvements in the public's understanding of mental illness over recent years, people with any form of mental illness are still subject to stigma, prejudice, and discrimination. Some cultures, particularly in developing countries, even actively hide mentally ill family members (Mental Health Commission of Canada, n.d.b). And whereas most people would have no qualms about saying, "Yes, I have pneumonia, and I'm taking antibiotics," few taking antidepressants would admit it. Likewise, when an individual is sick, friends and family often send cards and flowers, but when mental illness is the cause, the patient is often socially isolated.

In 2009, the MHCC launched Opening Minds, the largest organized initiative in the country's history to reduce stigma, improve how people think about mental illness, and promote fair and equitable treatment of those who suffer from it. Stigma affects all aspects of a person's life. Mindful of this, Opening Minds targets four main groups: health care providers to create positive, accepting, and caring attitudes; youth to identify those at risk and promote early intervention; the workforce to encourage understanding and tolerance at work; and the media to positively influence public views and attitudes (In the News: Clara's Big Ride).

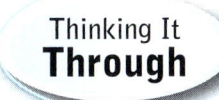

Thinking It Through

Many Canadians are reluctant to admit to being diagnosed with mental illness.

1. Would you be more likely to keep quiet about a mental illness than a physical disorder?
2. If you were on an antidepressant, would you feel comfortable telling anyone?
3. If a friend told you he or she was depressed and had thoughts of suicide, what would you do?

In the News — Clara's Big Ride

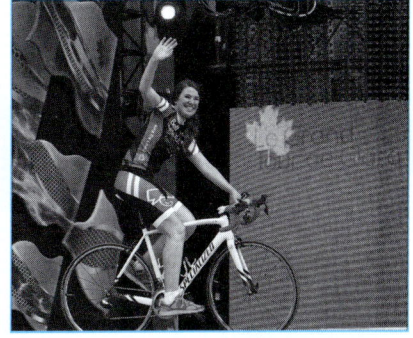

Clara Hughes, a six-time Olympic medallist, has shared her struggle with depression with the world. An active promoter of mental health awareness, she is a leading participant in Bell's Let's Talk mental health campaign. In the spring of 2014, she began cycling across Canada to raise awareness for mental health. She believes that the stigma attached to mental illness is lessening but still is very much present.

Sources: Stunt, V. (2014, March 14). Clara Hughes cycles across Canada to promote mental health. *CBC*. Retrieved from http://www.cbc.ca/news/canada/hamilton/news/clara-hughes-cycles-across-canada-to-promote-mental-health; MacDonald, G. (2014, March 13). On the eve of her cross-country bike tour, Clara Hughes speaks out about depression. *The Globe and Mail*. Retrieved from http://www.theglobeandmail.com/life/health-and-fitness/health/i-was-injured-in-body-and-spirit/article17476765/h-1.2573334x.

Photo Credit: The Canadian Press/Fred Chartrand.

COMMON MENTAL HEALTH DISORDERS

Alcohol and drug addiction and mood disorders (major depression, generalized anxiety disorder, and bipolar disorder) are among the most common mental health problems. Major depression is the most significant mood disorder and is expected to be the second leading cause of **disease burden** globally by 2020 (World Health Organization, 2001).

Suicide related to undiagnosed or poorly managed mental health problems is a significant concern. Approximately 4000 Canadians take their own lives each year, most of whom were confronting or dealing with a mental illness (Mental Health Commission of Canada, 2012).

Disease burden
The impact of a health problem, measured by financial cost, mortality, morbidity, or other indicators.

CHALLENGES

Any person with a mental health disorder or substance abuse issues is likely to face a number of challenges. Which ones and to what extent largely depend on the support the person has, for example, from family and friends, and the extent of effective medical intervention. Three of these challenges are discussed below.

Mental Illness and Homelessness

A large number of homeless people in Canada—25% to 50%—have a mental disorder or substance abuse problem, and many have a combination of disorders (Munn-Rivard, 2014). Homeless people report high stress levels, low self-esteem, and little or no social support. They also often experience poor physical health and have a high rate of suicide attempts. In fact, the Canadian Institute for Health Information (CIHI, as cited in CNW Group, 2007) reports that 35% of visits to emergency departments by homeless people relate to mental health and behavioural disorders.

The cost of homelessness to Canadians is estimated at $7 billion annually (Gaetz, Donaldson, Richter, et al., 2013). This figure includes health care costs, legal fees, and social services expenditures for this population. Individual communities bear most of the responsibility for looking after the homeless—some programs receive government funding; others rely entirely on volunteers. Rain City Housing and Support Society in Vancouver is a nonprofit organization that offers numerous services to mentally ill individuals who are homeless.

Mental Illness and the Justice System

Increasingly, people with mental health problems are involved with the criminal justice system. While incarceration provides a roof over their heads, mentally ill inmates receive only limited treatment. Additionally, few prison officials are trained how to recognize behaviours related to mental health disorders or how to respond appropriately to troublesome situations arising from such behaviours (e.g., negotiating, communicating, ensuring proper care). The consequences are drastic. As well as going without treatment, mentally ill inmates are placed into situations they can neither understand nor deal with. Sadly, suicide remains the leading cause of death in Canada's correctional facilities (Kirmayer, Brass, Holton, et al., 2007).

Of major concern is the increase in self-harm and acting-out incidents within prisons. These events have been under scrutiny since the case of Ashley Smith (see In The News: Inadequate Mental Health Care in Prisons: The Consequences). An investigation confirmed that staff members were ill-equipped to respond to the needs of inmates with mental illness (Office of the Correctional Investigator, 2013).

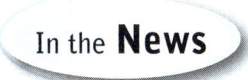

Inadequate Mental Health Care in Prisons: The Consequences

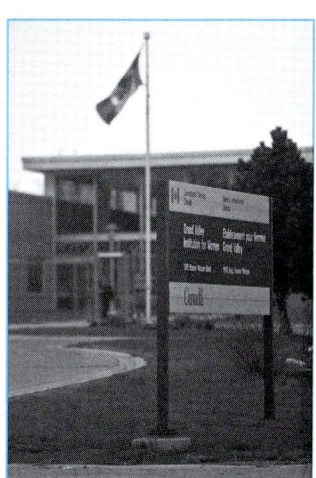

On October 19, 2007, 19-year-old Ashley Smith of New Brunswick was found unconscious after attempting to strangle herself in a segregation cell at the Grand Valley Institution for Women in Kitchener, Ontario. She died in hospital shortly after. Ashley's history showed that she had been involved with the court, correctional, and health care systems since she was 13 years old and had tried to harm herself on previous occasions, often by self-asphyxiation. Despite her mental health issues, Ashley had not had a psychological assessment during her 11.5 months in federal custody, nor had she had access to adequate mental health services. Guards watching Ashley trying to strangle herself had reportedly been instructed not to intervene as long as she was still breathing because these attempts were frequent—a decision that proved fatal. Ashley had been scheduled for transfer to a psychiatric hospital, but no beds had become available.

It was concluded that Ashley's death was both tragic and preventable and that it continued a "disturbing and well-documented pattern of deaths in custody" (Office of the Correctional Investigator, 2009). Reports on the inquest can be viewed online.

Sources: Canadian Broadcasting Corporation. (2008, June 24). Death of Moncton girl preventable, prison ombudsman says. *CBC News*. Retrieved from http://www.prisonjustice.ca/starkravenarticles/ashley_smith_Cl_0708.html; Office of the Correctional Investigator. (2009, March 3). *Backgrounder: "A preventable death."* Retrieved from http://www.oci-bec.gc.ca/cnt/rpt/oth-aut/oth-aut20080620-eng.aspx; Brennan, R. J. (2009, March 7). Mental illness rife in prisons. *The Toronto Star*. Retrieved from http://www.thestar.com/life/health_wellness/2009/03/07/mental_illness_rife_in_prisons.html.

Photo credit: The Canadian Press/Geoff Robins.

In collaboration with the MHCC, Correctional Service Canada is working to address the issue of mental illness within the prison system. The strategic document *Mental Health Strategies for Corrections in Canada* includes plans to implement a national process for screening offenders upon entry into the correctional system; train staff members at all levels; provide primary, intermediate, and more intensive mental health care in all facilities; and better prepare inmates for transition back into the community.

Mental Illness and Employment

People with mental illness suffer higher levels of unemployment and underemployment than the general population, with unemployment ranging from 70% to 90%, depending on the severity of the illness (Mental Health Commission of

Canada, 2012). Several studies highlight the huge economic impact of mental health issues:

- Mental health issues will cost Canadian businesses over $6 billion each year due to absenteeism and ineffective productiveness (Mental Health Commission of Canada, 2012).
- The private sector spends $180 million to $300 million on short-term disability benefits related to mental illnesses and $135 million on long-term disability benefits in a given year (Lopez-Pacheco, 2013).
- Mental illness is the fastest-growing claims category for workplace disability, affecting 21.4% of the working population (Lopez-Pacheco, 2013).

Some workplaces have taken steps to reduce occupational stress by providing support and implementing preventive strategies, such as flexible working hours, work-at-home days, access to counselling, "sleep rooms," exercise facilities, and measures to improve job satisfaction.

Increasingly, employers are held responsible for terminating workers who display behaviours incongruent with workplace standards and later have been diagnosed with mental illness. Human rights tribunals often rule in the plaintiff's favour, using a law known as the "duty to inquire," which puts the onus on the employer to investigate if odd behaviour is related to a mental health issue.

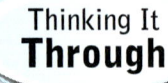

Pierre was exhibiting depressive behaviours at work. At times he was argumentative and defensive. His work productivity slipped, and he was often absent. After several warnings to "improve," he was terminated. Pierre filed a human rights complaint. His employer was found to have wrongly terminated him and without due process. The employer had to rehire Pierre, make accommodation for his depression while Pierre was under treatment, and reimburse him for lost wages.

1. Why do you think Pierre did not tell his employer about the depressive episode?
2. What steps should the employer have taken other than cautioning him to improve?
3. What can employers do to make the workplace less stressful and to deal with employees experiencing a mental health problem?

THE FUTURE OF MENTAL HEALTH CARE

Changing Directions, Changing Lives is the first national strategy for mental health. Released in 2012, the strategy primarily aims to improve care for people diagnosed with mental illness across the country and provide them and their families with the necessary resources and support. The strategy acknowledges that even the best and most coordinated treatments and services will fall short of reducing the impact of mental illness in Canada. As with physical health, therefore, the promotion of mental health and prevention of mental illness are fundamental.

Despite the system's problems, most experts believe the move away from institutionalized care was the right one. Current thinking leans toward integrating mental health services into existing primary care systems and improving interdisciplinary collaboration on the part of all health care providers.

HEALTH CARE COSTS AND AN AGING POPULATION

Advances in medical science and clinical practice have resulted in people living longer—some with good health, but many others with multiple health problems requiring medical intervention and support. Older Canadians use the health care system more often. For example, a person over the age of 80 is more likely than someone just 65 to have chronic health conditions, require a hip or knee replacement, or need cataract surgery. And as they age, the costs of services and care rise.

Associated Concerns

As Canadians retire, they take with them a vast amount of information, wisdom, and experience that guide workplace decisions. As well, having more retired Canadians means higher government spending on pensions. At the same time, concerns arise about how to sustain the health and wellness of our aging population while retaining the resources to care for the rest of the population.

Lower Taxation Base

Fewer working-age Canadians means a smaller workforce, along with a corresponding reduction in tax dollars for all levels of government, resulting in the government's having less money to spend on health care and social programs, such as the old-age pension.

Loss of Skilled Labour

The number of persons aged 65 years and over doubled between 1981 and 2009 and will double again by 2036 (Schwartz, 2010). The exit of so many people from the workforce will affect many sectors of society, including health care, a field in which shortages of many health care providers persists.

Physicians' Time

The Canadian Institute for Health Information (2011) reports that 95% of older Canadians have a family doctor. Although older Canadians do not appear to overuse physician time in terms of the number of visits, their visits do last longer than one from a younger person. Older adults rarely have just one problem—the main complaints may be joint pain, indigestion, and generalized aches, but isolating and dealing with a single complaint is difficult. As well, older Canadians are more likely to be on multiple medications that require constant updating and monitoring. Nurse practitioners (NPs) and physician assistants (PAs), however, have greatly improved access to primary care by assuming some of a physician's duties. NPs work independently but collaboratively with physicians, while PAs work directly with physicians and assume some physicians' duties.

As discussed in Chapter 9, Canada is suffering an acute shortage of specialists to care for older Canadians. In 2012, only 230–242 certified specialists in geriatric medicine cared for 4.3 million older Canadians (Hogan, Borrie, Basran, et al., 2012), a ratio of one geriatrician to as many as 18,695 patients. Although most jurisdictions are attempting to attract more physicians to this specialty, it is an uphill battle. Doctors are in short supply in general, and geriatrics does not boast a wide appeal. Furthermore, compensation for geriatricians typically falls below that for other specialists.

Training primary care physicians in geriatrics and introducing more clinics dedicated to caring for older adults could make a difference. Primary health care reform initiatives already in place are proving helpful. In particular, interdisciplinary health teams (dietitian, social worker, physiotherapist, chiropodist, physician, nurse, and pharmacists) are providing older Canadians with a much broader range of required health services.

Acute Care Hospital Beds

Older Canadians constitute 14% of the population but account for 40% of acute hospital stays, 85% of hospital-based continuing care, 82% of home care, and 95% of residential care (Canadian Institute for Health Information, 2011).

Many older Canadians admitted to hospital find that they cannot return home and live independently because of their medical condition. Hospital beds then often end up occupied by individuals not requiring active treatment. Finding space for and providing interim care to people in transition between the hospital and a nursing home are an ongoing problem. The term *alternate level of care* (ALC) is used to describe individuals who are occupying a bed in an active hospital setting but no longer require the related services and are just waiting for discharge to an appropriate facility or home (with appropriate support). For example, Mr. Smith had a hip replacement and no longer needs the care he received postoperatively, but he is waiting for a bed in a rehab facility. He would be referred to as an ALC patient or the less professional slang term, a bed-blocker (Canadian Institute for Health Information, 2011).

Emergency departments are used more by older Canadians (many from long-term care facilities) than by young or middle-aged Canadians, often for conditions that could be handled within the community, and more older Canadians are admitted to hospital from the ED. Falls are responsible for 34% of injury-related hospital admissions, and 40% of these result in a fractured hip (Public Health Agency of Canada, 2011). Others are admitted to acute care beds from home and wait for admission to alternative care facilities such as nursing homes. Although most jurisdictions have made improvements in the availability of alternative care accommodation, a shortage remains, contributing to a lack of acute care beds and backups in emergency departments, where people requiring ALC must wait for admission—over half of hospitalized older Canadians occupying acute care beds were discharged to some type of residential facility in 2012 (Canadian Institute for Health Information, 2012c). An emphasis on prevention, a team approach to health care, and better management of chronic conditions will reduce the number of hospital admissions and keep older Canadians healthier and in their homes longer.

Predictions for the Future

Although the health-related costs for older Canadians have remained relatively stable, they are expected to rise over the next decade as this age group increases in number. By 2031, projected estimates state that approximately $4.4 billion will be spent on direct health care costs for fall-related injuries among this age population (Scott, Wagar, & Elliott, 2010). Some of these costs include surgery, rehabilitation, and, all too often, placement of the injured party in long-term care.

Other issues confronting the health care system are more acute, such as the shortage of health care providers, funding shortfalls for community support, the need for long-term care beds, and the cost of prescription drugs. Careful planning now—for example, implementing team-based strategies to manage those with chronic diseases and disabilities associated with aging—can ease the situation.

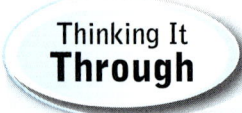

With an aging population, informal caregivers increasingly must provide care for older family members. Almost 17% of these caregivers report stress related to this role.

1. Do you think the use of informal caregivers is important to keeping down the costs of caring for older Canadians?

2. What supports do you think the health care system could or should provide to these caregivers?

HUMAN HEALTH RESOURCES

Shortages in human health resources exist in almost all areas of health care—doctors, nurses, dentists, laboratory technologists, physiotherapists, diagnostic test technicians, psychologists, chiropractors, and midwives.

AVAILABILITY OF REGULATED NURSES

It is difficult to actually determine whether there is a shortage of nurses Canada-wide. The CIHI, for example, has stated that the number of nurses in Canada is increasing (A. Porter-Chapman, personal communication, August 21, 2014). In addition, data released by the Canadian Association of Schools of Nursing showed that the number of nursing graduates has also increased, as have the number of programs and number of students. Nevertheless, shortages of regulated nurses exist in some regions across the country. Variations can be attributed to population needs, the mix of health care providers, the way health care is organized, and the collaboration of professionals. Geography also plays a role—the more remote the community, the more likely it is to need more nurses.

The History

A shortage of regulated nurses was first felt in the 1980s and 1990s, when funding cutbacks in health care services meant fewer jobs for nurses. As a result of these cutbacks, the number of nurses graduating from academic facilities decreased, and many nurses left the country for jobs elsewhere.

When the looming nursing shortage became apparent, nursing programs increased the number of seats they offered to students, and an interest in nursing resurfaced. Most jurisdictions have developed strategies both to recruit new nurses and to encourage existing nurses to stay in the profession. Despite these measures, a shortage persists. The Canadian Nurses Association reports that Canada is facing a shortfall of approximately 20,000 nurses right now and will need 60,000 more nurses by the year 2022. Attrition is a contributing factor, with the number of nurses approaching retirement continually increasing. A report by the CIHI (2012b) stated that, in 2011, one in four RNs were over the age of 55.

Working Conditions

Adverse working conditions remain an issue for many regulated nurses. The acuity of care has increased, and, in many regions, the patient-to-nurse ration has not. The result is stressful work situations, long hours, and tremendous levels of responsibility. A 2013 survey by *The Fifth Estate* (as cited by CBC News, n.d.) revealed that 60% of nurses claimed that there was insufficient staffing to do their jobs properly.

Contract and Part-Time Positions

In 2011, over 41.3% of registered nurses and 48.9% of licensed practical nurses were employed in part-time (i.e., contract or scheduled positions) or casual positions (Canadian Institute for Health Information, 2012b). Many, therefore, have two or more jobs to attain full-time hours. Casual positions are unpredictable and stressful due to lack of security, benefits, and workplace stability.

STRATEGIES TO ATTRACT AND RETAIN NURSES

A number of strategies have been employed over the past decade to increase the number of regulated nurses practising in Canada, such as increased government funding in nursing programs at colleges and universities. As well, some provinces (e.g., British Columbia and Ontario) have implemented condensed programs to fast-track the graduation of nurses prepared at the degree level. Nursing education has been changed to meet the increasing demand for skilled nursing services, resulting in nurses with a more extensive mix of skills and competencies. For example, across Canada, diploma programs for registered nurses are being eliminated in favour of degree programs: graduates receive a bachelor of science in nursing (BScN) or a bachelor of nursing (BN).

Licensed Practical Nurses

In 2011, there were 84,587 licensed practical nurses (LPNs) working in Canada. Nearly 43% were working in hospitals, and 39% in long-term care facilities, where most assume supervisory roles. Over 16% worked in rural settings or in northern regions (Canadian Institute for Health Information, 2012b). LPNs are closing the gap left by diploma-prepared RNs. Educational programs for LPNs have been lengthened in most jurisdictions to prepare people to assume a broader scope of practice, including much of the responsibility formerly assumed by diploma-prepared registered nurses. For example, LPNs (called *registered practical nurses* [RPNs] in Ontario) give medications, assume charge positions, look after intravenous drips (IVs), and do dressings in long-term, residential, and acute care settings.

Advanced Educational Opportunities

Many nurses are choosing to advance to other levels within their profession or to qualify for other designations, such as nurse practitioner, clinical specialist radiation therapist, anaesthesia assistant, and surgical first assist. In Quebec, the scope of practice of specialized registered nurses allows them to monitor patients with chronic diseases, adjust medications, and order diagnostic tests. It is hoped that these measures will address gaps in the health care continuum, particularly related to physician shortages.

Strategies to allow foreign graduates entry to practice are also in place. Many facilities are using a prior learning assessment tool to assess the competencies of internationally trained nurses.

SHORTAGE OF DOCTORS

The History

In the early 1990s, federal advisors in the federal, provincial, and territorial governments determined that Canada had too many doctors in proportion to the population growth. To address this trend, the federal government commissioned the Barer-Stoddart Report to study the causes of accelerating health care costs. Released in 1991, the report stated that an excess of human health resources (most notably, doctors) usurped a huge chunk of the health care budget and, consequently, recommended a decrease in medical school acceptances and limits on the admission of foreign physicians to the country. Medical schools across the country decreased enrollment by 10% to 20%, a reduction in seats that remained in effect for the next ten years. In addition, immigrating physicians were given no guarantee of acceptance into medical practice, and fewer foreign medical students received visas to complete training in Canada. Before long, the effects were felt, most acutely by Canadians who could not find a family doctor. If they moved or their physician retired or relocated, they were out of luck, relying on clinics and emergency departments for medical care. Rural Canada was hit hardest. In 2006, almost a third more family or general practice physicians practised in urban rather than rural Canada (Figure 10.1).

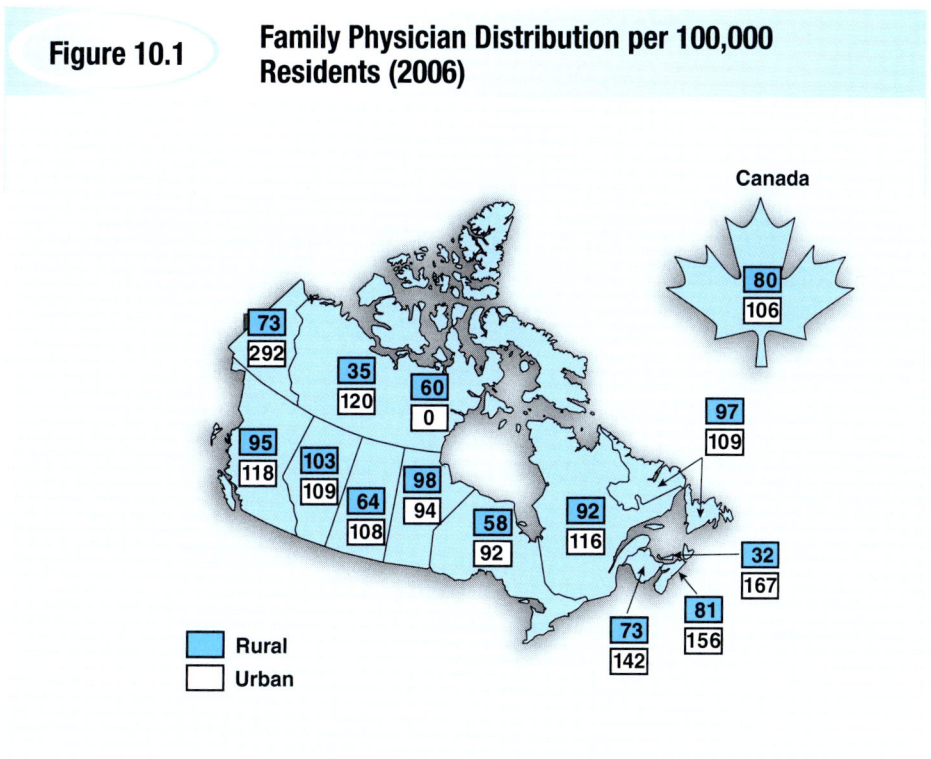

Figure 10.1 Family Physician Distribution per 100,000 Residents (2006)

Source: Canadian Institute for Health Information, *Health Care in Canada 2008* (Ottawa, Ont.: CIHI, 2008), p. 17.

Is There Still a Shortage?

As discussed in Chapter 8, the number of doctors in Canada has increased steadily over the past several years and is expected to continue to do so. Although the gap is closing, about 4.3 million Canadians still do not have a family doctor. Medical schools have increased enrollment, made it easier for foreign physicians to gain entry to practice, and are taking steps to make family medicine an attractive option compared to other specialties. For example, they are stressing that family doctors now have better work–life balance, with fewer on-call hours, more collaborative care options, and vacation time offered in most primary care group practices. Putting in fewer practice hours allows general practitioners of both genders the flexibility that allows for family time. Practices that are turnkey operations fully equipped with the latest technology, reducing the amount of paperwork and increasing the efficacy of the practice, have added appeal.

Although a significant number of doctors are at or nearing retirement age—a statistic that used to be a concern—a surprising number are continuing to practise at least until they can find a suitable replacement to assume responsibility for their patients (National Physician Survey, 2013).

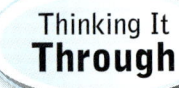 

Medical schools across Canada have been admitting increasing numbers of women, many of whom want to have families, meaning that they may at some point feel compelled to reduce their workload, their hours, or both.

1. In today's society, do you think that physicians who are also mothers can balance their family responsibilities with the demands of a full patient load?

2. What challenges do you see for physicians who are their children's primary caregivers?

HOME AND CONTINUING CARE

Home care services are both curative and restorative in nature and are provided by an interdisciplinary team of professionals and caregivers at home and in the community. Professional services may be offered by nurses, physiotherapists, speech-language therapists, or social workers. Other caregivers may provide housecleaning, meal preparation, personal care, or shopping services.

THE PROBLEM

The demand for home care services (both short-term and long-term) has grown. Across Canada, one in every six older adults is receiving some level of home care services (Canadian Home Care Association, 2013). Older Canadians want to maintain their independence for as long as possible, and living at home with the proper support is often a better option to living in long-term or continuing care. Home care is more cost-effective; however, many barriers exist: insufficient numbers of trained home care workers; limited provincial and territorial insurance coverage for these services; inconsistent, poorly coordinated, and poor-quality care; and scheduling or communication problems between caregivers (Canadian Home Care Association, 2013).

Recipients of Home Care

Home care patients include people of any age, but statistically, more older Canadians are using the service. Patients include those who are discharged early from hospital and require short-term support; those with chronic conditions who are not sick enough to remain in an institution or hospital but who cannot manage independently; and those who, because of age or a disability, cannot live independently but can get by with a little help. Home care offering specialized palliative support has also become a viable option for persons wishing to die at home.

Accessing Home Care Services

In most jurisdictions, people requiring home care need a referral, either from a physician or some other central agency, to determine the legitimate need for home care services. The home care agency will then conduct a needs assessment for the potential patient. Most jurisdictions use a standardized assessment tool called the Resident Assessment Instrument–Home Care, or RAI-HC. This tool allows the nurse or other designated health care provider to assess multiple domains of the patient's function and suggest protocols for care and service requirements.

Public funding for these services is not keeping up with the demand. Inadequate home care availability could result in older Canadians' being admitted to long-term care facilities before needing full-time care, increased demand on family members to provide care, significant limitations on what or how much care can be provided, and financial stress on families trying to pay for home care services (Canadian Home Care Association, 2013).

The Impact of Home Care

Home care is recognized as a critical component of primary health care. The current philosophy is that individuals can receive better and more cost-effective care at home. As well, people cared for in the home appear to recover faster and are less likely to acquire an institution-based infection.

Funding

The provision of home care is not mandated under the *Canada Health Act*. However, with the 2004 accord, all levels of government agreed to certain principles, including two weeks of provincial or territorial coverage of some services (e.g., pain control, IV therapy, dressing changes) for acute care patients discharged from hospital; two weeks of community care for people with acute mental illness; and two weeks' palliative care. Outside of these principles, provincial and territorial governments select the services and number of hours of home care a patient is entitled to under their respective plans.

In Canada, home care is provided by a mix of public (i.e., government), for-profit, and not-for-profit organizations. The number of funded hours a patient is eligible for is usually determined at the initial assessment. Most often, the individual requires more hours than provincial or territorial insurance will pay for. To receive the extra time and services, patients must pay the full amount for some services and a copayment for others. Home care, therefore, can be costly and out of reach for many Canadians. Even some volunteer-dominated services (e.g., Meals on Wheels) come with a cost to the patient. Growing numbers of private, for-profit organizations offer home care services. We Care, one of the largest, with branches across Canada, offers nursing, personal support, homemaking, cleaning, and companionship services 24 hours a day, 7 days a week.

The Future

Since the 2004 accord, the most progress has been made in funding and managing short-term home care. The growing necessity for family members to provide care comes with its own problems, including caregivers' needing care and support themselves. Many families or individuals have two or three children and yet have to provide ongoing daily home care for an aging parent or parents. Some jurisdictions have legislated a compassionate leave, which allows people to take time from their workplace to care for a loved one without fear of losing their job.

Organizations and stakeholders, including the Canadian Medical Association (CMA), have asked the federal government to expand medicare to include home care. As an alternative to reopening the *Canada Health Act*, which is unlikely, the CMA has proposed a *Canada Extended Health Services Act* to cover home care and other extended health care services. Currently, the government has shown no serious consideration of this request.

A study on safety at home found that ongoing problems with home care include medication errors, falls, infection, and miscommunication among agencies and professional and nonprofessional workers. The study indicated that 100,000 to 130,000 home care patients experienced preventable adverse events related to care (Canadian Institutes of Health Research, 2013). As a result, the Canadian Patient Safety Institute (CPSI), a not-for-profit organization funded by Health Canada, is forging ahead with educational initiatives to reduce infection rates and promote safer methodologies for medication administration.

Continuing Care and Home Care: The Relationship

Continuing care addresses the need for services similar to those delivered in the home but for people requiring more intense care. While not yet ready to manage outside of a hospital setting, candidates for continuing care no longer require acute care services. Also called *extended care* or *chronic* or *complex care*, continuing care is typically rendered in a facility separate from the hospital or attached to an acute or rehabilitative unit within a hospital.

A 2012 study found that 54% of older adults who waited in acute care beds (ALC patients)—some for a very long time—were discharged to a residential care facility (Canadian Institute for Health Information, 2012c). Research shows that during such a wait, older adults experience a decline in their general health, physically and cognitively. To facilitate faster transition from the acute care setting to suitable ALC environments, government bodies across the country are taking measures to increase the capacity of home care programs.

DRUG COVERAGE

Prescription drugs are the fastest-growing cost driver in the health care system today. As discussed in Chapter 8, Canadians' use of prescription drugs has increased in general, but particularly so among older Canadians, who tend to take more medications as they age.

Funding

Although the provinces and territories provide some coverage to vulnerable populations (e.g., low-income individuals, older adults), Canada has neither a universal pharmacare program nor a national catastrophic drug plan, leaving a large portion of Canadians unable to pay for the medications they need. As discussed in Chapter 6, the federal government finances drug plans through various agencies for First Nations and Inuit Canadians, veterans, the Royal Canadian Mounted Police, and federal offenders; Citizenship and Immigration Canada covers drug costs for specified refugee claimants, and the Department of National Defence, for members of the Canadian Forces. Still, many Canadians carry no private drug insurance and suffer financial hardship when they need medications.

The Future

Although the need for a national drug plan has long been recognized, no immediate strategy has resulted (see Chapter 1). A national pharmacare plan would offer many benefits including the creation of a central agency to control the price of drugs and to monitor the quality and price of new drugs introduced to the market.

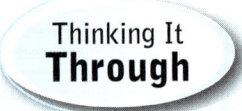

Thinking It Through

There are increasing calls for public health insurance plans to add comprehensive home care services and medications to insured services. However, these additions will cost enormous amounts of money that will compromise funding for other services.

1. Do you think funding home care services and prescription drugs is a good idea?

2. Can you see a workable compromise?

WAIT TIMES AND ACCESS TO MEDICAL CARE

One of Canada's biggest health care challenges is the long wait lists for selected health care services. In 2004, Canada's first ministers met to address the problem and agreed to implement measures aimed at reducing wait times in five priority areas: cancer treatment, cardiac care, diagnostic imaging, joint replacement, and sight restoration (cataract surgery).

The causes of the long waits vary across the country, although these common themes persist (Canadian Institute for Health Information, 2013b):

- An increase in the number (volume) of people requiring services
- A shortage of human health resources
- Limited access to required diagnostic services
- Lack of coordination of services
- Limited access to operating rooms and operating time for surgeons, often because of hospital operating costs (e.g., hospitals may close operating rooms as a cost-saving measure)

Canadians often have to wait to see specialists, have diagnostic tests (especially magnetic resonance imaging [MRI] and computed tomography [CT] scans), or visit a general practitioner for routine medical care. In general, wait times for these services range from 4 to 18 weeks, depending on the location and the service required. Most provinces and territories host Web sites that post the approximate wait for each service and, if long, may suggest seeking help elsewhere.

IMPROVING WAIT TIMES

In 2004, the federal government provided funding ($5 billion) to augment provincial and territorial investments through the Wait Times Reduction Fund. The provinces and territories were to establish "reasonable" guaranteed wait times for the five priority areas (see pages 353-355), following some general guidelines from the federal government. They began by collaborating to produce what they term "benchmark" time frames for guaranteed maximum wait times, which were adjusted throughout the process. For example, since 2012, a wait of no more than four weeks has been considered reasonable for radiation therapy for cancer patients; 182 days for hip and knee replacements, although emergencies such as hip fractures have a maximum wait of 48 hours (Case Example 10.1); and 112 days for cataract surgery for high-risk persons (Canadian Institute for Health Information, 2013b). Cardiac bypass surgery limits range from 2 to 26 weeks, depending on the patient's condition. No national benchmark time frame has been set for either MRI or CT scans, although Alberta, Ontario, and Prince Edward Island have developed their own wait time targets.

Case Example 10.1

John, age 82, is admitted to hospital through Emergency, where he was diagnosed with a hip fracture resulting from a fall. The hospital must complete a hip replacement within a 48-hour time frame. John will be made comfortable until his surgery takes place.

Individual jurisdictions are prioritizing these services according to need and adjusting guaranteed wait times accordingly. After determining the guaranteed wait times, each province and territory must provide patients with alternative treatment options in the case of the wait time guarantee being unmet (Case Example 10.2).

Case Example 10.2

Aisha, who lives in Alberta, has breast cancer. She was guaranteed a wait of no more than eight weeks to begin receiving her radiation treatments. After ten weeks without treatment, the Alberta government sought treatment for her in the United States and covered the cost.

Although some jurisdictions have shown improvement in wait times, the national results for 2013 revealed little progress. In 2012, for example, a record number of surgeries (especially joint replacements and cataract surgeries) were performed, but wait times did not improve significantly (Canadian Institute for Health Information, 2013a). In fact, radiation treatment is the only therapy that surpassed the ten-year target of treating 90% of patients requiring the therapy within a 28-day period. Although the ten-year plan for wait time reduction ended in 2013, provinces and territories continue working toward improving wait time performance.

It must be noted that people experiencing emergency or urgent medical situations are not subject to wait lists. Instead, with triage, they receive care as soon as possible. Across Canada, most Canadians report that when they urgently need care, they get it.

Improving Emergency Department Wait Times

Despite pan-Canadian efforts to improve the wait times in emergency departments, Canada has one of the worst records in terms of ED wait times when compared with 11 other countries (including U.K., Germany, and the Netherlands). In 2011–2012, there were approximately 16.2 million visits to hospital emergency departments across the country. Most were walk-ins (12% of which came by ambulance). In terms of waits, approximately one in ten individuals will wait about eight hours to be seen, with the median wait time currently being just over four hours (Canadian Institute for Health Information, 2012a). One in ten visits in 2011–2012 resulted in admission to hospital, the majority of those with chronic conditions (Canadian Institute for Health Information, 2012a). These patients and others requiring admission appear to wait longest in the ED, likely because of the time it takes to sort out their complex health problem(s) and organize treatment, tasks that also contribute to longer wait times overall.

Other reasons for longer wait times include the volume of visits from people using the ED for nonessential reasons (e.g., a cold, rash, headache), a persisting shortage of family doctors, and a shortage of ED staff. While many Canadians unfortunately view the ED as a reasonable place to seek after-hours health care, **orphan patients** may just not know where else to turn.

Orphan patient
A person without a family doctor.

The inability to access family doctors in a timely manner results in increasing numbers of nonacute cases being seen in the ED. To rectify this, at least in part, many physicians are moving toward a service model that accommodates patients the same day they call. First, however, doctors must clear any backlog of patients.

With the implementation of primary health care reform groups, after-hours access to family doctors has improved across Canada. Most of these groups offer after-hours telephone advice, as well as evening and Saturday clinics. Additionally, all jurisdictions have province- or territory-funded telephone access to health advice.

Physician shortages still result in reduced hours or rotating closure of some EDs, with coverage arranged with neighbouring hospitals. Usually, such situations are reversed as soon as staffing issues are resolved. To ease the problem, many EDs now hire nurse practitioners or physician assistants to see nonurgent cases.

Assessing and triaging patients as soon as they arrive at the ED is one of the most effective measures for reducing ED wait times. A standardized tool, the Canadian Triage and Acuity Scale (CTAS), has increased assessment effectiveness. Patients assessed at I or II on the scale are seen sooner than those assessed at III or IV. Many regions also have smartphone apps that will let a person know how long the wait time is in a particular ED, more evenly distributing patients who need care.

To free up space for those who come into the ED with complex conditions that require extended care, many hospitals have created transitional care beds for ALC patients.

Ontario's Emergency Room Wait Times Strategy sought to find ways to reduce waits. Solutions included offering hospitals dedicated financial incentives to shorten waits and increasing ED staffing. Nova Scotia has developed a program to train advanced-care paramedics to respond to calls in nursing homes, conduct geriatric assessments, and perform designated treatments (e.g., drawing blood and suturing), reducing the need to transfer many of these patients to the ED. A successful program in Alberta, the Emergency to Home: A Seniors Journey to the Right Care, has seniors assessed in the ED by emergency and home care staff, supported by a home care coordinator. When medically able, the patients are discharged to the appropriate community facility or home with the needed support, avoiding the use of ACL beds and reducing the number of individuals waiting in the ED for admission.

You have an extremely sore throat and a bad cough. You think you might need an antibiotic. It is Friday morning, you have plans to go away for the weekend, and you work until 5:00 P.M.—the time that your family doctor's office closes. What would you do?

ABORIGINAL HEALTH CARE

Aboriginal peoples in Canada comprise more than 50 distinct and diverse groups, each with its own language and traditional land base. For the most part, the plight of the Aboriginal population, although serious, makes headlines only when a significant event occurs, such as drinking water contamination on a reserve, a rash of suicides within a community, or a housing crisis. For example, in 2012, the Neskantaga First Nation declared a state of emergency after recording an average of ten suicide attempts per month during that year. Also in 2012, Chief Teresa Spence, who is widely known for her association with the Idle No More movement, thrust Aboriginal people into the spotlight when she went on a hunger strike to bring attention to the need for livable housing on the Attawapiskat First Nations **reserve** (a community north of Timmins, Ontario). The fact is that for many Aboriginal communities, the inequities they endure are ongoing.

Section 35 of the Canadian Constitution recognizes three distinct groups of Aboriginal people: First Nations (formerly known as Indians), the Inuit (formerly known as Eskimos), and Métis. According to the 2011 census, Aboriginal Canadians make up about 4.3% of the total population, a 20% increase over their representation in the 2006 census. Although Aboriginal Canadians can be found in every province and territory, most live in the Western provinces and Ontario.

Aboriginal communities face huge disparities in socioeconomic conditions, profoundly affecting the health and well-being of this population group. In addition, for many communities, the available health care is woefully inadequate, with gaps in both organization and delivery, especially in more remote communities.

The federal government is responsible for providing much of the health care and related funding for Canada's Aboriginal people. Delivering equitable, high-quality health care to these populations, however, presents several challenges. Some of these are addressed in this section along with a number of the most prevalent health-related issues Aboriginal Canadians currently face.

> **Reserve**
> Land set aside by the Crown and designated for the use and occupancy of Aboriginal people.

Status Versus Non-Status Indians

First Nations Canadians were more commonly known as Indians until the early 1980s. Although the term *First Nations* is deemed "politically correct" and widely used, it has no legal standing in Canada. First Nations include both status and non-status Indians.

Status Indians, sometimes referred to as *treaty Indians*, are persons registered in Canada's official record, which identifies all status Indians—requirements and criteria are outlined in the *Indian Act*. The list is administered by Aboriginal Affairs and Northern Development Canada (AANDC). **Non-status Indians** are any First Nations individuals who are not registered with the federal government or are not registered to a band that signed a treaty with the Crown.

Status Indians, as well as Inuit, are eligible for certain programs and services unavailable to non-status Indians. For example, status Indians can apply for

> **Status Indians**
> First Nations people registered in Canada's official record; sometimes referred to as *treaty Indians*.
>
> **Non-Status Indians**
> First Nations individuals who are not registered with the federal government.

postsecondary tuition support (in addition to help with living and travel expenses); on-reserve social programs that mirror provincial programs, such as income assistance and assisted living; and the Non-Insured Health Benefits program, which covers some prescription medication and health services that are not covered provincially. Status Indians are also not taxed on income earned on a reserve and are exempt from paying the goods and services tax on items purchased on a reserve.

Clearly, there are huge benefits to being registered as a status Indian in Canada. Non-status Indians (including the Métis) have battled for years to be recognized under the Constitution as Status Indians (In the News: Métis and Non-Status Indians Seek Recognition as Status Indians).

In the News — Métis and Non-Status Indians Seek Recognition as Status Indians

In 2011, a federal court judge ruled that all Métis and non-status Indians in Canada should be considered as "Indians" under the *Constitution Act* and thus fall under federal jurisdiction. The move would ensure that this sector of the Aboriginal population in Canada was eligible for the same rights, benefits, programs, and services awarded to status Indians under the law. These amenities include access to health care benefits and the rights to sustenance hunting and fishing that status Indians already have.

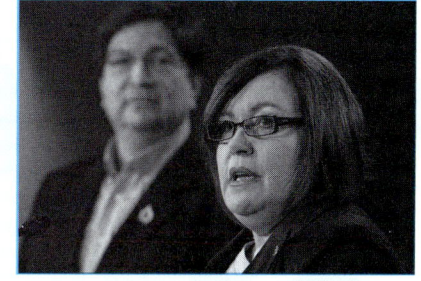

In April 2014, the Supreme Court of Canada upheld the decision in part, ruling that Métis should be recognized as Indians under the Constitution but that recognition to non-status Indians is different and should be decided on a case-by-case basis. The federal government can appeal this decision.

Sources: Roman, K. (2013, October 30). Métis and non-status Indians defend victory in court. *CBC*. Retrieved from http://www.cbc.ca/news/politics/m%C3%A9tis-and-non-status-indians-defend-victory-in-court-1.2287813; Gorman, M. (2013, January 21). 5 Questions: Métis chief hails ruling on status rights. *The Chronicle Herald* [Nova Scotia]. Retrieved from http://thechronicleherald.ca/novascotia/487807-5-questions-metis-chief-hails-ruling-on-status-rights; Canadian Press. (2014, April 17). Court of Appeal upholds landmark ruling on rights of Métis. *CBC*. Retrieved from http://www.cbc.ca/news/aboriginal/court-of-appeal-upholds-landmark-ruling-on-rights-of-m%C3%A9tis-1.2613834.

Photo Credit: The Canadian Press/Adrian Wyld.

THE CHALLENGES

As discussed in Chapter 3, the determinants of health impact the extent to which a person, a community, or a population possesses the requirements to be healthy and productive. Reviewing these determinants will provide insight into the impact they have on the health of many Aboriginal Canadians. Some sources also include as an Aboriginal determinant of health the continuing trauma suffered as a result of compulsory attendance at Indian residential schools and the forced separation from their families and homes (Aboriginal Healing Foundation, 2009; Public Health Agency of Canada, 2012). The effects of these determinants on the physical and mental health of this population are staggering, and an inequity with regard to one determinant leads to inequities in another. For example, unemployment leads to poverty; poverty leads to food insecurity, substandard housing, and overcrowding; related social problems include poor self-esteem, family violence, substance abuse, marginalization, and racism. The effects of these include but are not limited to a higher mortality and morbidity rate resulting from chronic diseases, infections, suicide, substance abuse, sexually transmitted infections (STIs), and teen pregnancies.

Unemployment

According to the 2011 National Household Survey, the overall unemployment rate for Aboriginal people in Canada was 15% (Statistics Canada, 2014). These people had an average annual income of approximately $16,000, which included money from government sources, such as child benefits, employment insurance, social assistance, old-age security benefits, and guaranteed income supplements. In contrast, the average for unemployed non-Aboriginals is $36,000 (Assembly of First Nations, 2011). In remote geographic locations, the unemployment rate can be upwards of 60% or 70%.

In 2011, about 43% of First Nations adults reported that they were unable to provide themselves and their families with basic amenities such as food, shelter (including utilities), and clothing (Assembly of First Nations, 2011). Poverty is a direct result of an inadequate income and affects almost every aspect of the lives and health of those affected.

Education

Schools for Inuit and First Nations people on reserves are the responsibility of the federal government. Many Aboriginal communities have complained about the chronic underfunding related to outdated funding formulas for education. Only 22% of First Nations children have access to preschool programs (Assembly of First Nations, n.d.). For First Nations, the problems are similar both on and off reserves (30% of Aboriginal youth attend provincial schools off reserves). Many on-reserve schools lack fundamental learning tools that schools in more populated regions take for granted, and some are in need of repair. In more remote communities without schools, youths must leave their communities to get any kind of education, a stressor for both the children and their families.

The Assembly of First Nations identified a secondary school graduation rate of just over 35% (Chiefs Assembly on Education, 2012). Off-reserve First Nations had a secondary school completion rate of 72% (42% of Inuit and 77% of Métis aged 18 to 44 had a high school diploma or equivalent in 2012) (Statistics Canada, 2013). That said, some communities boast a graduation rate close to 100%—for example, Membertou First Nation in Nova Scotia (Chiefs Assembly on Education, 2012). Lack of education limits employment opportunities, promotes financial and economic insecurity, and contributes to altered self-esteem and related social problems. To address inequities in education, in 2014, the federal government attempted to introduce a plan to reform First Nations education that met the needs of Aboriginal leaders.

Food Insecurity

Aboriginal households are more likely to experience **food insecurity** than non-Aboriginal households. Traditionally, Aboriginal people ate healthy diets high in animal protein and low in carbohydrates and fat, the sources of which are varied. For a variety of reasons—fear of environmental contamination of traditional food sources, lack of a hunter in the household, and increasingly limited resources—Western food, much of it with poor nutritional value, has largely replaced traditional food in many communities. Access to healthier market foods is restricted by their high cost and limited availability (Socha, Zahaf, Chambers, et al., 2012).

The results of food insecurity and consumption of food with little nutrition include malnutrition, developmental delays, low birth weights, obesity, cardiovascular disease, diabetes, and other chronic diseases.

According to Aboriginal Affairs and Northern Development Canada (2010), in the most isolated communities, a food basket with enough nutritious food for a family of four for one week costs between $360 and $450. The same basket in Southern Ontario costs $200 to $250. The federal program Nutrition North aims to increase the availability of healthy food in northern communities, but the program does not regulate food prices (Peritz, 2014). Various levels of government, however, provide food subsidies to offset the high cost of food in more remote regions, and the federal government has produced a food guide for Aboriginal people to educate them about nutrition. Evolve includes a link to an interactive map illustrating the cost of various food items in some northern communities.

Food insecurity
Poor or no physical or economic access to nutritious foods required to maintain a healthy state.

Housing

Adequate housing and quality housing are important determinants of health and a significant issue for a large proportion of Aboriginal people. Many existing houses are poorly constructed, ill designed to last through harsh conditions, and in need of structural, plumbing, and electrical repairs. Rodents, mould, and mildew add to the problems. In many communities, trailerlike accommodation is the norm, with 12 or more individuals crammed into a small space. Overcrowding promotes infectious diseases (e.g., respiratory diseases, tuberculosis, and hepatitis A, especially in children) as well as violence, stress, and other mental health issues. Often the skills required to make appropriate household repairs, as well as the financial and physical resources to do so, are lacking. The federal government does provide some assistance for on-reserve housing, but the community members usually must meet the costs of housing needs.

Mental Health and Substance Abuse

Substance abuse is an ongoing concern for Canada's Aboriginal people. It is perpetuated by several factors, ranging from socioeconomic problems such as isolation and poverty to the lingering effects of colonization and the residential school era. Traumatized adults who were abused physically, spiritually, emotionally, and sometimes sexually have passed the after-effects of that trauma down to subsequent generations.

Substance abuse often takes the form of overuse of alcohol, cannabis, speed, amphetamines, or solvent inhalants (e.g., glue, gasoline, paint). After cannabis, crack cocaine was the most used drug by Aboriginal people living in urban areas (First Nations Information Governance Centre, 2012).

The most frequently diagnosed mental health conditions are major depression and anxiety disorders. Major depression and feelings of hopelessness are often connected to suicide. While suicide rates for non-Aboriginal Canadians are dropping, the rate among Aboriginals has continued to rise. The suicide rate among Canada's Aboriginal population is two to three times higher than the Canadian average, with youth rates even worse, at five to seven times higher. The suicide rate among Inuit youth is a stunning 11%, with those between the ages of 10 and 29 proving most at risk (Kirmayer, Brass, Holton, et al., 2007).

Chronic Diseases

Sixty-two percent of Aboriginal adults report living with at least one chronic condition, and this rate increases with age. Over half the population over the age of 60 have up to four chronic conditions. Most commonly seen are hypertension, diabetes, arthritis, back pain, and respiratory disorders (e.g., asthma). Related risk factors, especially for diabetes and cardiorespiratory conditions, include a higher incidence of obesity, inactivity, and smoking. The obesity rate for Aboriginal adults is highest for First Nations and Inuit Canadians. The smoking rate for all three Aboriginal groups is twice that of the general population. Risk factors related to second-hand smoke also remain a concern.

Sexual Health and Pregnancies

Among First Nations and Inuit populations, 9% of teenage girls were mothers in 2006; on reserves, 12% of First Nations teenage girls had children. In the same year, about 4% of Métis teenage girls were mothers (O'Donnell & Wallace, 2011).

The incidence of STIs is also higher among this population as compared to non-Aboriginals, with human immunodeficiency virus (HIV) and acquired immune deficiency syndrome (AIDS) on the rise (First Nations Information Governance Centre, 2012). While Aboriginal people make up only about 3.8% of the Canadian population, they represented approximately 12.2% of new HIV cases across the country in 2011. Astoundingly, in Saskatchewan of that year, 81% of all newly diagnosed cases were in Aboriginal Canadians and those of related ethnicity. A significant number of the diagnosed HIV/AIDS cases are caused by drug injection with contaminated needles (Aboriginal Healing Foundation, 2009).

Some reasons cited for the increasing prevalence of STIs among the Aboriginal population include a general lack of knowledge and understanding about STIs, poverty, marginalization, and related social determinants (drug abuse, unprotected intercourse). The federal government is working on several projects with multiple departments including the Public Health Agency of Canada (PHAC), the National Aboriginal Council on HIV/AIDS, and Health Canada—particularly the First Nations and Inuit Health Branch (FNIHB)—to provide evidence-informed solutions to this problem (Aboriginal Healing Foundation, 2009).

Children

Aboriginal children are the fastest-growing segment of the population of all Canadian children, and, as with Aboriginal adults, they bear the burden of more inequities than any other group of Canadian children. They are affected by the same socioeconomic factors that impact the health of their parents—in particular, poverty, poor housing, and poor educational outcomes. Whether living on reserves or off reserves in urban settings, these children are vulnerable. Those off reserves often live in low-income housing. Overcrowded conditions are common both on and off reserves and affect 50% of Aboriginal children as opposed to 21% of non-Aboriginal children (First Nations Information Governance Centre, 2012).

Although improving, infant mortality rates among Aboriginals are three to seven times higher than the national average. Fewer Aboriginal children are properly immunized (the rate is 20% lower than the national average); therefore, Aboriginal children are at risk for contracting diseases that immunizations prevent (e.g., mumps, whooping cough, measles, chicken pox) (First Nations Information Governance Centre, 2012).

Among Aboriginal children, there is a higher rate of childhood obesity, which leads to diabetes, and a higher rate of children born with fetal alcohol spectrum disorder. These children are further affected if exposed to the higher incidence of substance abuse, suicide, and family violence their parents may experience; as they grow older, many abuse substances or suffer from depression or suicide ideation themselves or even take their own lives.

Older Aboriginal Canadians

As an Aboriginal Canadian ages, the risks become more pronounced. Those living in overcrowded, rundown houses are more susceptible to acquiring infectious diseases. And those dilapidated and overcrowded houses are also difficult to adapt to meet the needs of a disabled individual when necessary. In addition, limited finances make renovating a house for someone with a disability unlikely. Those receiving old-age security (OAS) pensions are often financially insecure, in part because they may be the only person in the household with a reliable income and so readily share their resources with others (a core value among the Aboriginal population), meaning that less of that income goes toward their own needs. Those unable to manage independently often have difficulty finding support: home care services are in short supply, particularly in more remote regions.

Many older Aboriginals suffer from emotional and mental issues that stem from colonization, fracturing of their cultural practices, their experiences in residential schools, loss of independence, grief over familial substance abuse, and family violence. A significant number of older Aboriginal Canadians delay seeking medical help because of a deep-rooted mistrust of institutions and Western health care practices and a fear of having to leave their community and loved ones for treatment. Individuals trained to care for older people in Aboriginal communities are limited.

All levels of government are making efforts to close the gaps in health care for older Aboriginal Canadians. For example, the First Nations Health Authority in British Columbia is a not-for-profit corporation working with B.C.'s regional health authorities (RHAs) to ensure that First Nations people—including seniors—will receive equitable care.

Morbidity and Mortality Rates

The life expectancy for Aboriginal Canadians is about four to seven years less on average than that for non-Aboriginal Canadians. Life expectancy for the Inuit population, in particular, is even less—approximately 15 years shorter than the average non-Aboriginal Canadian life expectancy (Canadian Baptists of Western Canada, 2013).

The most common cause of death for Aboriginal people between the ages of 1 and 44 is injuries—up to four times the national average. These include fires and motor vehicle collisions (including those involving ATVs and snowmobiles). Heart disease is the second leading cause of death, followed by cancer (First Nations Information Governance Centre, 2012).

Morbidity rates from cancer for Aboriginals are higher than in the general population. One contributing factor is that Aboriginals are, on average, diagnosed later, according to the Assembly of First Nations (2009). A compounding factor is that access to screening procedures for the Aboriginal population lags behind that for non-Aboriginals.

Systems of Health Care Delivery for Aboriginals

Health Canada and its First Nations and Inuit Health Branch assume most of the responsibilities for the health care of Aboriginal peoples, with intervention and additional services provided by other designated organizations and stakeholders, including provincial, territorial, and municipal governments and the PHAC. Unfortunately, a disruption of services can occur frequently because of a lack of both coordination and communication among the varying levels of governments, agencies, and other stakeholders.

There is yet to be a consensus on the best approach to delivering health care in an effective and culturally sensitive manner. Many feel that health care would be best controlled and managed locally, by bands in communities or on reservations. Depending on local and provincial or territorial agreements, some Aboriginal groups have the option of withdrawing from government control over their health matters and managing their own health care programs. Many communities have taken on this responsibility, with varying degrees of success. The concept bears a resemblance to regional health authorities (or their counterparts), which were founded on the belief that the people within a given community best understand the health care services required in that community. As well, individuals from the community can better motivate and direct fellow members of the community to accept help, adopt balanced lifestyles, and participate in disease prevention and health promotion.

Access

It must be noted that Aboriginal Canadians are eligible to access the same health care services as any other Canadian. Therefore, in an urban setting, or in a rural setting close to hospitals and clinics, access and universality are usually not a significant problem.

These two principles—access and universality—pose the greatest challenges for those living in more remote communities, especially in fly-in (no road access) regions. Almost all of these communities have nursing stations, small clinics, or hospitals with a limited number of beds. Those with roads to larger centres also have ambulance services, albeit sometimes limited. Nursing stations typically have one or two examination rooms, a treatment room, and two or three beds in case a patient requires a short-term stay or must wait for air ambulance transport to a larger centre. Although nursing stations and clinics tend to be well equipped by most standards, the extent of care provided is limited to less serious conditions and trauma cases.

All too often, individuals with serious trauma or more complex conditions or even those needing palliative care, screening procedures, specialists' visits, or delivery of babies must leave their community for treatment. Patients are transported by air ambulance to the closest facility that can meet their medical needs, usually without a choice of where they are sent.

These health care facilities are primarily staffed by registered and practical nurses, nurse practitioners, paramedics, or a combination of these professionals. Larger centres (and "larger" is a comparative term here) do have a limited number of doctors, usually general practitioners, who will visit neighbouring communities on a rotation or as-needed basis. Retaining medical and nursing staff is a challenge, however, and the turnover is high. Besides factors related to living in an isolated area, health care providers who remain also lack access to further training and professional development, although this situation is improving with electronic access to learning opportunities. Provincial and territorial governments offer financial and tax incentives to practitioners who work in northern regions.

Specialists from larger centres visit designated communities regularly, primarily those with hospitals or clinics where diagnostic equipment is available. Treatment, support, and consultations are also provided through video conferencing.

For individuals who have to be medevaced out, the process can be traumatic. Leaving one's community is difficult for any individual, but it is especially so when the evacuee has to leave family members and other support systems behind, particularly when facing an unknown health crisis. Some jurisdictions will provide funding for one support person—a friend or family member—to accompany a patient.

Western Versus Traditional Healing Practices

Another concern among many Aboriginals is the disparity between Western and traditional healing practices. For the most part, Aboriginal Canadians receive health care based on Western medical beliefs, practices, and procedures. However, a number of health centres, although serving a general population, now focus on the needs of Aboriginal people and incorporate traditional healing practices into their programs (Box 10.1).

Box 10.1 The Sioux Lookout Meno Ya Win Health Centre

Andaaw'iwewin egkwa Mushkiki (Traditional Healing Practices and Medicines) is a culturally sensitive program that incorporates traditional practices, principles, and spiritual healing ceremonies that usually take place in a specially designed ceremonial room and include vigils, smudging, and healing circles. The room has an open firepit with circular seating. Ya Win Health Centre has a roster of traditional practitioners who are available to patients requiring their services. These practitioners must go through a process of certification administered by a traditional practitioners committee. In addition, Aboriginal hospital patients can choose to be served traditional meals (game and fish) that are exempt from the inspection policies imposed on other food.

The hospital's diagnostic services include fluoroscopy, ultrasound, digital mammography, and CT scans. Attached to the health centre is an extended care facility and a medical withdrawal unit to treat patients withdrawing from drug and alcohol addiction.

Sources: Sioux Lookout Meno Ya Win Health Centre. (n.d.). Retrieved from http://www.slmhc.on.ca/; Ontario Nursing Jobs. (2010). Sioux Lookout Meno Ya Win Health Centre. Retrieved from http://ontarionursing.ca/featured-employer-401.html.

Many jurisdictions have introduced university programs geared toward graduate Native health care providers who will be more likely to work in northern communities and deliver health care that is sensitive to Aboriginal health practices, such as spiritual healing. Alberta was the first province to make recruiting Aboriginal students a priority. The University of British Columbia's Native physician program has set a target to graduate 50 physicians by 2020. Evidence suggests that Aboriginal people are more likely to follow the advice of an Aboriginal health care provider, resulting in better health outcomes.

In 2013, between 200 and 250 First Nations, Inuit, and Métis (FNIM) physicians were actively practising, but it is estimated that ten times that number are required to meet the health care needs of Canada's Aboriginal population (Lorenz, 2013). As part of the strategy to increase the numbers of Aboriginals in health care fields, the Indigenous Physicians Association of Canada (IPAC) and the Association of Faculties of Medicine of Canada (AFMC), in particular, have been working with Aboriginals to suggest careers in health care to Aboriginal youth. As well, training opportunities in all aspects of health care must be made more geographically accessible, a barrier that can be overcome through distance education, video conferencing, and the Internet. Such educational opportunities require the flexible financial support of federal, provincial, and territorial governments. In 2011, the federal government provided Nunavut with $4.9 million to support up to eight new family medicine residents in collaboration with

Memorial University's Faculty of Medicine in Newfoundland and Labrador. This investment also targeted the establishment of a family practice training centre in the Qikiqtani General Hospital in Iqaluit (Newfoundland and Labrador Medical Association, 2011).

The Indigenous Physicians Association of Canada and the Association of Faculties of Medicine of Canada are currently collaborating to introduce to universities programs that specifically address Aboriginal health concerns. In 2008, the groups launched the First Nations, Inuit, and Métis Health Core Competencies, a curriculum framework for undergraduate medical education. As well, the National Aboriginal Health Organization (NAHO), funded by Health Canada, implements strategies to improve the health of the people it represents through such activities as research, education, and the promotion of culturally relevant approaches to health care (Indigenous Physicians Association of Canada & Association of Faculties of Medicine of Canada, 2008).

STRATEGIES FOR IMPROVEMENT

Many stakeholders believe that the First Nations health care system has to become more integrated with provincial systems in order to deliver care that is comprehensive, patient-centred, and cost-effective. Some degree of integration would minimize duplication of services, gaps in services, and costly oversights.

The federal, provincial, territorial, and local governments have jointly initiated strategies to improve housing, sanitation, and access to prenatal care, as well as facilities and counselling to deal with substance abuse—but with limited success. All levels of government are working with Aboriginal leaders and communities to address issues affecting individual and regional inequities. More recently, stakeholders have collaboratively adopted a population health approach to better address the needs of each community. The first step has been to draft a tool for gathering essential health information, which will contribute to designing health care reforms. For this approach to prove successful, health care providers must show sensitivity to the needs of the population and consider the unique lifestyle, beliefs, culture, and traditions of Aboriginal peoples.

As well, Aboriginals themselves must be involved at all levels of health care—from identifying health problems to participating in solutions for appropriate care. It is well recognized that no short-term solution exists for Aboriginal health issues. To bring about progress, Aboriginals must, with the assistance and support of all Canadians, find a balance between a healthy and prosperous lifestyle and their culture, traditions, and way of life. As well, the independence and dignity of Aboriginal peoples must be restored and honoured.

The broader challenges are complex. At the forefront are a multilayered and multifaceted health care system managed by multiple partners and levels of government; a lack of trust, understanding, and vision among stakeholders; cultural complexities; resource limitations (financial and physical); and the length of time it takes to implement change. Progress will require a sound commitment from all stakeholders and a willingness to build trust, maintain open minds, and employ innovative thinking to meet the challenges.

This section on Aboriginal health is far from inclusive (for further information, see *The Health Status of Canada's First Nations, Métis and Inuit Peoples* on Evolve). It must be stressed that jurisdictions vary greatly with respect to the needs of the Aboriginal populations and the quantity and quality of health care available. The provinces and territories continue to develop partnerships, strategies, and programs to address shortfalls in delivering health care to Canada's Aboriginal population wherever they live—in cities, rural areas, or in more remote communities.

INFORMATION TECHNOLOGY AND ELECTRONIC HEALTH RECORDS

The electronic exchange of information has expanded enormously in the past decade, with computerization changing the face of health care, business, and industry worldwide. Yet the Canadian health care system has lagged behind technological advances, despite the high volume of health information created, accessed, and exchanged on a daily basis in medical offices and facilities across the country.

Connectivity in health care benefits both health care providers and patients. Digitalization offers all health care providers endless options, including the opportunity to view the charts, X-rays, scans, and test results of hospitalized and office patients from their home or office and the ability to fax and digitally share documents via computers, speeding up the process of information exchange, limiting the risk for misplaced documents, and reducing the carbon footprint.

Sending prescriptions electronically is now the norm rather than the exception. E-prescriptions reduce errors from illegible handwriting and store a patient's pharmacological history, allowing the pharmacist at any point-of-service to monitor the patient's medications to reduce harmful drug-to-drug reactions and prescription abuse.

Current Canada Health Infoway projects include expanding and improving the use of digitized diagnostic imaging and patient self-monitoring systems (e.g., for patients with diabetes or hypertension), expanding drug and laboratory information systems, and continuing development and use of the **interoperable EHR** program. (See Web Resources on Evolve for a link to a

Interoperable EHR
Connected electronic systems that will enable authorized health care providers to view and, in some cases, update a patient's essential health information.

graphic representation of how interoperable EHRs work.) In 2012, the CIHI implemented across all jurisdictions a peer-to-peer program that had physicians who are technologically educated and practising in highly computerized environments providing related support and educational resources (e.g., videos and supporting documents) to those who require it. The focus is on promoting the benefits of electronics in improving interdisciplinary collaborative care. Each province and territory has an organization that supports the implementation of electronic health records (EHRs) within its jurisdiction (i.e., provides direction and sometimes funding).

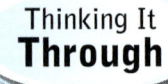

Mercedes, a 32-year-old New Brunswick resident, was brought into the emergency department at the Foot Hills Medical Centre in Calgary. She had been hit by a car and sustained a serious and painful leg injury. By the time Mercedes was seen in the ED, she was semiconscious and incoherent—a condition not congruent with her injury. The nurses located her provincial health card in her wallet and accessed her EHR, which revealed she was diabetic and allergic to codeine.

1. What information do you think was most important for the physician to have?

2. What possible problems might have occurred if the doctor did not have access to Mercedes's EHR?

Hospitals

Most hospitals in Canada either fully or partially use electronic systems. Laboratory and diagnostic tests are now ordered electronically. Patient charts, though primarily computerized, usually retain some hard-copy components (e.g., handwritten physicians' orders in patients' charts, progress notes, medication administration records, consent forms).

There is wide variation regarding which documents created in hospitals are allowed to be electronically sent to physicians' offices and other points of care. For example, in Ontario, Ontario MD has initiated the Hospital Report Manager, which can electronically send patients' hospital reports to the physician's office within 30 minutes of the report's being generated.

Doctors

Significantly more Canadian doctors have converted to electronic medical records (EMRs) over the past three years, up from 39% in 2010 to 62% in 2013

(National Physician Survey, 2013). The majority of these physicians do not practise in a fully electronic environment but use a mix of paper and electronic charts. EMRs have proven to vastly increase the efficiency or productivity of a medical practice, although initial acquisition of an electronic system is tedious and costly (between $30,000 and $40,000). Some 28% of Alberta's doctors are using EMR systems (the highest in the country); Ontario is next with 20%; and B.C. with 19%. The number of physicians using EMRs still lag behind that of the United Kingdom, where 89% of primary care physicians are considered "electronic," and the United States, which has a 28% usage rate (National Physician Survey, 2013). Although virtually all physicians are using computers for scheduling appointments, advances in software are now offering self-scheduling programs (used by just under 10% of primary care practitioners). Click4Time is a self-scheduling system that is growing in popularity and has won awards sponsored by the CIHI for its online appointment and resource booking system.

Fewer than 20% of all Canadian physicians have a practice website, offering patients access to their health information through secure portals. The patient can review their medication profile, lab and diagnostic test results, and immunization history, among other things. Some portals allow the patient to exchange secure e-mail with the health care team, change contact information, request prescription refills, and access educational materials.

The major laboratories in Canada now offer websites where patients can book appointments for lab tests online, making the process easier and more convenient for both physicians' offices and patients. Shortly after results are processed, most labs return them electronically to the physician. In 2012, Shoppers Drug Mart Corporation created Health Care Portal, designed to provide selected Canadian health care providers (e.g., doctors, nurse practitioners) with access to drug reimbursement information and other clinical tools (health information, handouts about selected conditions).

In underserviced areas, physicians are using secure e-mail and video conferencing to connect to patients, particularly in Canada's north. Even in urban settings, video conferencing is being used (see Case Example 10.3).

Case Example 10.3

Marc was diagnosed with cancer. He wanted a second opinion and insisted on one from a doctor he knew from the Mayo Clinic in the United States. A video consultation was arranged after the relevant diagnostic information was electronically sent to the specialist.

SECURITY AND EHRs

The security of electronic health information remains an uncertainty. Canadians have questions: Who is ultimately responsible for managing the information in an EHR? What is the proper protocol for obtaining patient consent to access the information? What measures are necessary to ensure that unauthorized persons do not have access? With multiple contributors to the EHR, how reliable is the information?

Jurisdictions are approaching the issue of consent differently. Where EHRs are used, strict access protocols are in place. In Alberta, for example, an authorized user who needs to access a patient's EHR must follow a strict procedure, logging in through two or more levels of authentication.

ADVANTAGES OF ELECTRONIC CHARTS

The pan-Canadian establishment of EHRs and EMRs will:

- Allow family doctors' offices to connect with specialists' offices, determine appointment availability, and choose the shortest wait time and most suitable appointment while the patient is still in the office
- Facilitate the prompt delivery of laboratory tests to a family doctor, hospital, specialist, or other health care provider, allowing physicians to adjust medications or order more blood work in a timely manner
- Enable patients to access their medical records through an electronic portal, allowing them to view lab reports and physician updates and to participate in their own health care management as directed by health care providers
- Improve access to home care facilities and services by using an integrated approach to prioritizing and organizing required care and by managing elements of medical treatment assisted by electronic information exchange
- Facilitate a drug information system that will allow a health care provider to view a patient's medications (e.g., in an ED, an attending physician or nurse can immediately access the drug profile of a recently admitted patient and provide prompt and more effective treatment while also avoiding drug-to-drug interactions, adverse effects, and overdoses)
- Enable implementation of public health tracking systems that will allow prompt identification of individuals who may have had contact with someone with an infectious disease, facilitating timely exchange of advice to those involved and the implementation of appropriate containment strategies, if appropriate (British Columbia is leading Canada in this area of electronic development)

CHALLENGES FOR EHR SUSTAINABILITY

The goal of providing Canada with a workable and nationwide system is ambitious. The initiative will require the following:

- Continued commitment of all stakeholders to share in the vision and embrace the technology
- Collaborative efforts by all levels of government and health care organizations
- Continual responsible financing for provincial and territorial initiatives, including funds to encourage all stakeholders to go electronic
- A public that trusts that their health information will be managed respectfully and securely
- Foolproof tracking and security systems that can identify who accesses what information in case of security breaches, and laws that specifically address privacy violations
- Computer software programs that message each other without connectivity difficulties
- Support systems at the federal, provincial, territorial, and municipal levels that work together to ensure seamless information exchange
- A uniform vocabulary of technical language to increase the effectiveness of system use
- Clearly defined laws governing the use and exchange of health information across provincial and territorial boundaries, including specific guidelines to clarify who bears responsibility for the information and what fees are charged for services provided

Connectivity to various points of care including physicians' offices, clinics, EDs, and pharmacies is one of the major obstacles of successfully implementing a pan-Canadian EHR system. Electronic systems must be capable of networking with local as well as provincial or territorial systems. Few jurisdictions have standardized options, so compatibility with other systems is also a concern.

Government funding to establish integrated EHR systems is limited in most provinces and territories, and some jurisdictions provide more funding than others and, therefore, are moving ahead more rapidly with system implementations. (See Evolve for a link to information about provincial EMR programs.) Computerization and EHRs will eventually exist across the country, and health care providers in all disciplines will ultimately have no choice but to join the movement. However, determining a definitive timeline to reach the goal of a fully electronic health care system is impossible. In fact, it may never be completely achieved. Hybrid systems (a mix of electronic and paper) will probably always co-exist with completely electronic environments.

THE FUTURE OF PRIMARY HEALTH CARE

The current trend toward community-based health care and the collaboration of health care groups to offer that care will continue. As discussed in Chapter 9, this team approach to health care embraces the objective of offering *all* Canadians timely access to primary health care services while trying to contain the soaring costs of delivering care. Health care teams are becoming more collaborative and interdisciplinary, providing numerous points of entry to care. More recently, population health studies are profiling the composition and needs of communities (proportion of older adults, prevalence of chronic diseases, life expectancy, percentage of people who are obese, needs of visible minorities, income, level of education) to create a tailored approach to health care. Consider chronic diseases: primary care providers in high-prevalence areas would aim to reduce the frequency and intensity of chronic diseases within the population, improve health outcomes, and reduce the cost of overall care by applying strategies for health promotion and disease prevention. Areas with a higher demographic of older Canadians might increase the emphasis on home care and community services to achieve better value for the health care dollar and better health outcomes for the patients.

Alternative health care providers are becoming a critical part of interdisciplinary teams, balancing a holistic lifestyle and treatments with the medical model of care. The focus on preventive care will become more clearly defined and efficiently implemented—for example, ensuring that, as recommended by current evidence-informed research, patients have access to mammograms, colorectal screening, immunizations, and Pap smears as appropriate. Increasing the use of the interdisciplinary team approach will improve patients' access to and quality of care as illustrated in Case Example 10.4.

Case Example 10.4

At the beginning of the chapter, you learned about Merle, who suffers from congestive heart failure, hypertension, diabetes, osteoarthritis, and chronic pain. Merle also wears glasses and must see an optometrist regularly because she has declining vision. Instead of relying on her family doctor to treat all of her medical problems, Merle would benefit from a team approach in the following ways:

- The dietitian could help monitor her blood sugar levels and provide diet counselling.

- The nurse practitioner could manage a significant portion of Merle's medical complaints, including, for example, her arthritis pain and hypertension.

- The nurse practitioner could also work with the dietitian to better regulate Merle's blood sugar levels, suggesting Merle visit her family doctor or referring her to a specialist if necessary.

- The optometrist can assess her vision at regular intervals, referring her to an ophthalmologist if the need arises.

- If Merle wishes to see a chiropractor, an acupuncturist, a massage therapist, or another alternative health care provider for pain control, for example, she can discuss the matter with her nurse practitioner or physician, a referral can be made, and Merle may be able to reduce the amount of pain medication she takes.

Through the health care team approach, a wider population base can access effective, high-quality health care from a variety of health care providers. The responsibility for keeping Merle as healthy as possible is more effectively distributed to individuals who have knowledge in specific areas.

THE FINANCIAL SUSTAINABILITY OF HEALTH CARE IN CANADA

The costs of our universal health care system are soaring, and the sustainability of the health care system is questionable. Containing costs is critical if Canadians are to continue to enjoy universal health care. Over the years, provinces, territories, and even individual communities have tried various methods to deliver quality health care in a cost-effective manner. Some strategies work; others don't. With mounting pressure on provinces and territories to contain costs while delivering quality health care, a business and manufacturing strategy known as *lean* has gained popularity in health care. Lean is a customer-oriented set of principles to achieve optimum productivity in a cost-effective manner. The strategy includes identifying wasteful and unproductive practices, services, and policies and eliminating them, adding value to the end product. The lean principles are now being used in hospitals, clinics, practice settings, and diagnostic facilities. Most jurisdictions are implementing or experimenting with lean to some degree. Saskatchewan, for example, uses it across the system; Alberta initially used it at the Tom Baker Cancer Centre to shorten wait times for radiation treatments; and British Columbia uses it in its health authorities. In 2011–2012, Manitoba adopted a province-wide five-year lean training and mentoring strategy for the province's RHAs and other stakeholders.

In health care, the customer is anyone who benefits from the lean strategy—patients and health care workers alike. Examples of nonvalued or wasteful entities in health care are long waits, inefficient use of the health care provider's time, duplicate or unnecessary tests, and the filling out of multiple forms with the same basic information. Waste can relate to the layout of a facility—poor planning and design impeding efficient patient flow, inefficient use of hospital beds, disorganization within a hospital unit (e.g., nurses wasting time searching for items they need), ineffective policies and policies not followed (e.g., noncompliance with infection control procedures), and inefficient use of operating rooms. Lean can also be applied to the realms of medical mistakes and hospital inefficiencies leading to errors in treatment and compromised patient safety and treatment outcomes.

The idea of lean is that a facility or service can be more efficient with less. For example, the answer for long waits in the ED is not to hire more staff and enlarge the department but to redirect resources, eliminate wasteful practices, re-evaluate policies, and implement value-added strategies. The lean strategy takes time to implement and requires skill and well-trained leaders to guide the process of conversion.

SUMMARY

10.1 Despite the implementation of strategies to address the issues of care of those with mental illness, problems remain. Mood disorders and substance and alcohol abuse are among the most common mental health disorders. Ensuring appropriate and timely treatment (including inside correctional facilities), reducing the stigma of mental illness, and addressing challenges such as suicide and homelessness remain priorities.

10.2 Older Canadians make up a significant proportion of the population. With advances in technology and the use of more effective medications, many are living longer but with one or more chronic conditions that require ongoing medical care. The cost to the health care system is a concern. Effectively adapting health care to meet the needs of an aging population while controlling costs remains a challenge.

10.3 Although the situation has improved greatly over the past five years, the shortage of human health resources across the country still affects every level and type of health care. Restructuring the way care is given and effectively using interdisciplinary teams have improved access for many Canadians to primary care professionals. The introduction of new levels of health care practitioners (e.g., physician assistant, nurse practitioners) and a redefinition of the roles of others have also proven effective.

10.4 There is an increased emphasis on caring for individuals in their homes rather than in hospitals, which prefer early discharge, or in long-term care facilities when patients can remain at home with some support. However, providing enough care is a challenge, in part because of a shortage of trained workers (e.g., personal support workers) and funding shortfalls.

10.5 Canada does not have a national drug plan. Provinces and territories do provide some coverage for Canadians over age 65 and for vulnerable groups (usually income related). Nevertheless, an overwhelming number of Canadians cannot afford prescription drugs.

10.6 In 2004, the first ministers met to address the issue of long waits for Canadians to access some health care services, including cancer treatment, cardiac care, diagnostic imaging, joint replacement, and cataract surgery. Although some progress has been made, in 2013, wait times in many areas were still unacceptably long. An increase in the volume of people seeking services is partly responsible.

10.7 Aboriginal Canadians face inequities not experienced by other Canadians. Largely reflected in the determinants of health, these include unemployment, poor living conditions, poverty, marginalization, and fragmented health care.

10.8 The implementation of electronic health records—a measure expected to improve health care at all levels—is currently under way in Canada.

10.9 Cost containment is a necessary reality if Canada's health care system is to survive. Applications such as the lean strategy are being implemented in health care facilities across the country.

Review Questions

1. Briefly identify three factors that affect a person's mental health.
2. What major challenges do we face in providing health care to Canada's increasing aging population?
3. Describe the reasons a shortage of regulated nurses may exist in one region and not another.
4. How is the government encouraging an increase in available home care services?
5. Why do some Canadians have no drug coverage?
6. Explain some of the major reasons behind unreasonable wait times for medical care.
7. Outline four areas in which the health of Aboriginal Canadians falls below national standards.
8. Discuss three benefits of the use of electronic health records.
9. What is the main focus of the lean strategy?

References

Aboriginal Affairs and Northern Development Canada. (2010, September 15). *Revised northern food basket—Highlights of price survey results for 2006, 2007 and 2008*. Retrieved from http://www.aadnc-aandc.gc.ca/eng/1100100035983/1100100035984.

Aboriginal Healing Foundation. (2009). *Residential schools, prisons, and HIV/AIDS among Aboriginal people in Canada: Exploring the connections*. Retrieved from http://www.ahf.ca/downloads/hivaids-report.pdf.

Assembly of First Nations. (n.d.). *A portrait of First Nations and education*. Retrieved from http://www.afn.ca/uploads/files/1_-_fact_sheet_-_a_portrait_of_first_nations_and_education.pdf.

Assembly of First Nations. (2009, July). *Access to cancer screening and First Nations*. Retrieved from http://64.26.129.156/cmslib/general/AFN%20Cancer%20Screening%20Review-final-ENG.pdf.

References

Assembly of First Nations. (2011, June). *Fact sheet: Quality of life of First Nations*. Retrieved from http://www.afn.ca/uploads/files/factsheets/quality_of_life_final_fe.pdf.

Canadian Baptists of Western Canada. (2013, May). *Fact sheet: Aboriginal people in Canada*. Retrieved from http://cbwc.ca/wp-content/uploads/2013/05/Fact-Sheet-Aboriginal-People.pdf.

Canadian Home Care Association. (2013, April 4). The picture is clear—Demand for home care in Canada exceeding resources. *CNW Group*. Retrieved from http://www.newswire.ca/en/story/1140439/the-picture-is-clear-demand-for-home-care-in-canada-exceeding-resources.

Canadian Institute for Health Information. (2011). *Health care in Canada, 2011: A focus on seniors and aging*. Ottawa: Author. Retrieved from https://secure.cihi.ca/free_products/HCIC_2011_seniors_report_en.pdf.

Canadian Institute for Health Information. (2012a). *Health care in Canada, 2012: A focus on wait times*. Ottawa: Author. Retrieved from https://secure.cihi.ca/free_products/HCIC2012-FullReport-ENweb.pdf.

Canadian Institute for Health Information. (2012b). *Regulated nurses: Canadian trends, 2007 to 2011*. Retrieved from https://secure.cihi.ca/free_products/Regulated_Nurses_EN.pdf.

Canadian Institute for Health Information. (2012c, November). *Seniors and alternate level of care: Building on our knowledge*. Retrieved from https://secure.cihi.ca/free_products/ALC_AIB_EN.pdf.

Canadian Institute for Health Information. (2013a, March 19). *More patients getting surgery, but wait times not improving*. Retrieved from http://www.cihi.ca/cihi-ext-portal/internet/en/document/health+system+performance/access+and+wait+times/release_19mar13.

Canadian Institute for Health Information. (2013b, February). *Wait times for priority procedures in Canada, 2013*. Retrieved from https://secure.cihi.ca/free_products/wait_times_2013_en.pdf.

Canadian Institutes of Health Research. (2013). *Safety at home: A pan-Canadian home care study 2013*. Retrieved from http://www.cihr-irsc.gc.ca/e/47023.html.

Canadian Mental Health Association. (n.d.). *Fast facts about mental illness*. Retrieved from http://www.cmha.ca/media/fast-facts-about-mental-illness/.

CBC News. (n.d.). *Inside a nurse's world: Where stress is status quo*. Retrieved from http://www.cbc.ca/news2/health/features/ratemyhospital/nurse-survey-results/.

Chiefs Assembly on Education. (2012, October 1–3). *A portrait of First Nations and education*. Gatineau, Quebec: Palais des Congrès de Gatineau. Retrieved from http://www.statcan.gc.ca/daily-quotidien/131125/dq131125b-eng.htm.

First Nations Information Governance Centre. (2012). *First Nations regional health survey. Phase 2 (2008/10): National report on adults, youth and children living in First Nations communities*. Retrieved from http://fnigc.ca/sites/default/files/First_Nations_Regional_Health_Survey_2008-10_National_Report.pdf.

Gaetz, S., Donaldson, J., Richter, T., et al. (2013). *The state of homelessness in Canada 2013*. Toronto: Canadian Homelessness Research Network Press. Retrieved from http://www.homelesshub.ca/SOHC2013.

Hogan, D. B., Borrie, M., Basran, J. F. S., et al. (2012, September 20). *Specialist physicians in geriatrics—Report of the Canadian Geriatrics Society Physician Resource Work Group*. doi:10.5770/cgi.15.41.

Indigenous Physicians Association of Canada & Association of Faculties of Medicine of Canada. (2008). *First Nations, Inuit, Métis health core competencies: A curriculum framework for undergraduate medical education*. Retrieved from http://www.afmc.ca/pdf/CoreCompetenciesEng.pdf.

Kirmayer, L. J., Brass, G. M., Holton, T., et al. (2007). Suicide among Aboriginal people in Canada. *Aboriginal Healing Foundation*. Retrieved from http://www.ahf.ca/downloads/suicide.pdf.

Lopez-Pacheco. (2013, February 5). Mental illness adversely affecting Canada's economic potential. *Financial Post*. Retrieved from http://business.financialpost.com/2013/02/05/the-economic-cost-of-mental-illness/.

References

Lorenz, D. (2013, February 12). Medical school application information for Aboriginal students. *TalentEgg.ca.* Retrieved from http://talentegg.ca/incubator/2013/02/12/medical-school-application-information-aboriginal-applicants/#sthash.mULAh6S9.dpuf.

Mental Health Commission of Canada. (n.d.a). *Making the case for investing in mental health in Canada.* Retrieved from http://www.mentalhealthcommission.ca/English/system/files/private/document/Investing_in_Mental_Health_FINAL_Version_ENG.pdf

Mental Health Commission of Canada. (n.d.b). *Opening minds.* Retrieved http://www.mentalhealthcommission.ca/English/initiatives-and-projects/opening-minds.

Mental Health Commission of Canada. (2012). *The facts.* Retrieved from http://strategy.mentalhealthcommission.ca/the-facts/.

Munn-Rivard, L. (2014, February 14). *Current issues in mental health in Canada: Homelessness and access to housing.* Ottawa: Library of Parliament. Retrieved from http://www.parl.gc.ca/Content/LOP/ResearchPublications/2014-11-e.htm.

National Physician Survey. (2013). *2013 national physician survey.* Retrieved from http://nationalphysiciansurvey.ca/surveys/2013-survey/.

Newfoundland and Labrador Medical Association. (2011). Federal funding expands family medicine residency program. *Nexus Online.* Retrieved from http://www.nlma.nl.ca/nexus/issues/spring_2011/articles/article_14.html.

O'Donnell, V., & Wallace, S. (2011, July). *Women in Canada: A gender-based statistical report: First Nations, Métis and Inuit women.* Ottawa: Statistics Canada. Retrieved from http://www.statcan.gc.ca/pub/89-503-x/2010001/article/11442-eng.htm#a14.

Office of the Correctional Investigator. (2013). *Annual report of the Office of the Correctional Investigator 2012–2013.* Retrieved from http://www.oci-bec.gc.ca/cnt/rpt/annrpt/annrpt20122013-eng.aspx.

Peritz, I. (2014, January 18). Speaking out against $600-a-week grocery bills. *The Globe and Mail.* Retrieved from http://www.theglobeandmail.com/news/national/the-north/why-is-food-so-expensive-in-nunavut-shop-for-yourself-and-find-out/article15915054/.

Public Health Agency of Canada. (2011, December 16). *The facts: Seniors and injury in Canada.* Retrieved from http://www.phac-aspc.gc.ca/seniors-aines/publications/public/injury-blessure/safelive-securite/chap2-eng.php.

Public Health Agency of Canada. (2012). *Fact sheet: Aboriginal peoples.* Retrieved from http://www.phac-aspc.gc.ca/aids-sida/pr/sec6-eng.php.

Schwartz, D. (2010, December 31). Will a retirement boom start in 2011? *CBC.* Retrieved from http://www.cbc.ca/news/canada/will-a-retirement-boom-start-in-2011-1.928398.

Scott, V., Wagar, L., & Elliott, S. (2010). *Falls & related injuries among older Canadians: Fall-related hospitalizations & intervention initiatives, p. 3.* Public Health Agency of Canada. Retrieved from http://www.hiphealth.ca/media/research_cem-fia_phac_epi_and_inventor_20100610.pdf.

Socha, T., Zahaf, M., Chambers, L., et al. (2012, March). Food security in a northern First Nations community: An exploratory study on food availability and accessibility. *Journal of Aboriginal Health, 8*(2), 5–14. Retrieved from http://www.naho.ca/jah/english/jah08_02/volume08_issue02.pdf.

Statistics, Canada (2013). *The education and employment experiences of First Nations people living off reserve, Inuit, and Métis: Selected findings from the 2012 Aboriginal peoples survey.* Retrieved from http://www.statcan.gc.ca/daily-quotidien/131125/dq131125b-eng.htm.

Statistics, Canada (2014). *National household survey.* Retrieved from http://www.statcan.gc.ca/eng/survey/household/5178.

World Health Organization. (2001). *Mental health: A call for action by world health ministers.* Geneva, Switzerland: Author. Retrieved from http://www.who.int/mental_health/advocacy/en/Call_for_Action_MoH_Intro.pdf.

Glossary

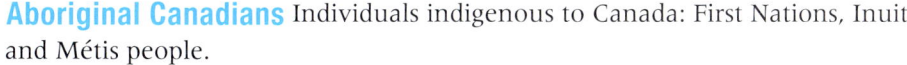

Aboriginal Canadians Individuals indigenous to Canada: First Nations, Inuit, and Métis people.

Accredited program A program that meets standards requisite for its graduates; usually, the standards are set by the profession's governing body, which may be national or provincial or territorial.

Act A usually comprehensive body of laws passed by Parliament or a provincial or territorial legislature.

Active euthanasia The taking of deliberate steps to end a dying person's life.

Active ingredients Those ingredients in a drug that have therapeutic value meant to cure, palliate, or otherwise treat a health problem.

Advance directive A legal document that specifies the nature and level of treatment a person would want to receive in the event of later being unable to make those decisions. Also called a *living will* or *treatment directive*.

Affiliating body An association that provides, among other things, direction, support, continuing education, and networking opportunities for its professional members (who may be regulated or nonregulated).

Age of majority The age at which a person is considered an adult; depending on the province or territory, age 18 or 19.

Allied health professional A health care provider other than a doctor, nurse, or, according to some sources, pharmacist or dentist who provides supportive health care, including direct patient care, technical care, therapeutic care, and support services.

Alternate levels of care (ALC) Inpatient care in a facility or part of a facility in which the level of care provided meets the physical, mental, and emotional needs of the patient.

Aseptic technique A procedure performed under sterile conditions to reduce the risk of infection.

Assisted suicide A person assists another who wishes to end his or her life but is unable to do so independently.

Autonomy The right to self-determination.

Beneficence The act of doing good or being kind.

Best practices Guidelines outlining treatments, procedures, or policies deemed to be most effective.

Block transfer One payment from the federal to the provincial and territorial governments to cover all services.

Branch A division of a main office offering extended or supportive functions.

Bureau Government department responsible for a specific entity or duty.

Canada Health Act Legislation passed in 1984 that governs and guides the delivery of equal, prepaid, and accessible health care to Canadians.

Capitation-based funding A funding formula to pay physicians who participate in some type of primary health care reform group. The doctor receives a set amount (determined by the age and health status of each patient) for each rostered patient per year.

Cardiovascular disease Disease that affects the heart and vascular system (i.e., blood vessels).

Catastrophic drug costs Prescription drug costs that cause undue burden on individuals with serious health conditions or illnesses.

Central agency An organization or department with the authority to direct or intervene in the activities of other departments. Central agencies aid with policy development and the coordination of activities.

Cerebrovascular disease A number of conditions that affect the flow of blood to the brain, the most serious of which is a stroke.

Circle of care The individuals and health care providers legitimately involved in rendering a patient's care.

Civil law A legal system in which laws governing civil rights and relationships within society, between people and property, and within families are written rather than being determined by judges.

Clinic A setting in which multiple health care providers work collaboratively, usually in a similar field, to provide cost-effective, patient-centred health care.

Code of ethics A set of values and responsibilities serving to guide the behaviour of the members of an organization or a profession.

Common law Laws established over time by judges based on decisions made on similar cases; sometimes referred to as *case law*.

Community-based care Care provided for the client in the home (e.g., incorporating visits from nurses or physiotherapists) or on an outpatient basis rather than in the hospital or another health care facility.

Compassionate interference The act of imposing treatment against a patient's will when deemed in the best interests of the patient.

Compensation That part of the health–illness continuum in which a person is neither in good nor poor health, is able to accommodate a malady, and is continuing on with daily life.

Confidential Kept private or shared only with authorized individuals (e.g., in health care, shared only with those authorized to have health information about a patient).

Conflict of interest The possible clash of two or more concerns. For example, a personal financial interest in a business may influence one's professional decisions.

Constitutional law The area of law dealing with legislation derived from or related to Canada's Constitution.

Consumer price index (CPI) A method of determining changes in the cost of goods and services through the monitoring of selected items (e.g., food, rent, mortgages, gasoline) across Canada. Used to measure inflation, the CPI may affect such payments as social security, spousal support, and rent, which are periodically adjusted to reflect the CPI.

Continuity of care Health care based on the treating practitioners' having all required information to optimize the care the patient receives. Having access to the individual's health records and maintaining excellent communication among all parties involved in the patient's care are ways to ensure continuity of care.

Contract law The branch of law dealing with agreements between parties, including the interpretation or enforcement of agreements when there is a dispute.

Controlled act An act that, as specified in the *Regulated Health Professions Act*, may be performed only by authorized regulated health care providers.

Controlled Drugs and Substances Act Federal legislation addressing Canada's drug laws, including a classification system for drugs.

Copayment A predetermined dollar amount or percentage of the cost of a health care service or medication that an individual must pay.

Criminal law The field of law dealing with crimes against the state or against society. Criminal law defines offences and controls the regulations concerning the apprehension, charging, and trying of those believed to have committed a criminal offence.

Culture Common elements of a social group, including its beliefs, practices, behaviours, values, and attitudes. Culture can relate to a society or to subgroups within a society.

Deductible The amount of money that an individual or family is required to pay toward health care costs before an insurance plan will take over.

Delegated act A controlled act that a physician authorizes another health care provider, either regulated or unregulated, to do in his or her stead and under supervision.

Delisted The removal of an item from a list or a registry. In Canada, the term is frequently used when a medical service is no longer considered medically necessary and is removed from the government's list of insured services.

Deontological theory An ethical theory that calls for a moral and honest action to be taken, regardless of the outcome.

Determinants of health The conditions (economic, social, environmental, etc.) in which people live that affect their current and future health.

Disability A physical or mental incapacity that differs from what is perceived as normal function. A disability can result from an illness or accident or be genetic in nature.

Disease A disorder or medical condition affecting a system or organ. The condition can be mental, physical, or genetic in origin. *Disease* also refers to a deviation from how the body normally functions.

Disease burden The impact of a health problem, measured by financial cost, mortality, morbidity, or other indicators.

Disease prevention Used in conjunction with health promotion. Information initiatives aimed at encouraging individuals, especially those in high-risk population groups (e.g., with a family history of diabetes or heart disease), to adopt strategies to prevent diseases.

Dispensing fee A service fee charged by a pharmacy for dispensing a prescription medication (i.e., reading the prescription and preparing the medication for the patient).

Divine command ethics An ethical theory believing that ethical philosophies and rules are set out by a higher power.

Double effect Acting in a manner that brings about the most good or the least harm.

Drug identification number (DIN) A unique number assigned to each medication approved by Health Canada for use in Canada.

Drug-seeking behaviour A behaviour or activity focused on obtaining access to addictive controlled substances.

Duties Obligations a person has in response to another's claims on them. A duty may result from a professional or personal obligation or may relate to one's own morals or values.

Duty of care The obligation to act in a competent manner according to the standards of practice.

Electronic health record (EHR) Health information collected by more than one facility and shared electronically among health care service providers (e.g., a doctor's office, emergency department, and pharmacy).

Electronic medical record (EMR) Health information obtained and stored at one facility, perhaps a dentist's, chiropractor's, or doctor's office.

Eligible Qualified for inclusion because of meeting certain criteria or requirements.

Enhanced services Optional health services, such as choice in hospital rooms, enhanced medical goods and services, and services not covered by the public health insurance system, offered to the patient at a cost.

Epidemiology The study of diseases in populations.

Ethical principle An acceptable, usually highly valued and moral, standard of human behaviour—for example, honesty, truthfulness, and fairness.

Ethical theory A framework of ideas that provides a template for making decisions to justify a set of actions.

Ethics The knowledge of and rules about behaving according to set values, duties, and moral principles.

Etiology The study of causes. In medicine, *etiology* refers to the origin or cause of a disease.

Evidence-informed Proven, through high-quality scientific studies, to be effective.

Exacerbation A period of time when a disease (usually chronic) is active and the person has symptoms. *Exacerbation* may also refer to an increase in the severity of a disease.

Extra billing An additional fee, considered a contravention of the *Canada Health Act*, charged to the user by a health care provider for a service covered under the terms of a provincial or territorial health insurance plan.

Fidelity The quality of being faithful.

Fiduciary duty A duty binding professionals to act with honesty and integrity, and in the best interests of their patients, with regard to their professional practice.

Fiduciary relationship A relationship based on trust.

First ministers The premiers of the provinces and territories.

First Nations A Canadian term of ethnicity referring to indigenous Canadians. The First Nations comprise 633 First Nations bands (usually registered as "Indians" under the *Indian Act*), representing 52 cultural groups and more than 50 languages. Other terms used include *Aboriginal*, *Native*, or *indigenous people*.

Food insecurity Poor or no physical or economic access to nutritious foods required to maintain a healthy state.

Forensic psychiatric hospitals Hospitals that assess and treat individuals referred by the Canadian courts and those requiring a secure inpatient facility due to a risk for harm to self or others.

Formulary list A list of prescription medications (often generic brands) selected for coverage by a public or private health insurance plan.

Geriatrics The branch of medicine dealing with the physiological characteristics of aging and the diagnosis and treatment of diseases affecting the aged.

Good Samaritan law A law protecting individuals who attempt to offer help to a person in distress.

Health accord A legal agreement between the federal and provincial and territorial governments on health care funding.

Health behaviour The activities a person engages in to acquire and maintain good physical and psychological health.

Health beliefs Things people believe to be true about their personal health and susceptibility to illness and about illness, prevention, and treatment in general.

Health care provider A person who has graduated from a health-related college or university program and is accredited by a professional or regulating body. Often, the person must be licensed by a provincial or territorial government.

Health–illness continuum A method of measuring one's state of health at any given point in time. A person's health state may range from optimum health at one end to death at the other end.

Health indicators Measurements that help to gauge the state of health and wellness of a population.

Health model A concept of an approach to care, including the development of a treatment plan and involvement and communication with a patient.

Health promotion Initiatives that inform people about things they can do to remain healthy and to prevent disease and illness.

Holistic Whole. In health care, a holistic approach treats the whole person, not an individual part of the person. For example, a holistic approach to treating a person with a heart condition would consider the patient's emotional state, diet, and fitness level, not just his or her heart problem.

Hospice A facility that provides supportive and compassionate care to individuals who are in the final stages of a terminal illness and their loved ones.

Hypoglycemic reaction A response to a drop in blood sugar levels. The symptoms may include mild weakness or dizziness; headache; cold, clammy, or sweaty skin; problems concentrating; shakiness; uncoordinated movements or staggering; blurred vision; irritability; hunger; fainting; and loss of consciousness.

Implied consent Consent assumed by the patient's actions, such as his or her seeking out the care of a health care provider or his or her failure to resist or protest.

Incident report A legal document outlining all relevant information concerning any negative occurrence in the workplace.

Inequities in health Unfair and unequal distribution of health resources in relation to resources available and the population involved.

Infant mortality The death of an infant (i.e., within the first year of life).

Informed consent A formal agreement signed by a patient consenting to a treatment, procedure, or test administered by a health care provider after the patient has been fully informed of all related risks and benefits.

Inpatient An individual remaining in a health care facility (e.g., an acute care hospital) overnight or longer.

Interoperable EHR Connected electronic systems that will enable authorized health care providers to view and, in some cases, update a patient's essential health information.

Interprofessional collaboration Multiple health care workers from a variety of professions working together to deliver evidence-informed, patient-centred health care.

Intersectoral cooperation Joint action among the public, the government, and nongovernment or community-based organizations.

Intubate The passing of a tube into a person's trachea to facilitate breathing.

Inuit Aboriginal people in northern Canada living generally above the tree line in the Northwest Territories, Northern Quebec, and Labrador.

Involuntary euthanasia A person's bringing about the death of a dying person with the dying person's consent.

Jurisdiction Authority or power over a designated region or geographic area.

Laparoscopic surgery A type of surgical procedure in which a small incision is made in the body, through which a viewing tube (laparoscope) is inserted. A small camera in the laparoscope allows the doctor to examine internal organs. Other small incisions may be made to insert instruments to perform surgery.

Legislation Laws made by a provincial or territorial legislature or by Parliament. To become law, a bill (i.e., proposed legislation) that has been introduced to Parliament requires the agreement of the House of Commons, the Senate, and the Crown (i.e., the Governor General, the representative of the British monarch in Canada).

Life expectancy The number of years a population or parts of a population are expected to live as determined by statistics.

Malpractice Illegal, negligent, or substandard treatment (failing to meet the treatment standards of one's profession) by a medical practitioner. Malpractice may be intentional or unintentional wrongdoing that may or may not result in injury to a patient.

Medically necessary A clinical judgement made by a physician regarding the necessity of a service provided under a provincial or territorial health plan to maintain, restore, or palliate (i.e., ease symptoms, such as pain, without curing the underlying disease).

Medicare The informal name for Canada's national health insurance plan. Note that the term's use in Canada differs from that in the United States, where *Medicare* refers to a federally sponsored program for individuals over the age of 65.

Methicillin-resistant *Staphylococcus aureus* (MRSA) A strain of *Staphylococcus aureus* that has become resistant to the antibiotic methicillin.

Minor A person under the age of majority in a particular province or territory.

Modalities Prescribed methods or techniques.

Morality A code of conduct defined by a group of people, culture, society, or religion. Individuals may have a moral code that governs the way they live, behave, and interact with others.

Morals A person's beliefs about right and wrong regarding how to treat others and how to behave in an organized society.

Morbidity The occurrence of disease or impairment resulting from accidents or environmental causes—for example, the number of people injured in a multiple-vehicle accident or the number of people who have a particular disease, such as cancer (but who have not died).

Mortality The occurrence of deaths resulting from disease, accidents, or environmental causes—for example, the number of people killed in a multiple-vehicle accident or the number of people who died from a particular disease, such as cancer.

Negligence The failure of a health care provider, whether intentional or unintentional, to meet the standards of care required of his or her profession; also sometimes referred to as *malpractice*, especially when resulting in harm or injury to the patient.

Nonmaleficence Doing no harm.

Nonprofit organizations (NPOs) Organizations that return surplus revenue (profits) back to the facility for purposes of maintaining or improving the facility and its operations; usually managed by a board as opposed to private owners.

Non-status Indians First Nations people registered in Canada's official record (the *Indian Act of Canada*), sometimes referred to as *treaty Indians*.

Nursing home A facility or part of a facility that provides accommodation to persons usually over the age of 16 requiring intensive personal care under the supervision of a registered nurse.

Oral consent Verbal agreement from a patient to undergo a treatment, procedure, or test performed by a health care provider.

Organisation for Economic Cooperation and Development (OECD)
Established in 1961 and now representing 30 countries, the OECD provides a setting in which member governments compare policy experiences, seek answers to common problems, identify best practices, and coordinate domestic and international policies.

Orphan patient A person without a family doctor.

Palliative care Care for the dying. Palliative care services, offered in the home or another facility (e.g., palliative care unit in a hospital or a hospice), may include nursing care, counselling, and pain management and may involve those close to the patient.

Pandemic A sustained, worldwide human-to-human transmission of disease.

Passive euthanasia The process of allowing a person to die by removing life support or other life-sustaining treatment.

Patented drugs Drugs that are legally protected from generic production for a period of 20 years from the date of filing.

Paternalism The attempt to control or influence another's decision regarding medical care. Paternalism does not honour the patient's right to autonomy.

Personal Information Protection and Electronic Documents Act (PIPEDA) A federal act ensuring the protection of personal information in the private sector.

Physician-assisted suicide The taking of one's own life with means provided by a doctor.

Population-based surveillance The collection and analysis of data that are needed to plan, implement, and evaluate population health initiatives.

Population health A framework for gathering and analyzing information about conditions that affect the health of a population. The aim is to both maintain and improve the health of the entire population and to reduce inequities in health status among population groups.

Positron emission tomography (PET) scanner A scanning device that uses nuclear imaging techniques to obtain 3-D images of parts of the body.

Power of attorney A legal document naming a specific person or persons to act on behalf of another in matters concerning personal care, personal estate, or both.

Practice setting The context and environment in which health care is delivered.

Prepaid health care Access to medically necessary hospital and physician services on a prepaid basis, and on uniform terms and conditions.

Primary care Front-line care, direction, and advice provided by multidisciplinary health care teams. Primary care also involves initiatives that seek to improve access to, quality of, and continuity of care; patient and health care provider satisfaction; and cost-effectiveness of health care services.

Primary care setting The organizational and physical environment in which a person receives point-of-entry care (e.g., a doctor's office, walk-in clinic).

Primary health care Health care with an emphasis on individuals and their communities. It includes essential medical and curative care received at the primary, secondary, or tertiary levels and involves health care providers, as well as community members, delivering, within the community, care that is cost-effective, comprehensive, and collaborative (i.e., uses a team approach).

Primary health care reform Changes to the delivery of primary health care with the goal of providing all Canadians access to an appropriate health care provider 24 hours a day, 7 days a week, no matter where they live.

Privacy The patient's right to control access to his or her body and personal information.

Professional misconduct Behaviour or some act or omission that falls short of what would be proper in the circumstances. Examples include deviating from a profession's standards of practice or violating the boundaries of a professional–patient relationship.

Proxy consent Consent given by a person authorized by a health care patient to give consent on his or her behalf.

Public health The use of health information from a variety of resources (e.g., Statistics Canada, the WHO, provincial, territorial, and regional sources) to improve the health of communities. Public health programs often carry out recommendations made by population health studies.

Publicly funded health care Health care services whose finances are managed by the government or a government agency for the good of the entire population.

Qualitative research A method of research that examines the way a population group thinks and behaves. The analysis is largely subjective in nature.

Quantitative research A method of objective research that deals with the measurement of data, such as the number of deaths from cancer.

Quarantine The enforced isolation of people having or suspected of having a contagious disease.

Quarantine Act Updated in 2005, this legislation gives the federal government powers to assess individuals and detain those who may pose a health risk to Canadians.

Rationalization of services Any changes that increase the effectiveness and efficiency of health care services—clinical, administrative, or financial.

Refraction Testing of the eyes to evaluate their ability to see. An ophthalmologist or optometrist does a refraction to determine the type of lens a patient needs in his or her glasses to maximize vision.

Refugee claimants People who, feeling unsafe in their home country, seek protection in another country.

Regulation A form of law, made by persons or organizations (e.g., an administrative agency) awarded such authority within an act (whether federal or provincial or territorial), that has the binding legal power of an act.

Regulatory law Laws made not by Parliament or by a legislature but by authorized persons or organizations to govern a particular group; these laws are ultimately subject to the provincial, territorial, or federal act that governs the administrative body, organization, or tribunal.

Remission A period of time during which a chronic disease is neither active nor acute and the person has no obvious symptoms.

Renal dialysis A process that filters waste and fluid from the blood similar to the way kidneys do. Individuals whose kidneys are not functioning must undergo this procedure several times a week to stay alive while waiting for a kidney transplant.

Reserve Land set aside by the Crown and designated for the use and occupancy of Aboriginal people.

Rights in health care Entitlements, or things that can and should be expected of health care providers and the health care system. Rights may be tangible (e.g., the right to receive a vaccination covered under the provincial or territorial plan) or intangible (e.g., the right to be treated with respect).

Risk assessment The assessment or examination of a condition or a situation to determine the potential harm or hazards (risk) related to it (e.g., the risk for having an accident if you drive a car in a snowstorm).

Role fidelity In health care, meeting the reasonable expectations of members of the health care team, patients, their families, and employers by being loyal, truthful, and faithful; by showing respect; and by earning and maintaining trust.

Rostering The registering of a patient in a primary health care reform group. Patients sign a nonbinding form stating that they will seek care only from a specific doctor or primary care group. Also called *patient attachment* or *formal registration*.

Royal assent The final stage a bill passes through before becoming law. Largely symbolic in nature, this approval is given by the Governor General as a representative of the Crown.

Scope of practice A range of skills, learned in school or through on-the-job training, that a practitioner can perform competently and safely. From a professional perspective, legal parameters usually, but not always, dictate what a practitioner may or may not do, based on the profession's education, training, and licensure.

Self-determination The freedom to make one's own decisions.

Self-imposed risk behaviours Actions (such as smoking tobacco) that a person willfully engages in despite knowing they pose a danger to his or her health.

Severe acute respiratory syndrome (SARS) A severe form of pneumonia that first swept across parts of Asia and the Far East before spreading worldwide in 2003.

Sick role behaviour A person's response to disease or illness. Removed from normal societal expectations and responsibilities, the sick person may respond to situations differently from when he or she is well. Sick role behaviour is usually temporary in nature.

Signs Those things related to an illness that a person or examiner can see (e.g., a rash).

Social movements Advancements by advocacy or interest groups to promote a common interest by acting together to influence public policy.

Socioeconomic gradient (SES gradient) A measurement of health or health inequalities as they relate to a person's or population's socioeconomic circumstances.

Specialist A physician trained in a specific field, usually concerning body systems or organs—for example, cardiology, internal medicine, orthopedic surgery—although some specialties (e.g., geriatrics) have a socioeconomic focus.

Status Indians Individuals recognized by the federal government as being registered under the *Indian Act*.

Statutory law Written law, formally created or established by the legislature.

Symptoms Those things that a person feels that may relate to an illness (e.g., fatigue, a headache). Symptoms are sometimes referred to as *clinical signs*.

Telehealth A telephone help system, usually available 24/7 and funded by the provincial or territorial government, used to provide professional health care advice to Canadians who cannot readily access a doctor or other primary care provider.

Teleological theory An ethical theory that defines an action as right or wrong depending on the results it produces; also called *consequence-based theory*.

Title protection Legal restrictions around and guidelines for the use of a professional title.

Tort A civil wrong committed against a person or his or her property.

Upstream investments Actions that can be taken to improve the health of a population or to prevent illness when the potential for a problem is first recognized.

Urodynamic Referring to tests and assessments done to measure the function of the bladder and urinary tract.

User charges A fee imposed for an insured health service that the provincial or territorial health care insurance plan does not cover.

Values Something a person holds dear, such as a quality or a standard by which to act or behave (e.g., loyalty, honesty).

Values history form A document that helps people think about the health care choices they would want made for them.

Vancomycin-resistant *Enterococcus* (VRE) A form of the bacteria *Enterococcus* that has become resistant to many antibiotics, including vancomycin—one of the most effective antibiotics to treat enterococcal infections.

Vancomycin-resistant *Staphylococcus aureus* (VRSA) A strain of *Staphylococcus aureus* that has become resistant to the antibiotic vancomycin.

Virtue ethics An ethical theory that operates under the belief that a person of moral character will act wisely, fairly, and honestly and will uphold ethical principles.

Voluntary euthanasia A person's bringing about the death of a dying person with the dying person's consent.

Wellness Good health and a sense of well-being on many levels (i.e., emotional as well as physical) as described or experienced by an individual.

Whistleblower An individual who assumes responsibility for publicly divulging information about a wrongdoing or misconduct by another individual or an organization.

Workplace Hazardous Materials Information Systems (WHMIS) legislation A group of laws, rules, or statutes enacted by a government (federal, provincial, territorial, or municipal).

Appendix

Declaration of Alma-Ata

Declaration of Alma-Ata: International Conference on Primary Health Care, Alma-Ata, USSR, 6–12 September 1978

The International Conference on Primary Health Care, meeting in Alma-Ata this twelfth day of September in the year nineteen hundred and seventy-eight, expressing the need for urgent action by all governments, all health and development workers, and the world community to protect and promote the health of all the people of the world, hereby makes the following Declaration:

I

The Conference strongly reaffirms that health, which is a state of complete physical, mental and social wellbeing, and not merely the absence of disease or infirmity, is a fundamental human right and that the attainment of the highest possible level of health is a most important world-wide social goal whose realization requires the action of many other social and economic sectors in addition to the health sector.

II

The existing gross inequality in the health status of the people particularly between developed and developing countries as well as within countries is politically, socially and economically unacceptable and is, therefore, of common concern to all countries.

III

Economic and social development, based on a New International Economic Order, is of basic importance to the fullest attainment of health for all and to the reduction of the gap between the health status of the developing and developed countries. The promotion and protection of the health of the people is essential to sustained economic and social development and contributes to a better quality of life and to world peace.

IV

The people have the right and duty to participate individually and collectively in the planning and implementation of their health care.

V

Governments have a responsibility for the health of their people, which can be fulfilled only by the provision of adequate health and social measures. A main social target of governments, international organizations and the whole world community in the coming decades should be the attainment by all peoples of the world by the year 2000 of a level of health that will permit them to lead a socially and economically productive life. Primary health care is the key to attaining this target as part of development in the spirit of social justice.

VI

Primary health care is essential health care based on practical, scientifically sound and socially acceptable methods and technology made universally accessible to individuals and families in the community through their full participation and at a cost that the community and country can afford to maintain at every stage of their development in the spirit of self-reliance and self-determination. It forms an integral part both of the country's health system, of which it is the central function and main focus, and of the overall social and economic development of the community. It is the first level of contact of individuals, the family and community with the national health system, bringing health care as close as possible to where people live and work, and constitutes the first element of a continuing health care process.

VII
Primary health care:

1. reflects and evolves from the economic conditions and sociocultural and political characteristics of the country and its communities and is based on the application of the relevant results of social, biomedical and health services research and public health experience;
2. addresses the main health problems in the community, providing promotive, preventive, curative and rehabilitative services accordingly;
3. includes at least: education concerning prevailing health problems and the methods of preventing and controlling them; promotion of food supply and proper nutrition; an adequate supply of safe water and basic sanitation; maternal and child health care, including family planning; immunization against the major infectious diseases; prevention and control of locally endemic diseases; appropriate treatment of common diseases and injuries; and provision of essential drugs;
4. involves, in addition to the health sector, all related sectors and aspects of national and community development, in particular agriculture, animal husbandry, food, industry, education, housing, public works, communications and other sectors; and demands the coordinated efforts of all those sectors;
5. requires and promotes maximum community and individual self-reliance and participation in the planning, organization, operation and control of

primary health care, making fullest use of local, national and other available resources; and to this end develops through appropriate education the ability of communities to participate;
6. should be sustained by integrated, functional and mutually supportive referral systems, leading to the progressive improvement of comprehensive health care for all and giving priority to those most in need;
7. relies, at local and referral levels, on health workers, including physicians, nurses, midwives, auxiliaries and community workers as applicable, as well as traditional practitioners as needed, suitably trained socially and technically to work as a health team and to respond to the expressed health needs of the community.

VIII

All governments should formulate national policies, strategies and plans of action to launch and sustain primary health care as part of a comprehensive national health system and in coordination with other sectors. To this end, it will be necessary to exercise political will, to mobilize the country's resources and to use available external resources rationally.

IX

All countries should cooperate in a spirit of partnership and service to ensure primary health care for all people since the attainment of health by people in any one country directly concerns and benefits every other country. In this context, the joint WHO/UNICEF report on primary health care constitutes a solid basis for the further development and operation of primary health care throughout the world.

X

An acceptable level of health for all the people of the world by the year 2000 can be attained through a fuller and better use of the world's resources, a considerable part of which is now spent on armaments and military conflicts. A genuine policy of independence, peace, détente and disarmament could and should release additional resources that could well be devoted to peaceful aims and in particular to the acceleration of social and economic development of which primary health care, as an essential part, should be allotted its proper share.

The International Conference on Primary Health Care calls for urgent and effective national and international action to develop and implement primary health care throughout the world and particularly in developing countries in a spirit of technical cooperation and in keeping with a New International Economic Order. It urges governments, WHO and UNICEF, and other international organizations, as well as multilateral and bilateral agencies, nongovernmental organizations, funding agencies, all health workers and the whole world community to support national and international commitment to primary health care and to channel increased technical and financial support to it, particularly in developing countries. The Conference calls on all the aforementioned to collaborate in introducing, developing and maintaining primary health care in accordance with the spirit and content of this Declaration.

Reproduced, with the permission of the publisher, from *Declaration of Alma-Ata: International conference on primary health care*, Alma-Ata, USSR, 6–12 September 1978. World Health Organization. (1978). Retrieved from http://www.who.int/publications/almaata_declaration_en.pdf.

Index

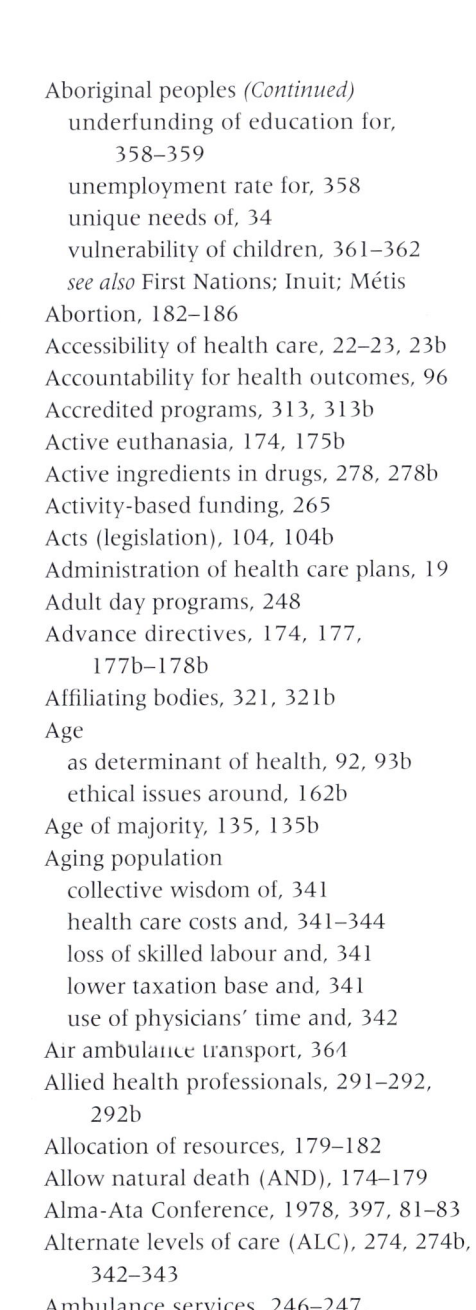

Numbers
10-province standard, 259
2004 Health Accord, 258
2014 Health Accord, 36, 260

A
Aboriginal Affairs and Northern Development Canada (AANDC), 356
Aboriginal health care
  access to, 182, 182b, 363–364
  challenges of, 357–363
  cultural sensitivity and, 5b, 168b
  improvements in, 232b
  inequities in, 92, 334, 355–367
  responsibility for, 3, 194
  strategies for improving, 366–367
  systems of delivery, 363–366
Aboriginal Health Transition Fund, 34
Aboriginal medicine
  Andaaw'iwewin egkwa Mushkiki (Traditional Healing Practices and Medicines), 365b
  in early Canada, 4
  history of, 4–5
  traditional healing practices, 364–366
  vs Western medicine, 364–366
Aboriginal peoples
  Canada's Food Guide for, 201, 202b
  collaboration with, 29, 88b
  defined, 63b, 194b
  drug plans for, 351
  food insecurity of, 359
  inadequate housing of, 359–360
  infant mortality rates of, 361
  mental health issues and, 360
  morbidity/mortality rates for, 362–363
  rate of chronic disease among, 360
  risks for elders, 362
  sexual health of, 361
  substance abuse issues and, 360
  suicide rate for, 360

Aboriginal peoples *(Continued)*
  underfunding of education for, 358–359
  unemployment rate for, 358
  unique needs of, 34
  vulnerability of children, 361–362
  see also First Nations; Inuit; Métis
Abortion, 182–186
Accessibility of health care, 22–23, 23b
Accountability for health outcomes, 96
Accredited programs, 313, 313b
Active euthanasia, 174, 175b
Active ingredients in drugs, 278, 278b
Activity-based funding, 265
Acts (legislation), 104, 104b
Administration of health care plans, 19
Adult day programs, 248
Advance directives, 174, 177, 177b–178b
Affiliating bodies, 321, 321b
Age
  as determinant of health, 92, 93b
  ethical issues around, 162b
Age of majority, 135, 135b
Aging population
  collective wisdom of, 341
  health care costs and, 341–344
  loss of skilled labour and, 341
  lower taxation base and, 341
  use of physicians' time and, 342
Air ambulance transport, 364
Allied health professionals, 291–292, 292b
Allocation of resources, 179–182
Allow natural death (AND), 174–179
Alma-Ata Conference, 1978, 397, 81–83
Alternate levels of care (ALC), 274, 274b, 342–343
Ambulance services, 246–247, 246b–247b
Ambulatory care clinics, 322, 324b

Note: Page numbers followed by "b," "f" and "t" indicate boxes, figures and tables, respectively.

401

Andaaw'iwewin egkwa Mushkiki (Traditional Healing Practices and Medicines), 365b
Apology laws, 141
Aseptic technique, 10, 10b
Assembly of First Nations, 359
Assisted Human Reproduction Canada (AHRC), 211
Assisted living accommodation, 248
Assisted suicide
  defined, 123, 123b
  legality of, 56b, 123–124
  purpose of, 174
  see also Physician-assisted suicide
Assistive devices, 248–249
Association of Faculties of Medicine of Canada (AFMC), 365–366
Audiologists, 316–317
Audit and Accountability Bureau (AAB), Health Canada, 197
Autonomy
  defined, 159, 159b
  as a right, 165–166, 166b, 170b

B

Barer-Stoddart Report, 346–347
Beneficence, 158, 158b
Best practices, 205, 205b
Biology as determinant of health, 78–79
Blended funding, 282
Block funding, 264
Block payments, 245, 246b
Block transfers, 16b, 32
Blood products, sale of, 7, 7b–8b
Blood Safety Surveillance and Health Care Acquired Infections Division, CIDPC, 210
Blueprint on Aboriginal Health, 35
Boundaries
  rationale for, 172–173
  in relationships with patients, 170–172, 171b
  at work, 171–172
Branches (Health Canada), 197–207, 197b
British North America Act, 3, 11, 111
Bureaus (Health Canada), 197, 197b

C

Canada Extended Health Services Act, 350
Canada Health Act
  application of, 120–124
  coverage of, 19–20, 20b
  criteria and conditions of, 19–23, 19b
  health care rights under, 161–163
  health insurance plans under, 223, 239
  history of, 18–26, 18b
  interpretation of, 24–25
  legislation leading to, 15–18
  opposition to, 26
  public administration of, 19
  reopening of, 350
  services insured under, 241–249
Canada Health Act Division, Programs Directorate, Health Canada, 206
Canada Health and Social Transfer (CHST), 32
Canada Health Infoway, 140, 284–285, 367–368
Canada Health Transfer (CHT), 32, 34, 258–260
Canada Social Transfer (CST), 32, 260
Canada's National–Provincial Health Program for the 1980s, 17
Canadian Blood Services, 7
Canadian Centre for Occupational Health and Safety (CCOHS), 111–112
Canadian Charter of Rights and Freedoms
  assisted suicide and, 123
  health care rights under, 103–104, 121–123, 161–162
Canadian Classification of Health Interventions (CCI), 213
Canadian Health Information Management Association (CHIMA), 140, 319–320
Canadian Health Network, 210
Canadian Hospice Palliative Care Association, 272
Canadian Institute for Advanced Research (CIFAR), 71–72, 83–84, 88
Canadian Institute for Health Information (CIHI), 89–92, 213

Canadian Institutes of Health Research (CIHR), 87–88, 88b, 208, 208b
Canadian Interprofessional Health Collaborative (CIHC), 306
Canadian Medical Association, 26
Canadian Medical Protective Association, 135, 141
Canadian Mental Health Association, 336
Canadian National Association of Trained Nurses (CNATN), 9
Canadian Paediatric Society, 217
Canadian Pandemic Influenza Plan, 216
Canadian Policy Research Networks (CPRN), 89
Canadian Practical Nurse Registration Examination (CPNRE), 312
Canadian Red Cross Society, 6–8
Canadian Triage and Acuity Scale (CTAS), 355
Cancer as cause of death, 63–65
Capitation-based funding, 265, 281–282, 281b
Cardiologists, 307
Cardiovascular disease (CVD)
    as cause of death, 65
    defined, 65b
Caregivers, 344b
Case-mix approach, 264
Catastrophic drug costs
    defined, 31b
    first ministers on, 34–35
    lack of coverage for, 32, 334
    provincial/territorial coverage of, 278, 335
    Romanow Report on, 29b–31b
    see also Drug insurance plans
Causes of death (Canada), 63–66, 64f
Central agencies, 197–199, 199b
Centre for Infectious Disease Prevention and Control (CIDPC), 210
Centre of Emergency Preparedness and Response, 216
Cerebrovascular disease
    as cause of death, 66
    defined, 66b

Charting
    by exception, 133
    narrative, 133
Chief Financial Officer Branch (CFOB), Health Canada, 197–199
Children's Aid Society, 9
Chiropodists, 315
Chiropractic medicine, 294–296, 295b–296b
Chronic care, 351
Chronic diseases, health care costs of, 262
Circle of care, 130, 130b
Civil law, 105, 105b, 110b
Clinics
    effectiveness of, 323
    types of, 322–324
    see also Private clinics
Codes of ethics, 170–174
    defined, 141b
    professional, 141
Coding systems, 213
Common (case) law, 105, 105b
Communications disorders assistants (CDAs), 317
Community Acquired Infections Division, CIDPC, 210
Community health centres (CHCs), 273, 329
Community-based health care, 271–273, 291
Community-based mental health care, 336
Compassionate care benefits, 34
Compassionate interference, 169, 169b–170b
Compensation, 55, 55b
Compensatory justice, 160–161
Complaint processes, regulated professions and, 140–142, 304
Complementary and alternative medicine (CAM), 293–296, 294b
Complementary and alternative practitioners, 291–292, 292t
Complex care, 351
Comprehensive care organizations, 329
Computed tomography (CT) scanners, 283–284

Confidentiality
  breach of, 138, 138b
  concept of, 136–138, 137b
  defined, 136b–137b
Conflict of interest, 126, 126b
Consent
  express, 129
  implied, 130, 130b
  informed, 127–132, 127b
  oral, 130, 130b
  for release of records, 134
  written, 129–130, 129b
Consequence-based theory, 156b
Constitution Act
  equalization payments under, 259, 259b
  health care under, 3, 111–119, 223, 223b
  status Indians under, 357b
Constitutional law, 103–104, 103b
Consumer price index (CPI), 209, 209b
Continuing care, 351
Continuity of care, 162–163, 163b
Contract law, 108, 108b
Controlled acts, 301–302, 301b–302b
Controlled drugs
  in hospitals, 113
  illegal use of, 115, 115b
  legislation covering, 113–115
  prescribing, 113–115
  supervised use of, 117b
Controlled Drugs and Substances Act, 112–118, 112b, 204
Convention on the Rights of Persons With Disabilities, 48b
Conventional health care providers, 291–292, 292t, 306–321
Conventional medicine, 293
Copayment
  for ambulance services, 246, 246b
  defined, 246b
  for long-term care, 274–275, 275b–276b
Coping skills as determinant of health, 77–78
Core health professionals, 291–292
Corporate Services Branch (CSB), Health Canada, 199

Cottage hospital system, 10b
Criminal law, 109–111, 109b–110b
Culturally sensitive health care, 5b, 59, 168b
Culture
  defined, 54b
  as determinant of health, 80
  influence on health beliefs, 54
  and response to hospitalization, 59, 60b

D

Data quality, 320
Databases, 213
Day care, 82b, 83
Day surgery, 270–271
Deductibles, 249–250, 250b
Delegated acts, 302–304, 302b–303b
Delisted services, 17b
Delivery of health care, 257
Deontological theory, 156, 156b
Department of Agriculture, 4
Department of Health, 4
Department of National Health and Welfare, 4
Department of Pensions and National Health, 4
Departmental Secretariat, Health Canada, 197
Determinants of health, 72f
  analysis of, 93
  defined, 71–80, 71b
  linking of, 83–84
Direct health care, provincial/territorial costs for, 261–262
Disability
  defined, 47–48, 47b
  rights of people with, 48b
Discharge Abstract Database (DAD), 213
Disease
  defined, 46–47, 46b
  prevention of, 71, 71b
Disease burden, 337, 337b
Dispensing fees, 249–250, 250b
Distributive justice, 160–161
Divine command ethics, 157–158, 157b

DNR (Do Not Resuscitate) orders, 174, 177, 177b
Doctors
　in early Canada, 4
　shortage of, 346–348, 279–280, 342, 354–355
　use of electronic medical records (EMRs), 368–370
　see also Physicians
Doctors' strikes, 14, 26, 26b
Double effect, 158, 158b
Douglas, Tommy, 13–15
Drug identification numbers (DINs), 251b
Drug insurance plans
　applying for, 250
　coverage of, 250
　funding of, 351
　lack of national plan, 278, 351
　provincial/territorial plans, 277–278
　public vs private, 249–250
　spending on, 249
　see also Catastrophic drug costs
Drug laws, 112–118
Drug Strategy and Controlled Substances Program, Health Canada, 204
Drugs
　active ingredients in, 278, 278b
　advertising, 118
　brand-name, 278–279
　controlled, 113–115
　generic, 209, 210b–211b, 278–279
　illegal, 115–118
　injection, 117b
　patented, 209–210, 209b, 211b, 279
　prescription, 118, 351–352, 352b
　rising cost of, 277–279, 334
Drug-seeking behaviour, 113–114, 113b–115b
Duties, 155, 155b, 164
Duty of care
　defined, 108b
　professional standard of, 108, 155, 155b

E

Ebola virus, 211–212
Economic and social development, 397
Education as determinant of health, 75
Electronic health information, 320
Electronic health records (EHRs)
　advantages of, 367, 368b, 370
　challenges with, 371
　cost of, 284–285
　defined, 139b
　expansion of, 367–371
　in hospitals, 368–370, 368b
　information requirements of, 138–140
　interoperable EHRs, 367–368, 367b
　recommended, 29b–31b
　security of, 370
　see also Health records
Electronic medical records (EMRs)
　advantages of, 285, 370
　defined, 139b
　doctors' use of, 368–370
　information requirements of, 138–140
　see also Health records
Eligibility for health care, 18b
Emancipated minors, 131
Emergencies, 118–119
Emergency departments, wait times in, 354–355
Emergency Preparedness Act (EPA), 216
Emergentologists, 307
Emotional wellness, 44–45
Employment
　as determinant of health, 75, 75b–76b
　mental illness and, 339–340, 340b
Employment and Social Insurance Act, 11
End-of-life issues, 123–124, 174–179
Enhanced services, 243b, 243b
Environmental wellness, 46
Epidemiology, 92, 92b
Epp, Jake, 83
Epp Report, 1986, 83
Equality of care, 106b
Equalization payments, 34, 259, 259b
Established Programs and Financing (EPF) Act, 15b–16b, 17–18
Ethical principles
　autonomy, 159, 159b, 165–166, 166b
　beneficence, 158, 158b
　breach of, 159b

Ethical principles *(Continued)*
   defined, 158–161, 158b
   double effect, 158, 158b
   fidelity, 160, 160b
   justice, 160–161
   nonmaleficence, 158, 158b
   respect, 158–159, 159b
   truthfulness, 159–160, 166–167, 167b
Ethical theories, 155, 155b–156b
Ethics
   codes of, 141, 141b, 170–174
   consequence-based theory of, 156, 156b–157b
   defined, 151–155, 151b
   deontological theory of, 156, 156b
   divine command ethics, 157–158, 157b
   teleological theory of, 155b–156b, 156
   virtue ethics, 156–157, 156b
   in the workplace, 169–174
Ethics committees, 173–174
Etiology, 45, 45b
Euthanasia
   active, 174b–175b
   involuntary, 174b–175b
   legality of, 56b, 175b
   passive, 174b
   purpose of, 174–176
   voluntary, 174b
Evidence-informed treatment, 293, 293b
Exacerbation, 47, 47b
Express consent, 129
Extended health care services, 25–26, 247–248, 351
Extra billing, 17, 17b, 25, 27

F

Family physicians, 306–307, 347f
Federal government
   health transfer payments, 258–260
   role in health care, 192
   health department. *see* Health Canada
Fee-for-service (FFS), 280–281
Fidelity, 160, 160b
Fiduciary duty, 126, 126b
Fiduciary relationship, 159–160, 159b

First ministers, 28–29, 28b
First ministers' accords, 33–36
First Ministers' Accord on Health Care Renewal, 2003, 33–34
First Ministers' Meeting on the Future of Health Care, 2004, 34
First Nations
   defined, 194b, 356
   improved health services for, 232b
   programs available to, 194, 356–357
   responsibility for health care of, 194, 199–200, 260
   see also Aboriginal peoples
First Nations and Inuit Health Branch, Health Canada, 199–200, 363
First Nations, Inuit, and Métis (FNIM) physicians, 365–366
First Nations, Inuit, and Métis Health Core Competencies, 366
Fiscal capacity, 259
Food Directorate, Health Canada, 201
Food insecurity, 359, 359b
Forensic psychiatric hospitals, 335, 335b
Formulary lists, 250, 250b
Fox, Terry, 43b
Funding for health care. *see* Health care funding

G

Gender as determinant of health, 79–80
General practitioners, 306–307
Generic drugs, 209, 210b–211b, 278–279
Genes, patenting of, 185–186, 186b
Genetic counselling, 185
Genetic endowment as determinant of health, 78–79, 79b
Genetic testing, 79b, 184–185, 185b
Geriatricians, 307
Geriatrics, 307, 307b
Gifts, accepting, 173
Global budget funding, 282
Good Samaritan laws, 143–144, 143b–144b
Griffiths, Susan, 56b
Group health centres, 329
Group homes, 248

Guardianship, 131
Gynecologists and Obstetricians (OB/GYNs), 307

H1N1 virus, 193, 200, 216–217
Hall, Emmett, 13–14, 17
Hall Report, 15b–16b, 17
Hard-to-serve communities and populations, 329
Hawking, Stephen, 56
Hazardous Materials Information Review Commission (HMIRC), 209
Hazardous Products Act, 112
Health
 defined, 41, 42b
 determinants of, 71–80, 71b, 72f, 83–84, 93
 inequities in, 397, 81, 81b, 92
 lifestyle's impact on, 50–52
 perceptions of, 50–52
 as a right, 397
Health accords, 33–36, 33b, 260
Health behaviour, 52–55, 52b
Health belief model, 52–55
Health beliefs, 53, 53b–54b, 80
Health Canada
 agencies of, 208–211
 Audit and Accountability Bureau (AAB), 197
 branches of, 197–207, 197b
 bureaus of, 197, 197b
 Canada's Food Guide, 201, 202b
 central agencies of, 197–199
 Chief Financial Officer Branch (CFOB), 197–199
 Corporate Services Branch (CSB), 199
 Departmental Secretariat, 197
 Drug Strategy and Controlled Substances Program, 204
 emergency powers, 118–119
 external services of, 199–207
 First Nations and Inuit Health Branch, 199–200, 363
 Food Directorate, 201
 Health Care Policy Directorate, 200

Health Canada *(Continued)*
 Health Products and Food Branch (HPFB), 201–204
 Healthy Environments and Consumer Safety Branch (HECSB), 204–205
 history of, 4
 internal services of, 197–199
 international collaboration of, 211–218
 Legal Services, 199
 Marketed Health Products Directorate, 202–203
 Marketing and Communications Services Directorate, 207
 mission statement, 193
 Natural Health Products Directorate, 203–204
 Office of Nursing Policy, 200–201
 Office of Nutrition Policy and Promotion, 201
 Office of the Chief Scientist, 200
 organization of, 195–197, 198f
 Pest Management Regulatory Agency (PMRA), 207
 Product Safety Program, 205
 Programs Directorate, 206
 Public Affairs and Strategic Communications Directorate, 206–207
 Public Affairs, Consultation and Communications Branch (PACCB), 206–207
 Regions and Programs Branch, 205–206
 responsibilities of, 87, 193–195
 Safe Environments Program (SEP), 204
 as source of information, 194
 Special Access Program, 279
 Strategic Policy Branch (SPB), 200–201
 Therapeutic Products Directorate, 201–202
 Tobacco Control Program, 204–205
 unelected employees of, 196, 196b
 Workplace Health and Public Safety Program, 205–206
Health card fraud, 241
Health cards, 240–241

Health care
  accessibility of, 22–23, 23b
  allocation of resources in, 179–182
  barriers to accessing, 80, 344
  community-based, 271
  culturally sensitive, 47b, 59
  current issues in, 341–343
  ethical issues in, 182–186
  ethical theories in, 155–158
  evolution of, 3–10
  federal responsibility for, 260
  financial sustainability of, 373–374
  government jurisdiction over, 111–119
  northern access to, 182, 182b
  planning of, 397
  regionalization of, 226–234
  as a right, 120–124, 121b–122b
  rights in, 161–169, 161b, 168b
  social movements and, 12
  values in, 153–155
Health care administration, 320–321
Health care assistants, 315–316
Health care attendants, 315–316
Health care costs, 16b, 257
  aging population and, 341–344
  of chronic diseases, 262
  drivers of, 283–285
  indirect costs, 262–263
  provincial/territorial costs, 261–262, 261t
  for technology, 283–284
Health care delivery, 257
Health care expenditures
  for hospitals, 263–274
  by use of funds, 263f
Health care funding
  bargaining for, 260
  Canada Health Transfer, 258–260
  competition for, 181, 182b
  vs delivery, 257
  distribution of, 236–237
  of home care, 349–350
  of hospitals, 264–269
  levels of, 257–263
  methods of, 234–237
  priorities, 180

Health care funding *(Continued)*
  private, 258
  public, 12, 14, 120, 256–257, 257b
  sources of, 236
  via premiums, 237b, 257–258
Health care legislation, 103–111
  civil law, 105
  common (case) law, 105
  constitutional law, 103–104
  regulatory law, 104
  statutory law, 104
Health care organizations, 329
Health care plans
  accessibility of, 22–23
  administration of, 19
  coverage of, 19–20
  funding of, 234–237
  portability of, 21–22, 21b–22b, 240b
  provincial and territorial, 223–226
  structure of, 224–226
  universality of, 20–21, 20b
  see also Health insurance
Health care policy, objective of, 18b
Health Care Policy Directorate, Health Canada, 200
Health care premiums, 234–235, 237b
Health care providers
  allied health professionals, 291–292, 292b
  categories of, 291–296, 292t
  complementary and alternative practitioners, 291–292, 292t
  conventional, 291–292, 292t, 306–321
  core health professionals, 291–292
  defined, 292b
  ethical principles guiding, 158–161
  insured, 247
  liability insurance for, 140
  nonregulated, 142
  regulation of, 140–142, 296–305, 297t–299t
  relationships with colleagues, 171–172
  relationships with patients, 170–172, 171b
Health care resources
  allocation of, 179–182
  demand for, 180

Health care teams, 27, 273
Health Council of Canada, 32, 34
Health emergency preparedness, 216
Health–illness continuum, 55–62, 55f, 55b, 57f, 57b
Health indicators, 90–92, 90b
Health information
   disposal of, 134–135
   ownership of, 133–134
   release of, 137–138
   security of, 138
   storage of, 134–135
Health information management (HIM) professionals
   domains of practice of, 320
   training of, 319–320
Health insurance
   introduction of, 11–15
   private, 237
   provincial and territorial, 223–226, 237–241
   third-party, 237
   Tommy Douglas and, 36
   types of, 237–249
   see also Health care plans
Health models, 48–50, 48b
Health outcomes, accountability for, 96
Health planning, public engagement in, 95
Health prerequisites, 83
Health Products and Food Branch (HPFB), Health Canada, 201–204, 203b
Health promotion, 71, 71b
Health records
   components of, 132–140
   ownership of, 133–134
   see also Electronic health records (EHRs); Electronic medical records (EMRs)
Health Reform Fund, 34
Health Regulations, International, 119
Health service organizations (HSOs), 329
Health services
   as determinant of health, 79
   insured/uninsured, 241–249
Health watch activities, 210
Healthy child development as determinant of health, 78

Healthy Environments and Consumer Safety Branch (HECSB), Health Canada, 204–205
Herbal medications, use of, 204b
Hippocratic Oath, 137b, 165b–166b
Holistic model, 49, 49b
Home care
   accessing, 322b, 349
   defined, 248
   demand for, 348
   funding of, 334, 349–350, 352b
   future of, 350–351
   impact of, 349
   as priority, 27
   recipients of, 349
   safety issues with, 350
Home care support workers, 315–316
Homelessness, mental illness and, 338
Hospices, 248, 290, 290b–291b
Hospital administration, cost of, 268
Hospital care
   cost of, 266–268, 266b, 267t
   cost-reduction strategies, 269–274
Hospital funding
   activity-based funding, 265
   block funding, 264
   capitated funding, 265
   case-mix approach, 264–265
   line-by-line funding, 264
   mechanisms for, 264–269
   population-based funding, 265
   requirements for, 265–266
   service-based funding, 264–265
Hospital Insurance and Diagnostic Services Act, 13, 18
Hospitalists, 308
Hospitals
   adaptation to, 59–60
   aging population and, 342–343
   cost of services, 268
   day surgery in, 270–271
   development of, 9–10
   electronic health records (EHRs) in, 368–370, 368b
   expenditures for, 263–274
   insured services, 244

Hospitals *(Continued)*
  length of stay in, 269–274
  mergers of, 273–274
  palliative care in, 272
  private rooms in, 269, 270b
  rationalization of services, 273–274
  same-day admissions, 270
  timely discharge from, 271
Hughes, Clara, 337b
Human health resources (HHR)
  cost of, 279–280
  defined, 279–283
  shortages in, 344–348
Hypoglycemic reaction, 203, 203b

I

ICD-10 (International Classification of Diseases-10), 213
ICD-10-CA, 213
Illegal drugs, permission to use, 115–118
Illness
  defined, 46
  signs of, 60, 60b
  stages of, 60–61, 60b–61b
  symptoms of, 60, 60b
Immigration, 92, 222b–223b
Immigration and Refugee Protection Act, 238
Immunization, 398, 94, 180–181, 361
  see also Vaccinations
Implied consent, 130, 130b
Incident reports, 109b–110b
Indian Act, 356
Indigenous Physicians Association of Canada (IPAC), 365–366
Indirect capitation funding, 282
Inequities in health, 81, 81b, 92
Infant mortality
  among Aboriginal peoples, 361
  defined, 63
  rate of, 63
Influenza vaccines, 217
Informal caregivers, 344b
Informed consent
  components of, 127–132
  defined, 127b
Injection drugs, supervised use of, 117b

Inpatients, 143, 143b
Insite (clinic), 117b
Insured health care providers, 247
Insured services
  Canada Health Act and, 241–249
  hospitals, 244
  medically necessary procedures, 244–246
  vs uninsured services, 245b
Integrated health organizations (IHOs), 329
Intellectual wellness, 45
Intentional torts, 106–107
Interdisciplinary team approach, 372, 372b–373b
Interim Federal Health Program (IFHP), 3, 194
International Classification of Diseases-10 (ICD-10), 213
International Classification of Functioning Disability and Health (ICF), 50
International Conference on Primary Health Care. *see* Alma-Ata Conference, 1978
International Health Regulations, 119
Internists, 308
Interoperable EHRs, 367–368, 367b
Interprofessional collaboration, 290–291
Intersectoral cooperation, 86–90, 86b, 95
Intubate, 317–318, 318b
Inuit
  defined, 194b
  lack of health care for, 182, 182b
  programs available to, 194, 356–357
  responsibility for health care of, 194, 199–200, 260
  see also Aboriginal peoples.
Involuntary confinement, 142
Involuntary euthanasia, 174, 175b
It's Your Health (bulletin), 207

J

Job protection, 34
Jolie, Angelina, 79b
Jurisdiction, 111, 111b
Justice, 160–161

K

Kelowna Accord, 2006, 35
Kirby Report, 29b–31b, 35, 85–86
Krever Inquiry, 7

L

Laboratory and diagnostic services, 321, 369
Laboratory Centre for Disease Control, 4
Laboratory of Hygiene, 4
Lalonde, Marc, 81
Lalonde Report, 81, 83, 85–86
Laparoscopic surgery, 270–271, 270b
Latimer, Robert, 175–176, 175b
Lean strategy, 258, 373
Legal problems, avoiding, 109b–110b
Legal Services, Health Canada, 199
Legislation
   defined, 103b
   in health care, 103
   privacy, 135–136
Liability insurance, 140
Licensed practical nurses (LPNs), 345–346, 312
Life expectancy, 62, 62t, 62b
Lifestyle, impact on health of, 50–52
Limited use list (LU), 251
Line-by-line funding, 264
Literacy as determinant of health, 75
Living wills, 174, 177
Long-term care accommodation
   copayment for, 274–275, 275b–276b
   demand for, 276
   funding of, 274–276
   mental health issues in, 276
   provincial/territorial management of, 274–275
   quality of, 276
   services offered by, 247–248

M

Magnetic resonance imaging (MRI), 283–284
Malpractice, 107, 107b
Marijuana
   medical, 115, 116b
   synthetic, 116–118
Marketed Health Products Directorate, Health Canada, 202–203
Marketing and Communications Services Directorate, Health Canada, 207
Mature minors, 131
Mazankowski Report, 29b–31b
Medical Care Act, 15b–16b, 17–18
Medical marijuana, 115, 116b
Medical model, 49–51
Medical products, funding of, 248–249
Medical schools, 4, 347, 348b
Medically necessary procedures
   Canada Health Act on, 242, 244–246
   defined, 24b, 120
   prohibition on private insurance for, 120, 124
   rare conditions and, 181b
   subjective nature of, 24–25, 24b
Medicare, 13–15, 13b, 223
Mental competence and rights in health care, 169
Mental Health Acts, 142
Mental health care
   future of, 340–341
   in prisons, 338–339, 339b
   structure of services for, 335–341
Mental Health Commission of Canada (MHCC), 35–36, 94, 336
Mental Health Strategies for Corrections in Canada, 339
Mental illness
   challenges of, 45, 338–340
   common disorders, 337–338
   employment and, 339–340, 340b
   homelessness and, 338
   justice system and, 35b–36b, 338–339, 339b
   as significant public health problem, 335–341
   stigma of, 336–337, 337b
   underfunding for, 334
Methicillin-resistant *Staphylococcus aureus* (MRSA), 251, 251b
Métis, 63b, 357b
   see also Aboriginal peoples

Midwives, 313–314
Minister of health, responsibilities of, 196, 224
Minors
  and consent, 131
  defined, 131b
  emancipated, 131
  mature, 131
Modalities, 291–292, 292b
Morality, 151–153, 151b
Morals, 151–153, 151b
Morbidity, 40–41, 41b
Mortality, 40–41, 41b
Most responsible physician (MRP), 281

N

Narrative charting, 133
National Aboriginal Health Organization (NAHO), 366
National Advisory Committee on Immunization, 217
National Ambulatory Care Reporting System (NACRS), 213
National Counter-Terrorism Plan, 216
National drug plan, 29b–32b, 351–352
National Forum on Health, 1994–1997, 85–86
National Health Grants Program, 12–13
National Security Policy and National Emergency Response System (NERS), 216
Natural health products, use of, 204b
Natural Health Products Directorate, Health Canada, 203–204
Negligence, 107–108, 107b
Neurologists, 308
New International Economic Order, 397, 399–400
Non-Insured Health Benefits program, 356–357
Nonmaleficence, 158, 158b
Nonprofit organizations (NPOs), 257, 272, 272b
Nonregulated health care providers, 142, 304–305, 306b
Non-status Indians, 356, 356b–357b

Northern regions
  delivery of health care to, 261
  health care plan, 231–234
Nurse practitioner–led clinics, 323
Nurse practitioners (NPs), 311–312, 311b
Nurses
  in early Canada, 9
  educational opportunities for, 346
  regulation of, 296
  shortage of, 279–280
  training of, 310–311
  see also Registered nurses; Regulated nurses
Nursing homes, 274, 274b–276b
Nursing schools, 9
Nursing services, cost of, 268
Nursing stations, 364

O

Obstetricians and Gynecologists (OB/GYNs), 307
Occupational health and safety, 111–112
Occupational therapists (OTs), 318–319
Occupational therapy assistants (OTAs), 319
Occupational wellness, 46
Office of Nursing Policy, Health Canada, 200–201
Office of Nutrition Policy and Promotion, Health Canada, 201
Office of the Chief Scientist, Health Canada, 200
Oncologists, 308
Ophthalmologists, 308
Opted-out physicians, 17, 125
Opticians, 314
Optional services, 25
Optometrists, 314
Oral consent, 130, 130b
Order of St. John, 6
Orderlies, 315–316
Organ transplantation, 179–180, 179b
Organisation for Economic Co-operation and Development (OECD), 218, 280, 280b

Orphan patients, 354, 354b
Osteopathic physicians, 314–315
Ottawa Charter for Health Promotion, 1986, 83
Outpatient clinics, 272, 322–323
Outsourcing, 284
OxyContin, addictive properties of, 114b

Palliative care
 community-based, 272
 defined, 31b
 importance of, 178–179
 provincial/territorial services in, 248
 Romanow Report on, 29b–31b
Pan-American Health Organization (PAHO), 218
Pandemics
 alerts for, 214–217, 214b
 defined, 214b
Parental rights, 167–169, 168b
ParticipACTION, 51
Passive euthanasia, 174
Patent Act, 209, 278
Patent protection, 211b
Patented drugs, 209–210
 controlling the cost of, 209, 279
 defined, 209b
 vs generic drugs, 211b
 see also Drugs
Patented Medicine Prices Review Board (PMPRB), 209–210, 279
Patenting genes, 185–186, 186b
Paternalism, 165, 165b–166b
Patient service associates, 315–316
Patient–physician relationship, termination of, 141–142
Patients' bills of rights, 163
Patient's Medical Home (PMH), 290–291
Payroll taxes, 235–236
Personal health practices as determinant of health, 77–78
Personal Information Protection and Electronic Documents Act, 2004 *(PIPEDA)*, 135–136, 135b, 139–140
Personal support workers (PSWs), 315–316

Pharmacare plan. *see* Drug insurance plans; National drug plan
Pharmacists, 313
Physiatrists, 309
Physical environment as determinant of health, 77
Physical wellness, 44
Physician assistants (PAs), 312–313
Physician-assisted suicide, 174, 174b, 176
 see also Assisted suicide
Physician–patient relationship, termination of, 141–142
Physicians
 blended funding of, 282
 capitation-based funding of, 281–282, 281b
 fee-for-service (FFS) funding of, 280–281
 First Nations, Inuit, and Métis (FNIM) physicians, 365–366
 global budget funding of, 282
 indirect capitation funding of, 282
 most responsible physician (MRP), 281
 opted-out, 17, 125
 payment methods, 280–283
 salaries for, 282
 specialists' compensation, 282–283
 training of, 306–310
 video conferencing by, 369, 369b
 see also Doctors
Physiotherapists, 318
Physiotherapy assistants (PTAs), 319
Podiatrists, 315–316
Population-based funding, 265, 281
Population-based surveillance, 92, 92b–93b
Population health
 defined, 70–71, 70b–71b
 in developing nations, 98
 introduction of, 80–86
 partners in implementation of, 97–98
 Public Health Agency of Canada (PHAC) template for, 90–96, 91f
 strategies, 94–95

Population health promotion model, 97, 96–97
Portability, 21–22
Positron emission tomography (PET) scanners, 284, 284b
Power, balance of, in therapeutic relationship, 172–173
Power of attorney, 131–132, 131b
Practice settings, 290, 290b–291b, 321–324
Prepaid medical care, 13–15, 13b
Prescription drugs
  advertising, 118
  as cost driver, 351–352
  insurance for, 351, 352b
Primary care
  access to, 79, 225f
  defined, 79b, 224–225
  vs primary health care, 224–225
Primary care physicians, 306–307
Primary care settings, 290
Primary health care
  characteristics of, 398–399
  defined, 398, 81b
  future of, 372–374
  international collaboration towards, 399
  vs primary care, 224–225
  WHO and, 82b
Primary health care groups, 327b
  examples of, 325
  patient enrollment in (rostering), 326–327
  payment mechanisms for, 326
  structure and function of, 325–327
Primary health care reform
  and aging population, 342
  beginnings of, 27, 324–329
  defined, 27b
  framework for, 29b–31b
  funding of, 200, 281
  goals of, 28t
Primary health care reform groups, 326b–327b, 327
Privacy, 136–137, 136b–137b, 320
Privacy Act (1983), 135
Privacy legislation, 135–136

Private clinics
  concerns about, 243b
  examples of, 126–127
  government funding of, 124–125
  legality of, 242
  see also Clinics
Private health care
  access to, 123, 125b
  commissioned reports on, 29b–31b
  existence of, 242
  legality of, 124–127
  legislation covering, 103, 126
  vs public health care, 120, 121b–122b
Private health insurance, 121b–122b, 123–124, 237
Private law, 105–111
Procedural justice, 160–161
Product Safety Program, Health Canada, 205
Professional misconduct, 107, 107b
Programs Directorate, Health Canada, 206
Protection motivation theory, 53
Provincial insurance plans
  applying for, 238–240, 238b
  eligibility for, 237–238, 239b
  portability of, 240b
  reciprocal agreement, 240b
  see also Provincial/territorial health care plans
Provincial/territorial drug benefits, 250, 251b
Provincial/territorial governments
  role in health care, 223
  structure of health care systems, 223–226
Provincial/territorial health care plans
  Alberta, 227–228
  British Columbia, 227
  categories of care, 224
  funding of, 234–237
  Manitoba, 228
  New Brunswick, 229–230
  Newfoundland and Labrador, 231
  northern regions, 231–234
  Northwest Territories, 232–233

Provincial/territorial health care plans *(Continued)*
  Nova Scotia, 230
  Nunavut, 233–234
  Ontario, 228–229
  Prince Edward Island, 230–231
  Quebec, 229
  regionalization initiatives, 226–234
  Saskatchewan, 228
  wait time for coverage, 240b
  Yukon, 233
  see also Provincial insurance plans
Proxy consent, 132, 132b
Psychiatrists, 308–309
Psychologists, 316
Public Affairs and Strategic Communications Directorate, Health Canada, 206–207
Public Affairs, Consultation and Communications Branch (PACCB), Health Canada, 206–207
Public health
  defined, 71b
  history of, 5–6
Public Health Agency of Canada (PHAC), 87, 210–211, 216
Public Health Agency of Canada (PHAC) template, 90–96, 91f
Public Health Program Initiative, 83–84
Public health units, 6
Public law, 105–111
Public Safety Canada, 216
Publicly funded health care, 12, 14, 120, 256–257, 257b

Q

Qualitative research, 93–94, 93b
Quantitative research, 93–94, 93b
Quarantine, 3, 3b, 5
Quarantine Act, 118–119, 118b
Quebec Charter of Human Rights and Freedoms, 121b–122b

R

Radiologists, 309
Rationalization of services, 264, 264b
Reasonable access, 22

Reciprocal agreement, 240b
Refraction, 308, 308b
Refugee claimants
  defined, 3b, 257
  drug costs for, 351
  health care for, 195b, 257, 260
  health insurance for, 3
Regional health authorities (RHAs), 226–234
Regionalization, 226–234
Regions and Programs Branch, Health Canada, 205–206
Registered nurses
  practice settings of, 268
  regulation of, 296
  shortage of, 344
  training of, 310–311
  see also Nurses
Registered practical nurses (RPNs), 312
Registered psychiatric nurses (RPNs), 312
Regulated health care providers
  codes of ethics for, 141
  common elements among, 300b
  complaint processes for, 140–142, 304
  educational standards for, 304
  licensing of, 304, 305b
  provincial/territorial differences between, 297t–299t
Regulated Health Professions Act (RHPA) (ON), 301
Regulated nurses
  availability of, 344–345
  lack of job security for, 345
  shortage of, 344–345
  strategies to increase numbers of, 345–346
  working conditions for, 345
Regulations, 104, 104b
Regulatory law, 104, 104b
Religion
  influence on health beliefs, 54
  and response to hospitalization, 59
Remission, 47, 47b
Renal dialysis, 268b

Report on the Health of Canadians, 1996, 84–85, 85b
Reserves, 355–356, 356b
Resident care aides, 315–316
Residential schools, 357–358
Respect, 158–159, 159b
Respiratory therapists (RTs), 317–318
Respirologists, 309
Respite care, 248
Restraints, legal issues around use of, 142–143
Right to consent, 176
Right to die, 176–178, 176b
Right to refuse treatment, 128, 128b
Rights in health care
  categories of, 162
  controversies around, 161–169, 162b, 168b
  defined, 161b
  duties and, 164
  individual rights, 168b
  mental competence and, 169
  parental rights, 167–169
Risk assessment, 215b, 215
Rodriguez, Sue, 123, 176
Role fidelity, 160b, 160
Romanow Report, 29b–31b, 32–33, 85–86
Rostering, 326–327, 326b–327b
Royal assent, 18b
Royal Commission on Health Services, 15b–16b

S

Safe Environments Program (SEP), Health Canada, 204
SARS (severe acute respiratory syndrome), 193, 193b, 200, 215–216
Scope of practice, 300b
Secondary care
  access to, 225f
  defined, 224
Self-determination, 152, 152b
Self-discharge from hospital, 143
Self-imposed risk behaviours, 49–50, 49b, 61–62, 61b, 77
Service-based funding, 265

Severe acute respiratory syndrome (SARS), 193, 193b, 200, 215–216
Shamans, 4–5
Sick building syndrome, 77
Sick role behaviour
  defined, 57–60, 57b
  in hospital, 58b, 59–60
  and stage of illness, 60–61
Signs (of illness), 60, 60b
Smallpox vaccinations, 5–6
Smith, Ashley, 339b
Social environment as determinant of health, 76–77
Social movements, 12, 12b
Social support networks as determinant of health, 74–75, 74b, 78b
Social union, 28–29
Social wellness, 45–46
Social–ecological model, 53
Socioeconomic gradient (SES gradient), 72–73, 73b, 84
Socioeconomic status as determinant of health, 72–74, 73b, 84b
Specialists
  compensation for, 282–283
  shortage of, 342
  training of, 306, 306b
  wait times for, 352
Speech-language pathologists, 316–317
Spiritual wellness, 45, 45b
St. John Ambulance, 6
Staffing shortages, 27
Stages of illness, 60–61, 60b–61b
Standards of care, 33–34
Statistics Canada
  health data gathered by, 89
  measurement of health status by, 90–92
Status Indians, 356, 356b–357b
Statutory law, 104, 104b
Strategic Policy Branch (SPB), Health Canada, 200–201
Surgeons, 309–310, 310b
Swine flu. *see* H1N1 virus
Symptoms (of illness), 60, 60b
Synthetic marijuana, 116–118

T

Taxation
  increasing levels of, 29b–31b
  tax points, 16b
Taylor, Gloria, 123
Telehealth, 327–329, 328b
Teleological theory, 155b–156b, 156
Telephone helplines, 327–329, 328b
Territorial Formula Financing (TFF), 259
Territorial health care plans. *see* Provincial/territorial health care plans
Tertiary care
  access to, 225f
  defined, 224
Therapeutic Products Directorate, Health Canada, 201–202
Therapeutic relationship
  balance of power in, 172–173
  transference in, 172–173
  trust in, 172
  vulnerability in, 172
Third-party health insurance, 237, 245
Title protection, 300–301, 300b
Tobacco Control Program, Health Canada, 204–205
Tort law, 106–108, 106b
Transference in therapeutic relationship, 172–173
Transtheoretical model, 52–53
Treaty Indians, 356
Trust in therapeutic relationship, 172
Truthfulness, 159–160, 166–167, 167b
Tuberculosis sanitariums, 10
Two-tier system, 124, 243b

U

Unemployment insurance program, 11
Uninsured services
  block payment plan for, 246b
  Canada Health Act and, 241–249
  vs insured services, 245b
Uninsured services plans, 245
Unintentional tort, 107
Universality, 20–21
Upstream investments, 94, 94b

Urgent care clinics, 322
Urodynamic, 322–323, 323b
User charges, 25, 25b

V

Vaccinations, 5–6, 86b, 217, 262b
  see also Immunization
Values
  defined, 153b
  in health care, 153–155, 154b
  influence on behaviour, 153b
Values history form, 177, 177b
Vancomycin-resistant *Enterococcus* (VRE), 251, 251b
Vancomycin-resistant *Staphylococcus aureus* (VRSA), 251, 251b
Victorian Order of Nurses (VON), 8–9
Video conferencing, 369, 369b
Virtue ethics, 156–157, 156b
Voluntary euthanasia, 174, 174b
Volunteer caregivers, 321
Volunteer organizations, health care provided by, 6–9, 8b
Volunteerism as determinant of health, 76, 76b
Vulnerability in therapeutic relationship, 172

W

Wait times
  causes of, 352–355
  in emergency departments, 334, 354–355
  funding to reduce, 352–354
  guaranteed maximum wait times, 352–353, 353b
  reasonable wait times, 123b, 163
  right to health care and, 121, 121b–122b, 164b
Wait Times Reduction Fund, 352–353
Walk-in clinics, 322
Wellness
  defined, 41–46, 41b
  dimensions of, 42–46, 44f
  emotional, 44–45
  environmental, 46

Wellness *(Continued)*
  intellectual, 45
  occupational, 46
  physical, 44
  social, 45–46
  spiritual, 45, 45b
Wellness model, 49–50
Whistleblowers, 144, 144b
Workers' Compensation Board (WCB), 111–112
Working conditions as determinant of health, 75
Workplace Hazardous Materials Information System (WHMIS), 111–112, 112b, 209
Workplace Health and Public Safety Program, Health Canada, 205–206

World Health Assembly, 217–218
World Health Organization (WHO)
  agenda of, 212b
  Alma-Ata Conference, 1978, 81
  collaborative approach of, 95
  on concept of health, 41, 42b
  and H1N1 virus, 217
  International Classification of Functioning Disability and Health (ICF), 50
  International Health Regulations, 119
  leadership of, 211–212
  pandemic alert system, 214–217, 214b
  and SARS crisis, 215–216
  in support of primary health care, 82b
Written consent, 129–130, 129b